Stroke Rehabilitation

Editors

JOHN CHAE
PABLO A. CELNIK

PHYSICAL MEDICINE AND REHABILITATION CLINICS OF NORTH AMERICA

www.pmr.theclinics.com

Consulting Editor
GREGORY T. CARTER

November 2015 • Volume 26 • Number 4

ELSEVIER

1600 John F. Kennedy Boulevard • Suite 1800 • Philadelphia, Pennsylvania, 19103-2899

http://www.theclinics.com

PHYSICAL MEDICINE AND REHABILITATION CLINICS OF NORTH AMERICA Volume 26, Number 4
November 2015 ISSN 1047-9651, ISBN 978-0-323-41348-0

Editor: Jennifer Flynn-Briggs
Developmental Editor: Donald Mumford

Photocopying
Single photocopies of single articles may be made for personal use as allowed by national copyright laws. Permission of the Publisher and payment of a fee is required for all other photocopying, including multiple or systematic copying, copying for advertising or promotional purposes, resale, and all forms of document delivery. Special rates are available for educational institutions that wish to make photocopies for non-profit educational classroom use. For information on how to seek permission visit www.elsevier.com/permissions or call: (+44) 1865 843830 (UK)/(+1) 215 239 3804 (USA).

Derivative Works
Subscribers may reproduce tables of contents or prepare lists of articles including abstracts for internal circulation within their institutions. Permission of the Publisher is required for resale or distribution outside the institution. Permission of the Publisher is required for all other derivative works, including compilations and translations (please consult www.elsevier.com/permissions).

Electronic Storage or Usage
Permission of the Publisher is required to store or use electronically any material contained in this periodical, including any article or part of an article (please consult www.elsevier.com/permissions). Except as outlined above, no part of this publication may be reproduced, stored in a retrieval system or transmitted in any form or by any means, electronic, mechanical, photocopying, recording or otherwise, without prior written permission of the Publisher.

Notice
No responsibility is assumed by the Publisher for any injury and/or damage to persons or property as a matter of products liability, negligence or otherwise, or from any use or operation of any methods, products, instructions or ideas contained in the material herein. Because of rapid advances in the medical sciences, in particular, independent verification of diagnoses and drug dosages should be made.

Although all advertising material is expected to conform to ethical (medical) standards, inclusion in this publication does not constitute a guarantee or endorsement of the quality or value of such product or of the claims made of it by its manufacturer.

Reprints. For copies of 100 or more of articles in this publication, please contact the Commercial Reprints Department, Elsevier Inc., 360 Park Avenue South, New York, NY 10010-1710. Tel.: 212-633-3874; Fax: 212-633-3820; E-mail: reprints@elsevier.com.

Physical Medicine and Rehabilitation Clinics of North America (ISSN 1047-9651) is published quarterly by Elsevier Inc., 360 Park Avenue South, New York, NY 10010-1710. Months of issue are February, May, August, and November. Business and Editorial Offices: 1600 John F. Kennedy Blvd., Suite 1800, Philadelphia, PA 19103-2899. Customer Service Office: 3251 Riverport Lane, Maryland Heights, MO 63043. Periodicals postage paid at New York, NY and additional mailing offices. Subscription price per year is $275.00 (US individuals), $486.00 (US institutions), $145.00 (US students), $335.00 (Canadian individuals), $640.00 (Canadian institutions), $210.00 (Canadian students), $415.00 (foreign individuals), $640.00 (foreign institutions), and $210.00 (foreign students). Foreign air speed delivery is included in all *Clinics* subscription prices. All prices are subject to change without notice. **POSTMASTER:** Send address changes to *Physical Medicine and Rehabilitation Clinics of North America*, Customer Service Office: Elsevier Health Sciences Division, Subscription Customer Service, 3251 Riverport Lane, Maryland Heights, MO 63043. **Customer Service: 1-800-654-2452 (US). From outside of the United States, call 314-447-8871. Fax: 314-447-8029. E-mail: JournalsCustomer Service-usa@elsevier.com (for print support); JournalsOnlineSupport-usa@elsevier.com (for online support).**

Physical Medicine and Rehabilitation Clinics of North America is indexed in *Excerpta Medica, MEDLINE/ PubMed (Index Medicus), Cinahl,* and *Cumulative Index to Nursing and Allied Health Literature.*

Contributors

CONSULTING EDITOR

GREGORY T. CARTER, MD, MS
Consulting Medical Editor; Medical Director, St Luke's Rehabilitation Institute, Spokane, Washington; University of Washington, School of Medicine, Seattle, Washington

EDITORS

JOHN CHAE, MD
Professor and Chair, Physical Medicine and Rehabilitation; Professor, Biomedical Engineering, Case Western Reserve University; Medical Director, Neuromusculoskeletal Service Line, MetroHealth System, Cleveland, Ohio

PABLO A. CELNIK, MD
Interim Director and Vice Chair for Research, Department of Physical Medicine and Rehabilitation; Medical Director, Outpatient Neurorehabilitation Program; Director, Human Brain Physiology and Stimulation Laboratory; Professor, Departments of Physical Medicine and Rehabilitation, Neurology and Neuroscience, Johns Hopkins University, Baltimore, Maryland

AUTHORS

FRANCOIS BETHOUX, MD
Associate Staff; Director, Mellen Center Rehabilitation Services, The Cleveland Clinic, Cleveland, Ohio

MARTIN B. BRODSKY, PhD, ScM, CCC-SLP
Assistant Professor, Department of Physical Medicine and Rehabilitation, Johns Hopkins University School of Medicine, Baltimore, Maryland

PABLO A. CELNIK, MD
Interim Director and Vice Chair for Research, Department of Physical Medicine and Rehabilitation; Medical Director, Outpatient Neurorehabilitation Program; Director, Human Brain Physiology and Stimulation Laboratory; Professor, Departments of Physical Medicine and Rehabilitation, Neurology and Neuroscience, Johns Hopkins University, Baltimore, Maryland

JOHN CHAE, MD
Professor and Chair, Physical Medicine and Rehabilitation; Professor, Biomedical Engineering, Case Western Reserve University; Medical Director, Neuromusculoskeletal Service Line, MetroHealth System, Cleveland, Ohio

DAVID A. CUNNINGHAM, MSc
Department of Biomedical Engineering, Lerner Research Institute, Cleveland Clinic, Cleveland; School of Biomedical Sciences, Kent State University, Kent, Ohio

GERARD E. FRANCISCO, MD
Chairman and Clinical Professor, Department of Physical Medicine and Rehabilitation, University of Texas Health Science Center (UTHealth); Director, The NeuroRecovery Research Center; Chief Medical Officer, TIRR Memorial Hermann, Houston, Texas

MICHAEL J. FU, PhD
Research Assistant Professor, Department of Electrical Engineering and Computer Science, Case Western Reserve University; Cleveland FES Center, Louis Stokes Department of Veterans Affairs Medical Center, Case Western Reserve University; MetroHealth Rehabilitation Institute, MetroHealth System, Cleveland, Ohio

MARLÍS GONZÁLEZ-FERNÁNDEZ, MD, PhD
Associate Professor, Department of Physical Medicine and Rehabilitation, Johns Hopkins University School of Medicine, Baltimore, Maryland

RICHARD L. HARVEY, MD
The Rehabilitation Institute of Chicago, Chicago, Illinois

ERIN E. HELM, DPT
Biomechanics and Movement Science Program, University of Delaware, Newark, Delaware

NEVILLE HOGAN, PhD
Professor, Departments of Mechanical Engineering, and Brain and Cognitive Sciences, Massachusetts Institute of Technology, Cambridge, Massachusetts

ZAFER KESER, MD
Department of Physical Medicine and Rehabilitation, University of Texas Health Science Center (UTHealth); The NeuroRecovery Research Center Houston, TIRR Memorial Hermann, Houston, Texas

JAYME S. KNUTSON, PhD
MetroHealth Medical Center, MetroHealth Rehabilitation Institute, MetroHealth System; Assistant Professor, Department of Physical Medicine and Rehabilitation, Case Western Reserve University; Assistant Professor, Cleveland Functional Electrical Stimulation Center, Louis Stokes Department of Veterans Affairs Medical Center, Cleveland, Ohio

HERMANO IGO KREBS, PhD
Principal Research Scientist and Lecturer, Department of Mechanical Engineering, Massachusetts Institute of Technology, Cambridge, Massachusetts; Department of Neurology, University of Maryland, School of Medicine, Baltimore, Maryland; Department of Rehabilitation Medicine I, School of Medicine, Fujita Health University, Toyoake, Aichi, Japan; Institute of Neuroscience, Newcastle University, Framlington Place, Newcastle upon Tyne, United Kingdom; Department of Mechanical Engineering, Osaka University, Suita, Osaka, Japan

ANDRE G. MACHADO, MD, PhD
Director, Center for Neurological Restoration, Neurological Institute; The Charles and Christine Carroll Family Endowed Chair in Functional Neurosurgery; Staff, Department of Neurosurgery, Neurological Institute; Staff, Department of Neuroscience and Biomedical Engineering, Lerner Research Institute, Cleveland, Ohio

STEPHEN J. PAGE, PhD, MS, OTR/L, FAHA, FACRM
Associate Professor, B.R.A.I.N. Laboratory (Better Rehabilitation and Assessment for Improved Neuro-recovery), Department of Occupational Therapy, The Ohio State University, Columbus, Ohio

JEFFREY B. PALMER, MD
Professor, Department of Physical Medicine and Rehabilitation, Johns Hopkins University School of Medicine, Baltimore, Maryland

HEATHER T. PETERS, MOT, OTR/L
Graduate Research Associate, PhD student, B.R.A.I.N. Laboratory (Better Rehabilitation and Assessment for Improved Neuro-recovery), Department of Occupational Therapy, The Ohio State University, Columbus, Ohio

ELA B. PLOW, PhD, PT
Assistant Staff, Department of Biomedical Engineering, Lerner Research Institute; Department of Physical Medicine and Rehabiliation, Neurological Institute, Cleveland Clinic, Cleveland, Ohio

KELSEY A. POTTER-BAKER, PhD
Department of Biomedical Engineering, Lerner Research Institute, Cleveland Clinic, Cleveland, Ohio

PREETI RAGHAVAN, MD
Assistant Professor of Rehabilitation Medicine and Physical Therapy; Director, Motor Recovery Research Laboratory, Department of Rehabilitation Medicine, Rusk Rehabilitation, New York University School of Medicine, New York, New York

DARCY S. REISMAN, PT, PhD
Biomechanics and Movement Science Program, Department of Physical Therapy, University of Delaware, Newark, Delaware

EIICHI SAITOH, MD
Professor and Chairperson, Department of Rehabilitation Medicine I, School of Medicine, Fujita Health University, Toyoake, Aichi, Japan

VISHWANATH SANKARASUBRAMANIAN, PhD
Department of Biomedical Engineering, Lerner Research Institute, Cleveland Clinic, Cleveland, Ohio

LYNNE R. SHEFFLER, MD
Assistant Professor, Department of Physical Medicine and Rehabilitation, Case Western Reserve University; MetroHealth Rehabilitation Institute of Ohio, MetroHealth System; Cleveland Functional Electrical Stimulation Center, Louis Stokes Department of Veterans Affairs Medical Center, Cleveland, Ohio

RICHARD D. WILSON, MD
Assistant Professor, Physical Medicine and Rehabilitation; Director of Stroke and Inpatient Rehabilitation, MetroHealth Medical Center, MetroHealth Rehabilitation Institute, Case Western Reserve University, Cleveland, Ohio

Contents

Foreword: An Expression of Gratitude   xiii

Gregory T. Carter

Preface: Stroke Rehabilitation   xv

John Chae and Pablo A. Celnik

Predictors of Functional Outcome Following Stroke   583

Richard L. Harvey

> Predicting functional outcome in stroke is challenging to most clinicians, partly because of the complexity of the condition and also because of the lack of validated prognostic models. The strongest predictors of functional outcome are age and motor function at stroke onset. There is a growing literature on predicting recovery of upper limb after stroke; however, literature on prediction of language recovery remains sparse. This review covers the current status of predicting functional outcome after stroke focusing on recovery of activities of daily living, ambulation, upper limb use, and aphasia. Use of clinical factors, imaging, and neurophysiological measures are discussed.

Upper Limb Motor Impairment After Stroke   599

Preeti Raghavan

> Understanding poststroke upper limb impairment is essential to planning therapeutic efforts to restore function. However, determining which upper limb impairment to treat and how is complex because the impairments are not static and multiple impairments may be present simultaneously. How impairments contribute to upper limb dysfunction may be understood by examining them from the perspective of their functional consequences. There are 3 main functional consequences of impairments on upper limb function: (1) learned nonuse, (2) learned bad use, and (3) forgetting as determined by behavioral analysis of tasks. The impairments that contribute to each of these functional limitations are described.

Hemiparetic Gait   611

Lynne R. Sheffler and John Chae

> The most common pattern of walking impairment poststroke is hemiparetic gait, which is characterized by asymmetry associated with an extensor synergy pattern of hip extension and adduction, knee extension, and ankle plantar flexion and inversion. There are characteristic changes in the spatiotemporal, kinematic and kinetic parameters, and dynamic electromyography patterns in hemiparesis, which may be assessed most accurately in a motion studies laboratory. An understanding of normal human gait is necessary to assess the complex interplay of motor, sensory, and proprioceptive loss; spasticity; and/or ataxia on hemiparetic gait.

Spasticity Management After Stroke   625

Francois Bethoux

Many poststroke survivors develop spasticity. Spasticity is usually associated with other neurologic impairments, in particular paresis, which complicate the evaluation of its consequences and of treatment outcomes. The diagnosis and the assessment of spasticity are based on clinical examination, in particular resistance to passive movement and abnormal involuntary muscle contraction. Nonpharmacologic and pharmacologic treatments are commonly combined to manage spasticity, based on prespecified goals. There is evidence supporting the effectiveness and safety of most medications commonly used to treat spasticity; however, more evidence is needed regarding functional outcomes and the impact of combining treatment modalities.

Hemiplegic Shoulder Pain   641

Richard D. Wilson and John Chae

Hemiplegic shoulder pain is a common complaint for stroke survivors. Many pathologies are included in the diagnosis of hemiplegic shoulder pain, and many with shoulder pain have a multifactorial cause. This article provides rehabilitation specialists with an approach to evaluation and management of those with hemiplegic shoulder pain.

Poststroke Communication Disorders and Dysphagia   657

Marlís González-Fernández, Martin B. Brodsky, and Jeffrey B. Palmer

Communication and swallowing disorders are common after stroke. Targeted surveillance followed by prompt evaluation and treatment is of paramount importance. The overall goals of rehabilitation for impaired swallowing and communication and swallowing deficits may differ based on the specific deficits caused by the stroke but the main goal is always to improve the patient's everyday interpersonal interactions and optimize participation in society. Fortunately, therapeutic or compensatory interventions can decrease the effects that communication and swallowing deficits have on the quality of life of stroke survivors.

Neuropharmacology of Poststroke Motor and Speech Recovery   671

Zafer Keser and Gerard E. Francisco

Almost 7 million adult Americans have had a stroke. There is a growing need for more effective treatment options as add-ons to conventional therapies. This article summarizes the published literature for pharmacologic agents used for the enhancement of motor and speech recovery after stroke. Amphetamine, levodopa, selective serotonin reuptake inhibitors, and piracetam were the most commonly used drugs. Pharmacologic augmentation of stroke motor and speech recovery seems promising but systematic, adequately powered, randomized, and double-blind clinical trials are needed. At this point, the use of these pharmacologic agents is not supported by class I evidence.

Robotic Therapy and the Paradox of the Diminishing Number of Degrees of Freedom 691

Hermano Igo Krebs, Eiichi Saitoh, and Neville Hogan

There has been remarkable growth in the development and application of robotics to ameliorate or remediate impairment. This growth is associated with a) the understanding that plasticity is a fundamental property of the adult human brain and might be harnessed to remap or create new neural pathways and b) the development of robots that can safely interact with humans and assist human performance. This article discusses whether robotic therapy has achieved a level of maturity to justify its broad adoption as a rehabilitative tool. How to improve outcomes further and how to select degrees of freedom to optimize care to particular patients is also discussed.

The Split-Belt Walking Paradigm: Exploring Motor Learning and Spatiotemporal Asymmetry Poststroke 703

Erin E. Helm and Darcy S. Reisman

Although significant effort is concentrated toward gait retraining during stroke rehabilitation; 33% of community-dwelling individuals following stroke continue to demonstrate gait asymmetries following participation in conventional rehabilitation. Recent studies utilizing the split-belt treadmill indicate that subjects after stroke retain the ability to learn a novel locomotor pattern. Through the use of error augmentation, this locomotor pattern can provide a temporary improvement in symmetry, which can be exploited through repetitive task specific locomotor training. This article reviews findings from this experimental paradigm in chronic stroke survivors and discusses the future questions to be addressed in order to provide optimal rehabilitation interventions.

Integrating Mental Practice with Task-specific Training and Behavioral Supports in Poststroke Rehabilitation: Evidence, Components, and Augmentative Opportunities 715

Heather T. Peters and Stephen J. Page

Stroke remains a leading cause of death, with most survivors experiencing long-term deficits in motor function. Upper extremity (UE) hemiparesis constitutes one of the most common and disabling poststroke impairments. Many contemporary rehabilitative methods target reacquisition of UE motor skills. One such intervention is mental practice (MP), which involves mental rehearsal without physical execution of the movement. MP has not been consistently integrated into clinical environments. This article discusses the scientific rationale for MPs, highlights evidence supporting their use, discusses components of the repetitive task-specific practice regimens accompanying MP, and discusses possible augmentative strategies and areas for research.

Neuromuscular Electrical Stimulation for Motor Restoration in Hemiplegia 729

Jayme S. Knutson, Michael J. Fu, Lynne R. Sheffler, and John Chae

This article reviews the most common therapeutic and neuroprosthetic applications of neuromuscular electrical stimulation (NMES) for upper and lower extremity stroke rehabilitation. Fundamental NMES principles and purposes in stroke rehabilitation are explained. NMES modalities used for upper and lower limb rehabilitation are described, and efficacy studies are summarized. The evidence for peripheral and central mechanisms of action is also summarized.

Stroke Rehabilitation Using Virtual Environments   747

Michael J. Fu, Jayme S. Knutson, and John Chae

This review covers the rationale, mechanisms, and availability of commercially available virtual environment-based interventions for stroke rehabilitation. It describes interventions for motor, speech, cognitive, and sensory dysfunction. Also discussed are the important features and mechanisms that allow virtual environments to facilitate motor relearning. A common challenge is the inability to translate success in small trials to efficacy in larger populations. The heterogeneity of stroke pathophysiology has been blamed, and experts advocate for the study of multimodal approaches. Therefore, this article also introduces a framework to help define new therapy combinations that may be necessary to address stroke heterogeneity.

Tailoring Brain Stimulation to the Nature of Rehabilitative Therapies in Stroke: A Conceptual Framework Based on their Unique Mechanisms of Recovery   759

David A. Cunningham, Kelsey A. Potter-Baker, Jayme S. Knutson, Vishwanath Sankarasubramanian, Andre G. Machado, and Ela B. Plow

Despite showing early promise, several recent clinical trials of noninvasive brain stimulation (NIBS) failed to augment rehabilitative outcomes of the paretic upper limb. This article addresses why pairing NIBS with unilateral approaches is weakly generalizable to patients in all ranges of impairments. The article also addresses whether alternate therapies are better suited for the more impaired patients, where they may be more feasible and offer neurophysiologic advantages not offered with unilateral therapies. The article concludes by providing insight on how to create NIBS paradigms that are tailored to distinctly augment the effects of therapies across patients with varying degrees of impairment.

Index   775

PHYSICAL MEDICINE AND REHABILITATION CLINICS OF NORTH AMERICA

FORTHCOMING ISSUES

February 2016
Running Injuries
Michael Fredericson and
Adam Tenforde, *Editors*

May 2016
Concussion in Sports
Scott R. Laker, *Editor*

August 2016
**Outpatient Ultrasound-Guided
Musculoskeletal Techniques**
Evan Peck, *Editor*

RECENT ISSUES

August 2015
**Evidence-Based Treatment Guidelines for
Treating Injured Workers**
Andrew S. Friedman and
Gary M. Franklin, *Editors*

May 2015
Chronic Pain
James P. Robinson and
Virtaj Singh, *Editors*

February 2015
Pediatric Rehabilitation
Andrew J. Skalsky, *Editor*

RELATED INTEREST

Cardiology Clinics of North America, February 2015 (Vol. 33, Issue 1)
Vascular Disease
Leonardo C. Clavijo, *Editor*

VISIT THE CLINICS ONLINE!
Access your subscription at:
www.theclinics.com

Foreword

An Expression of Gratitude

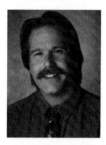

Gregory T. Carter, MD, MS
Consulting Editor

> *One looks back with appreciation to the brilliant teachers, but with gratitude to those who touched our human feelings. The curriculum is so much necessary raw material, but warmth is the vital element for the growing plant and for the soul of the child.*
>
> —*Carl Jung*

As my tenure as medical editor of the *Physical Medicine and Rehabilitation Clinics of North America* comes to an end, I want to extend my sincerest thanks to Elsevier for granting me the privilege of holding this position for many years now. In particular, I would like to acknowledge the hard work and dedicated excellence of senior *Physical Medicine and Rehabilitation Clinics of North America* editor Jennifer Flynn-Briggs, who helped me in more ways than I can list here. In addition, I want to acknowledge Donald Mumford of Elsevier for his patience and persistence in helping me meet publishing deadlines. There are many others I would like to thank, too many to mention individually. However, I would be amiss to not formally recognize all of the guest editors and countless authors of the articles that were published during my time as medical editor. The *Clinics* has very high standards. Publishing an article in these volumes represents a considerable amount of time and work, often done after clinic and on weekends. When reading a *Clinics* volume, realize that you are holding the product of untold hours of effort. In that light, I offer my heartfelt appreciation to Dr John Chae and the many excellent authors he recruited for this issue.

In closing, I would like to acknowledge my dear friend and mentor, Dr George H. Kraft, who was the medical editor for several decades before me. Under Dr Kraft's leadership, the *Physical Medicine and Rehabilitation Clinics of North America* grew to be one of the

Phys Med Rehabil Clin N Am 26 (2015) xiii–xiv
http://dx.doi.org/10.1016/j.pmr.2015.09.001
1047-9651/15/$ – see front matter © 2015 Published by Elsevier Inc.

pmr.theclinics.com

best, Medline-referenced, sources of up-to-date cutting-edge clinical reviews. When Dr Kraft decided to step down, I was deeply honored to assume his position.

    Respectfully submitted,

Gregory T. Carter, MD, MS
St Luke's Rehabilitation Institute
711 South Cowley Street
Spokane, WA 99202, USA

E-mail address:
gtcarter@uw.edu

Preface

Stroke Rehabilitation

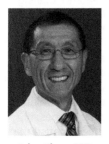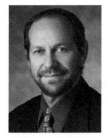

John Chae, MD   Pablo A. Celnik, MD
Editors

We are pleased to present this latest issue of *Physical Medicine and Rehabilitation Clinics of North America* dedicated to stroke rehabilitation. We thank Greg Carter for giving us the opportunity to provide this update to our colleagues, especially the clinicians on the frontline of clinical care. The goals of stroke rehabilitation should be to reduce impairment and maximize the function, societal participation, and quality of life of stroke survivors. In light of these goal, we launch this issue with a comprehensive review of predictors of functional outcome to help us focus on those specific issues that impact clinically meaningful recovery following stroke. This is then followed by a series of articles that focuses on specific manifestations of stroke with major implications on outcomes. The phenomena of "nonuse," learned "bad-use," and "forgetting" are presented to help inform the formulation of treatment plans for the restoration of upper limb motor function. These same phenomena are present in the lower limb, but with a different set of implications leading to the characteristic hemiplegic gait and associated impact on mobility. As stroke recovery enters the chronic phase, nearly half of all stroke survivors develop spasticity. There is now emerging evidence that some treatments for spasticity not only reduce spasticity but also improve upper and lower limb functional performance. A musculoskeletal pain syndrome that uniquely impacts stroke survivors is shoulder pain. While the initial inciting factor is likely glenohumeral instability or biomechanical compromise, central mechanisms may be more dominant in the chronic phase with their unique implications on treatment strategies. The section concludes with a review of poststroke communication disorders and dysphagia, manifestations of stroke that have major learning, relational, nutrition, and societal participation implications.

The second set of articles focuses on treatment modalities that are presently not yet part of the standard treatment armamentarium. Our goal is to provide the practicing clinician an update on these modalities. Neuropharmacology has been a focus of investigation for decades. However, due to inconsistent results or limited internal and external validity of the various studies, firm clinical recommendations cannot be

Phys Med Rehabil Clin N Am 26 (2015) xv–xvi
http://dx.doi.org/10.1016/j.pmr.2015.08.013
1047-9651/15/$ – see front matter © 2015 Published by Elsevier Inc.

pmr.theclinics.com

presented. In contrast, there are more robust data in support of robotic therapy, especially with respect to upper limb applications. However, the rehabilitation community needs to decide whether the data are compelling enough to integrate this approach into the "standard of practice." A novel treatment paradigm for hemiplegic gait that many practicing clinicians may not be familiar with is split-belt treadmill training. Although the technique is not ready for clinical implementation, it is an intriguing approach to address step length asymmetry, which reduces propulsive force of the paretic limb, resulting in increased walking speed and efficiency. We then provide updates on mental practice, neuromuscular electrical stimulation, and virtual reality environments, which generally show improvements at the level of impairment but less robust translation to activities. Yet, these interventions may have a role in the treatment of specific stroke survivors, and readers are invited to critically evaluate these approaches and determine relevance to their respective clinical practices.

We conclude this issue with an article on brain stimulation, primarily because the approach represents a necessary shift in the treatment paradigm in stroke rehabilitation. To date, the development of interventions, for the most part, has focused on single-treatment approaches. However, in the face of only modest improvements, at best, there is a growing consensus that more meaningful clinical outcomes can only be achieved through combination therapies. Stimulating the brain via a variety of approaches may prepare the neural substrate for relearning strategies and serve as the prime candidate for testing this hypothesis.

We are very appreciative of all the contributors to this issue and their willingness to share their respective expertise. It is our hope that our colleagues in the field will find this issue helpful as they explore new treatment approaches for their patients. For some, this issue may also lead to insights regarding research ideas that will translate to the development of new clinically relevant diagnostic or treatment options.

John Chae, MD
Case Western Reserve University
MetroHealth Rehabilitation Institute
4229 Pearl Road
Cleveland, OH 44109, USA

Pablo A. Celnik, MD
Departments of Physical Medicine and
Rehabilitation, Neurology and Neuroscience
Johns Hopkins Hospital
Johns Hopkins University
600 North Wolfe Street
Baltimore, MD 21287, USA

E-mail addresses:
jchae@metrohealth.org (J. Chae)
pcelnik@jhmi.edu (P.A. Celnik)

Predictors of Functional Outcome Following Stroke

Richard L. Harvey, MD

KEYWORDS

- Stroke • Motor function • Language recovery • Functional outcome prediction

KEY POINTS

- Motor function at baseline and age are the strongest clinical predictors of stroke recovery. Bedside examination, such as Medical Research Counsel testing, can provide the clinician with enough information to predict long-term recovery.
- Ambulation ability is a strong predictor of long-term independence. Ability to regain walking ability can be predicted by balance ability at onset.
- Arm and hand recovery can be predicted by motor function at onset, but actual use of hand in functional activities requires significant recovery of motor speed and manipulative skill.
- Language recovery can be predicted by language ability at stroke onset. A good ability to comprehend language and intact repetition predict better language outcome.
- Combining motor ability, neurophysiological measures such as preservation of motor-evoked potentials by transcranial magnetic stimulation, and imaging may provide useful predictive value if current available models can be validated in large patient cohorts.

INTRODUCTION

Accurate prediction of functional outcome in patients with stroke has the potential to enhance clinical care as well as improve the quality of stroke research. Prognostic models can facilitate education and counseling of patients and families, and stream-line planning for rehabilitation and discharge. Specific predictors can help target treatment options to the patients who will most benefit, and avoid treatments in those who are unlikely to respond. Such models can improve research analysis when adjusting for baseline characteristics in study cohorts and comparing different randomized trials for meta-analysis.[1]

The use of formal prognostic models to predict functional outcome have not been used in clinical stroke rehabilitation because large representative cohorts have not been studied and existing models are not well validated.[2] Thus, prognosis has been limited to a handful of "clinical pearls" and the clinician's personal experience, with

The Rehabilitation Institute of Chicago, 345 East Superior Street, Chicago, IL 60611, USA
E-mail address: rharvey@ric.org

Phys Med Rehabil Clin N Am 26 (2015) 583–598
http://dx.doi.org/10.1016/j.pmr.2015.07.002
1047-9651/15/$ – see front matter © 2015 Elsevier Inc. All rights reserved.

the help of existing literature. It is important to note that the literature on prognosis has provided some useful information on recovery of impairment and activity, but fewer data on participation. Additionally, there is a paucity of research on the impact of cognitive and perceptual dysfunction and recovery. Most of the available literature is composed of small cohort studies and systematic reviews. Although formalized and validated predictive models would be an improvement over current practice, there remains much value in the use of "rules of thumb" for prognosis of functional outcome. The purpose of this review was to attempt to list those rules of thumb based on existing prognostic models, current epidemiologic evidence, and my own experience as a stroke rehabilitation specialist.

PATTERNS OF RECOVERY FROM STROKE AND KEY MEASURES OF OUTCOME

Motor recovery has been extensively studied in stroke due to the availability of reliable and valid measures. The first rules of thumb were provided by Twitchell[3] in 1951 when he described the patterns of natural recovery from stroke. In observing a cohort of stroke survivors he concluded the following sequential processes of recovery:

- Initial loss of voluntary movement and reflexes
- Rapid restoration of reflexes proceeding to hyperreflexia
- Development of increased muscle tone
- First voluntary movements in shoulder and hip
- Appearance of further voluntary movement with flexor pattern in upper limb and extensor pattern in lower limb
- Both flexor and extensor movements appear in upper and lower limbs
- Spasticity is reduced as isolated joint and finger movements emerge

Twitchell[3] noted that patients can progress quite quickly through this recovery pattern or stop recovering at any given level depending on stroke severity. Signe Brunnstrom[4] used Twitchell's findings[3] to develop a scale of motor impairment after stroke.[5] Later, Axel Fugl-Meyer and colleagues[6] used Twitchell's principles[3] to design a more detailed scale of motor impairment using an elegant scoring system. The upper limb portion of the Fugl-Meyer assessment (FMA) is now considered a standard outcome measure in clinical stroke recovery research.

Although the lower limb portion of the FMA also has been used in stroke research, recent clinical trials have used walking speed as an ideal measure of lower limb recovery. Walking speed is associated with lower limb impairment, aerobic capacity, and functional ambulation.[7–10] Improvements in walking speed also correlate with improved overall ability, as measured by the Modified Rankin Scale (**Table 1**).[11]

Although it is a fairly insensitive measure of functional activity, the Modified Rankin Scale (MRS) is a standard measure of outcome in acute stroke research and has been used in studies on early prediction of outcome.[12] Along with ambulation, overall severity of motor function is related to MRS, with minimal motor impairment being associated with favorable outcome, typically defined as an MRS ≤ 2 (slight disability or better).[13] But it is important to recognize that a favorable outcome on the MRS is not strongly related to recovery of the affected arm and hand. Aphasia, on the other hand, is associated with greater dependence as measured by MRS.[14,15] This is not surprising, given that significant residual deficits in comprehension predict a lower probability of return home following acute rehabilitation and are associated with lower motor and cognitive scores on the Functional Independence Measure (FIM).[16,17]

Thus, severity of impairment after stroke is related to overall functional ability. Better motor recovery in the arm and leg, faster walking speed, and good language

Table 1	
Modified Rankin scale	
0	No symptoms.
1	No significant disability. Able to carry out all usual activities, despite some symptoms.
2	Slight disability. Able to look after own affairs without assistance, but unable to carry out all previous activities.
3	Moderate disability. Requires some help, but able to walk unassisted.
4	Moderately severe disability. Unable to attend to own bodily needs without assistance, and unable to walk unassisted.
5	Severe disability. Requires constant nursing care and attention, bedridden, incontinent.
6	Dead.

From van Swieten JC, Koudstaal PJ, Visser MC, et al. Interobserver agreement for the assessment of handicap in stroke patients. Stroke 1988;19:605; with permission.

comprehension result in greater long-term independence. With these principles as a foundation, the current literature on prediction of functional outcome following stroke is reviewed. The focus is primarily on clinical factors that are predictive of stroke outcome, but the more recent use of imaging and neurophysiological measures also is briefly discussed.

PREDICTORS OF FUNCTIONAL OUTCOME AFTER STROKE

Following Twitchell's[3] description of natural motor recovery in stroke, he described factors that were positive and negative predictors of outcome:

- Predictors of better recovery
  - Only mild spasticity at its worst and none at shoulder
  - Rapid progression through synergy to isolated movement
- Predictors of worse recovery
  - Late return of reflexes
  - Late onset of voluntary movement
  - Increasing severity of spasticity

In practice, these principles seem to hold true. From here, research on outcome for general recovery of activities of daily living, walking ability, upper limb skill, and language function is presented.

Activities of Daily Living

Most studies examining overall recovery of independence in activities of daily living (ADLs) use the Barthel Index (BI) or the MRS.[2,18] The clinical measurements that are strongly associated with long-term (>3 months) independence in ADLs are age, the National Institutes of Health stroke scale (NIHSS) and the early BI score.[2,18–25] Younger age consistently predicts favorable ADL outcome, defined as an MRS ≤ 2 or a BI ≥ 95.[2,19–21,24–26] A lower score on NIHSS at admission (<10) predicts a favorable outcome; however, the closer the NIHSS is to zero, the better the prediction of independence.[20,21,25] Higher scores on BI measured early after stroke are associated with favorable outcomes.[19,22,27] But unlike the NIHSS, which has a good predictive strength at 48 hours after stroke, the BI is a better predictor of long-term ADL when measured at 5 days or later.[22,23] The unreliability of BI within the first 48 hours is likely due to the challenge of accurately determining functional ability early after stroke admission.[18]

Male gender has been associated with better functional outcome in several studies,[20,25,28] but in a large systematic review, gender was found to have no relation to ADL outcome.[2] Other less consistently reported clinical predictors of long-term ADL independence include urinary continence, good sitting balance, absence of aphasia, and absence of diabetes mellitus.[20,24,26,28,29] Diabetic patients, especially those who are older, face a higher risk of severe stroke leading to worse outcome.[24] No other medical comorbidities have been associated with functional outcome.[2] Jongbloed[26] noted in a systematic review that longer time before hospital admission was associated with worse functional ability at discharge, suggesting that earlier hospital arrival provided for more effective acute treatment. In contrast, Tei and associates[25] found that longer time before hospital admission was associated with favorable outcome at 3 months after stroke, suggesting that persons with very mild stroke symptoms are less likely to initiate timely emergency care. Recently, Ntaios and colleagues[30] developed the ASTRAL score, which uses patient age, NIHSS, time from stroke to admission, visual field deficit, admission glucose, and level of consciousness on admission to predict mortality and poor outcome (>2 on MRS) at 3 months or later (**Table 2**). This score has been validated in several populations.[30–32]

There is an expanding use of cranial imaging for the prediction functional outcome after stroke. But it is not yet clear whether prognosis based on imaging can exceed that of clinical assessment. For example, larger stroke volume on anatomic imaging is associated with worse functional outcome, but early motor strength and BI have stronger predictive value.[24,33,34] Stroke volume measured on acute diffusion-weighted imaging (DWI) is not superior to NIHSS or age in predicting late MRS.[35,36] However, Zaidi and colleagues[37] found that small final infarct volume on DWI following thrombolysis in a cohort of patients with middle cerebral artery stroke predicted better MRS score (<2) at 90 days after stroke. Very large strokes result in poor outcome, but the impact of small-volume and moderate-volume strokes is dependent on the structures involved. For example, strokes that injure the posterior limb of internal capsule (PLIC) predict motor outcome better than overall stroke volume.[38]

Analysis of cortical spinal tract (CST) structure using diffusion tensor imaging (DTI) and tractography improves prediction of outcome. DTI is a magnetic resonance technique that measures the directional movement of water molecules along white matter tracts and is an anatomic measure of tract connectivity. Measures of the water flow along a tract (anisotropy) versus in no particular direction (isotropy) are useful for differentiating intact versus injured portions of white matter, respectively. Using DTI after stroke,

Table 2
ASTRAL Score for calculation of unfavorable outcome following acute ischemic stroke

Clinical Factors	Points
Age: for every 5 y (from 0)	1
Severity: for every NIHSS point	1
Time delay: time from onset >3 h	2
Any visual field deficit	2
Acute glucose >7.3 or <3.7 mmols/L	1
Level of consciousness decreased on NIHSS	3

Higher ASTRAL score is associated with higher probability of unfavorable outcome as measured by an MRS >2 at 3 months after stroke.

Abbreviation: NIHSS, National Institutes of Health stroke scale.

From Ntaios G, Faouzi M, Ferrari J, et al. An integer-based score to predict functional outcome in acute ischemic stroke. Neurology 2012;78:1916–22; with permission.

Radlinska and colleagues[39] showed that a lower tract volume and lower fractional anisotropy (FA) were associated with worse functional performance at 6-month follow-up.

In conclusion, neurologic status, motor ability, and function at stroke onset best predict long-term outcome on ADLs. Younger age predicts better outcome, whereas injury to PLIC on cranial imaging is associated with worse outcome.

Ambulation

Prognosis for ambulation after stroke is fairly good, such that 70% to 80% of chronic stroke survivors have the ability to walk.[40] On the negative side, only approximately 30% to 50% return to community ambulation, with gait speed being a key determinant of success.[8,41] There have been no systematic reviews to identify predictors for walking after stroke. Two small studies have shown that sitting balance 2 weeks after stroke onset can predict 6-month ambulation ability.[20,42] In particular, a score of ≤50 on the Trunk Control Test 14 days after stroke predicts that walking is unlikely at 6-month follow-up (**Table 3**).[20] Better trunk control on admission to rehabilitation also predicts better discharge motor FIM[43] and better ADL performance 6 month after stroke.[44] Age, NIHSS, baseline FIM score, and motor strength are also correlated with walking outcome, but none of these are as strong a predictor as balance.[20] Although early sitting balance can predict later walking, only gains in dynamic (walking) balance are associated with improvements in long-distance ambulation.[45]

Reding and Potes[46] plotted life tables showing that probability of walking after stroke is related to stroke severity. In particular they showed that more than 90% of patients with stroke will walk again, with or without an assistive device or some assistance after stroke. This goal was achieved for patients with pure motor hemiplegia at approximately 14 weeks after stroke, at 22 weeks for those with motor and sensory deficits, and at 28 weeks for those with motor, sensory, and visual deficits. Thus, it is not whether patients can walk with or without assistance after stroke, but when. When considering fully independent ambulation, the rates of recovery were as follows: 90% of those with only motor deficits are independent walkers at 14 weeks after stroke, 35% with motor and sensory deficits walk at 22 weeks, and only 3% of those with motor, sensory, and visual deficits are walking on their own even at 30 weeks after stroke.

As mentioned previously, there is a clear relationship between gait speed and overall functional independence. Both higher gait speed and timed distance walking are equally predictive of community ambulation after stroke.[47] Higher gait speeds are

Table 3 Trunk control test
Activity
Rolling to weak side
Rolling to strong side
Sitting up from lying down Balance in Sitting position
Scoring for Each Activity
0 = Unable to do on own
12 = Able to do but only by pulling on rail bedsheets and or stabilizing on arm
25 = Normal
Total = 100 points

From Collin C, Wade D. Assessing motor impairment after stroke: a pilot reliability study. J Neurol Neurosurg Psychiatry 1990;53:576–9; with permission.

related to better aerobic endurance, leg strength, balance, and a low fear of falling.[10,47] Although studies assessing early predictors of later community ambulation after stroke are lacking, one small study showed that early (<3 months) ability to walk at a speed of just over 0.4 m/s, and a low fear of falling, can predict community ambulation at 6 months. These associations suggest, as has recent clinical research, that high-intensity gait training at aerobic levels of effort, focusing on walking speed, might improve timed gait distance and potentially facilitate return to community ambulation.[48]

There has been limited research on predicting ambulation outcome with imaging. Lesion size and location have been associated with gait severity, but the level of injury to CST after stroke does not predict later walking speed or response to gait training.[49,50] There has recently been a growing interest in the use transcranial magnetic stimulation (TMS) for predicting motor outcomes because of its ability to measure the integrity (or conductivity) of motor systems in the central nervous system. The absence of TMS-induced motor-evoked potentials (MEPs) in the tibialis anterior muscle of a hemiplegic limb is associated with poor recovery of transfer ability and walking, but the predictive value TMS for functional recovery in lower limb has not been verified.[51,52]

Upper Limb Dexterity

The recovery of motor control and function in the upper limb follows a similar rate and pattern as the lower limb using standardized tests of both impairment and activity.[53,54] But actual functional use of the upper limb after stroke demands the return of a high degree of fine motor skill. For example, Flemming and colleagues[55] found in a small cohort of stroke survivors that a dexterity score of $\geq$54 of the maximum 57 on the Action Research Arm Test (ARAT) was necessary for patients to report that they use their impaired upper limb half as much or better as before stroke. The amount of recovered hand skill has also been shown to have a strong impact on patients' reported health-related quality of life.[56,57] In 2001, Coupar and others[58] reported findings from a meta-analysis that included 58 studies examining recovery of upper limb function after stroke. Not surprisingly, this analysis was hampered by the large variety of outcome measures used to assess performance. Still, they were able to conclude that the only clinical predictors that were strongly associated with upper limb recovery were baseline arm and hand motor ability and function. Lower motor performance at baseline results in a lower arm and hand ability 3 to 12 months after stroke. These findings were consistent with a previous systematic review by Chen and Winstein.[59] The measures used for baseline motor function in these studies included the Medical Research Council (MRC) strength testing, motricity index, NIHSS arm motor score, Scandinavian stroke scale arm impairment score, FMA, ARAT, Rivermeed arm score, BI, the motor assessment scale and others. Limited upper limb recovery was also associated with baseline lower limb motor function, but to a lesser degree. Thus, even simple bedside tests, such as manual muscle grade (MRC) or motricity index, which is composite score of the MRC for both upper and lower limb, are the simplest tools clinicians can use to predict later arm recovery (**Table 4**).[60–62] Au-Yeung and Hui-Chan[63] determined that a motricity index score of 64 of 100 or better in the impaired upper limb at 4 weeks after stroke predicts an ARAT of $\geq$35 at 6 months. If 2-point discrimination on the affected limb is normal at 2 weeks, then an upper limb motricity index of 45 or better predicts the same outcome. Of note, younger patients with low motor scores at baseline have the potential to recover hand dexterity even beyond 6 months after stroke.[64] Sensorimotor testing likely has its limitations. Strength does predict better outcome on standardized tests of upper limb dexterity and function, but even a detailed sensorimotor assessment of impaired upper limb explains only 25% of the variance when measuring the quality of a

Table 4	
Motricity Index is a composite score of both upper and lower limb	
ARM	**Pinch Grip Scoring**
Pinch grip	0 = No movement
2.5-cm cube between thumb and forefinger	11 = Beginning of prehension
Elbow flexion	19 = Grips cube but cannot hold against gravity
From 90° flexion at elbow	22 = Grips cube, held against gravity but not against weak pull
Shoulder abduction	26 = Grips cube against pull but weaker than unaffected side
From against chest	33 = Normal pinch grip
LEG	**Muscle Grading**[a]
Ankle dorsiflexion	0 = No movement
From plantar-flexed position	9 = Palpable contraction in muscle but no movement
Knee extension	14 = Movement seen but not full range against gravity
From 90° flexion of knee	19 = Full range against gravity, not against resistance
Hip flexion	25 = Movement against resistance but weaker than other side
From 90° flexion at hip	33 = Normal power

The scores for each limb have a maximum value of 99 + 1 = 100 points. The index is scored with patient in sitting position.

[a] Scored for elbow, shoulder, ankle, knee, and hip testing. Muscle grading is the same as MRC, but scored on a 33-point scale.

From Collin C, Wade D. Assessing motor impairment after stroke: a pilot reliability study. J Neurol Neurosurg Psychiatry 1990;53:576–9; with permission.

reaching task, such as speed, accuracy, and efficiency.[65] Thus, there is far more involved in recovering skilled movement than motor strength alone.

More specific predictors of hand recovery and function include early shoulder and finger movement. For example, the ability for a patient to shrug or abduct the affected shoulder on admission to a rehabilitation unit (1–6 weeks after stroke) predicts hand recovery and function at discharge and 3 months after stroke.[66,67] Similarly, the presence of active finger extension at 7 days after stroke predicts higher BI scores and better hand ability at 6 months as measured by 9-hole peg test, FMA, and motricity index.[68,69] Nijland and colleagues[70] found that patients with active shoulder abduction (MRC grade $\geq$1) and some active finger extension after mass finger grasp within 72 hours of stroke onset have a 98% probability of improving by at least 10 points or more on the ARAT at 6-month follow-up. Stinear and colleagues[71] showed that a combined MRC score of 8 or better in testing shoulder abduction and finger extension early after stroke predicts a score of 54 or better on ARAT at 12 weeks after stroke.

Steve Wolf and Binder-Macleod[72] noted in 1983 following a series of experiments they conducted on electromyographic biofeedback for upper limb recovery after stroke that patients with active wrist and finger extension are more likely to recover hand function. Thus, the ability to partially extend wrist and fingers became key entry criteria for participation in the EXCITE (EXtremity Constraint Induced Therapy Evaluation) trial that showed the efficacy of constraint-induced movement therapy (CIMT) for upper limb recovery after stroke.[73] In the context of therapy, hand control and finger extension predict superior response to CIMT treatment.[74,75]

The Fugl-Meyer assessment is a more detailed measure of motor control and requires more time to perform in the clinical setting, and yet it has a strong predictive value for upper limb recovery.[76] Prabhakaran and others[77] provided a model for predicting 6-month upper limb FMA based on FMA measured within 72 hours of stroke.

$$\text{Predicted } \Delta\text{FMA upper limb} \approx 0.7 \text{ (66-baseline FMA upper limb)} + 0.4$$

The model suggests that patients will improve to 70% of the difference between their baseline FMA and their maximum potential (ie, 66 points) on the FMA. This proportional recovery model holds true for nearly all patients, with the exception of those with the most severe arm impairment at onset. Approximately two-thirds of patients with a baseline FMA of approximately 18 or less will fail to achieve the 70% predicted recovery. Those who do worse than predicted have no finger extension, a facial palsy (on the NIHSS), severe lower limb impairment (on the FMA), and total or partial anterior circulation infarction.[78]

Imaging can assist in prediction of upper limb recovery, but clinical motor function remains a better predictor.[76] Still, there is a strong relationship between the presence of a subcortical stroke lesion and worse long-term hand recovery as measured by FMA.[79-81] This is particularly true when the lesion is located in the PLIC.[80,81] Pure cortical strokes, especially those that do not involve motor cortex or adjacent centrum semiovale, predict good recovery of FMA both acutely and at 1 year after stroke.[79,80] Using DTI, Schaechter and colleagues[82] demonstrated a positive correlation between FA of ipsilesional CST and motor hand skills in patients with chronic stroke. Patients with lesions involving extrapyramidal tracts in addition to CST have inferior performance on FMA and the Wolf Motor Function Test compared with those with CST involvement alone on DTI.[83]

The use of TMS to predict upper limb recovery based on motor tract integrity does have some clinical value in patients with complete arm and hand paralysis. The ability to evoke a motor response in the abductor digiti minimi of the affected upper limb in paralyzed patients (MRC<2) 1 week after stroke is a strong predictor of some recovery of upper limb movement 1 year after stroke.[84] The predictive ability for upper limb recovery with an MEP is quite specific (99%), meaning there are no false positives. The sensitivity on the other hand ranges from 62% to 94%, because some patients without an MEP will still regain some motor function.[85] Thus, MEPs have an excellent positive predictive value for arm recovery in patients with total arm paralysis, but recovery of 3 or more points on the upper limb FMA 1 week after onset has an equivalent positive predictive value.[86] Still, it is important to note that several systematic reviews have reported that, along with voluntary motor ability, neurophysiological measures, such as the presence of an MEP early after stroke, are the strongest predictors of later recovery.[58,59,87]

Stinear[88] proposed an algorithm for predicting arm recovery after stroke that is clinically promising. Predicting recovery potential (PREP) uses clinical evaluation, TMS, and MRI to separate patients with acute stroke into 4 categories of expected recovery based on ARAT performance at 12 weeks (**Fig. 1**). PREP uses shoulder abduction and finger extension MRC grades (SAFE) to determine probability of *complete* recovery, as was proposed by Nijland and colleagues.[70] The presence of an MEP using TMS over injured motor cortex determines *notable* recovery. Finally, to identify patients who will have *limited* versus *no* recovery, MRI analysis of FA asymmetry is required. Asymmetry of FA compares the FA measurement of PLIC within both the injured and uninjured hemispheres. An FA asymmetry of 0 indicates no injury to PLIC of the affected hemisphere and a value of 1 indicates no preserved white matter tracts on the injured side. An FA asymmetry of greater than 0.15 is a point of no return, predicting no recovery. In a sample of 40 patients with a wide range of initial impairment assessed within 2 weeks of stroke, PREP had a positive predictive value of complete recovery of 88% and a negative predictive value of 83%.[71] The other recovery categories were well separated across possible 12-week ARAT performance. With further study and refinement, PREP could be useful for planning rehabilitation care and functional goals.

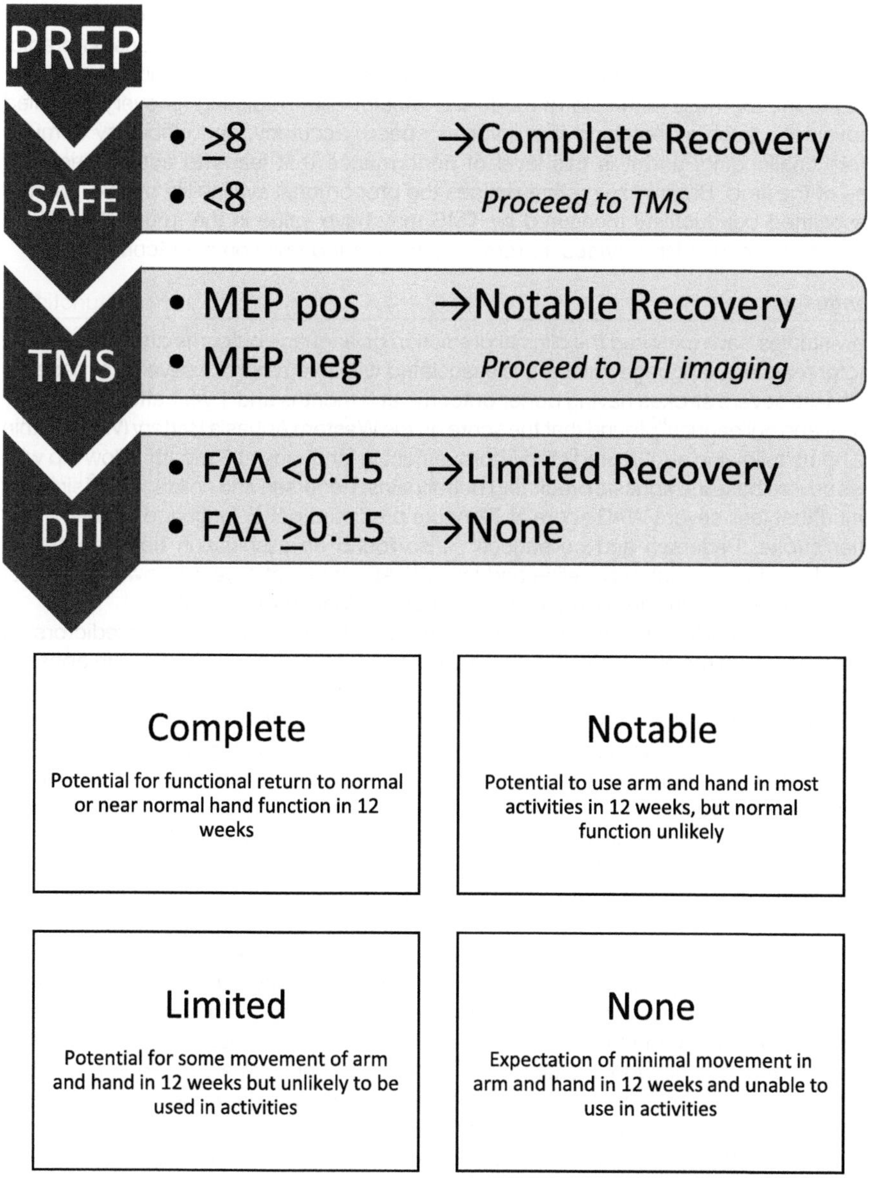

PREP

SAFE
- ≥8   →Complete Recovery
- <8   *Proceed to TMS*

TMS
- MEP pos   →Notable Recovery
- MEP neg   *Proceed to DTI imaging*

DTI
- FAA <0.15   →Limited Recovery
- FAA ≥0.15   →None

Complete

Potential for functional return to normal or near normal hand function in 12 weeks

Notable

Potential to use arm and hand in most activities in 12 weeks, but normal function unlikely

Limited

Potential for some movement of arm and hand in 12 weeks but unlikely to be used in activities

None

Expectation of minimal movement in arm and hand in 12 weeks and unable to use in activities

Fig. 1. The PREP algorithm predicts arm and hand recovery using clinical, TMS, and MRI (DTI) assessments. SAFE is added MRC score from shoulder abduction and finger extension (maximum = 10). MEP is positive (pos) or negative (neg) for MEPs in extensor digitorum communis muscle of affected upper limb with TMS over injured motor cortex. FAA is the fractional anisotropy asymmetry of bilateral poster limb of the internal capsule measured as (FA noninjured side − FA injured side)/(FA noninjured side + FA injured side). The algorithm predicts motor recovery that is complete, notable, limited, or none, as measured by the ARAT and can be defined functionally as shown. (*Adapted from* Stinear C, Barber PA, Petoe M, et al. The prep algorithm predicts potential for upper limb recovery after stroke. Brain 2012;135:2527–35.)

Presently it can be concluded that motor strength is a strong predictor of arm and hand recovery, and that early active shoulder movement and finger extension predict later hand function. FMA has a very good predictive value using the proportional recovery model, for those with mild to moderate impairment. Predicting recovery of skilled movement, such as reaching that involves speed, accuracy, and efficiency is much more challenging, and it is this level of performance that leads to actual functional use of the limb. Brain imaging that defines the proportional availability of CST and the associated conductivity measured by TMS may have value in the future. The PREP algorithm in particular provides a promising model for prediction of outcome.

Language

Few studies have explored the clinical prediction of language outcome after stroke. Like motor recovery, language outcome is associated with overall stroke severity at baseline with less severe strokes having better outcome at 3 months and 1 year after stroke.[89,90] Lazar and colleagues[89] found that the score on the Western Aphasia Battery (WAB) within 72 hours following stroke predicted improvement in language at 3 month follow-up with less severe baseline aphasia predicting better gains. Pedersen and colleagues[90] similarly found that less severe WAB score at 72 hours predicted better language scores 1 year after stroke. Pedersen and colleagues[90] also found an association between severe neurologic impairment at baseline and lower WAB scores at 1-year follow-up. A lower baseline BI score similarly predicts worse language function 1 year later.

Only one study has examined the components of language as predictors of outcome. Hachioui and others[91] followed 147 patients with acute stroke with aphasia. They measured 3 language components 4 days after stroke, including semantics (word meaning), phonology (word sound), and syntax (sentence structure). At 1-year follow-up, phonology was the best independent predictor of language outcome. Predictive strength improved if 6-week phonological performance was included in the model. Phonology tested repetition, reading aloud, judging same/different spoken word pairs, and matching the first phoneme of a spoken word with its grapheme. Thus, phonological ability required skill with repetition and comprehension more so than verbal fluency and oral expression. This group also found that younger age and higher education were associated with better language outcome. Others have also found a similar association with age and language outcome.[89,90]

Cranial imaging provides very inconsistent predictability for language outcome. Although large lesions involving the entire left hemisphere language network and poor baseline language function predict poor late outcome, localized involvement of specific language network locations (eg, Broca and Wernicke areas) do not correlate with outcomes or rates of recovery.[92] Using lesion data from large samples of aphasic patients along with information on recovery and outcome could potentially provide accurate prediction. A data bank called "Predicting Language Outcome and Recovery after Stroke" (PLORAS) is currently being developed for this purpose. With such a data-led system, a new patient with aphasia could have acute brain imaging compared with many others with similar lesions, providing a likelihood of recovery.[92] Saur and colleagues[93] tested a similar concept using functional MRI 2 weeks after stroke where clinical factors plus analysis of blood oxygen-level dependent (BOLD) activity in the right inferior frontal cortex improves prediction of language recovery at 6 months. Other imaging modalities may be helpful. Regional blood flow to angular gyrus and lower insular ribbon on admission computed tomography angiography can predict improvement on NIHSS language score by acute hospital discharge.[94] DTI imaging of the right and left arcuate fasciculus shows promise for predicting language recovery.[95,96]

In conclusion, severity of language performance at onset of stroke is the strongest predictor of long-term language recovery. Phonological skill that is clinically evident by a patient's ability to comprehend spoken language and repeat sentences is predictive of better recovery. Cranial imaging is not yet a reliable tool for prediction of language outcomes.

SUMMARY

The field of rehabilitation medicine currently lacks universally accepted, well-validated models for predicting recovery after stroke. But there are certain clinical pearls we can use at the bedside. Shoulder abduction and finger extension at stroke onset predict arm recovery. Good sitting balance at onset predicts return to independent walking. Ability to comprehend and repeat spoken language predicts better language recovery. But with better and more precise cranial imaging techniques, which will allow improved analysis of brain structure, and with neurophysiological techniques, such as TMS, that allow measure of motor tract integrity, useful clinical algorithms may be possible. To test these models, data banks are needed that contain clinical, imaging, and neurophysiological information from large cohorts of patients with stroke. National and global stroke rehabilitation consortiums that use standardized measures and diagnostic technologies are needed to develop reliable predictive models for stroke care and research.

REFERENCES

1. Counsell C, Dennis M, McDowall M, et al. Predicting outcome after acute and subacute stroke—development and validation of new prognostic models. Stroke 2002;33:1041–7.
2. Veerbeek JM, Kwakkel G, van Wegen EE, et al. Early prediction of outcome of activities of daily living after stroke: a systematic review. Stroke 2011;42:1482–8.
3. Twitchell TE. The restoration of motor function following hemiplegia in man. Brain 1951;64:443–80.
4. Brunnstrom S. Movement therapy in hemiplegia: a neurophysiological approach. New York: Harper & Row; 1970.
5. Sawner K, LaVigne J. Brunnstrom's movement therapy in hemiplegia: a neurophysiological approach. Philadelphia: JB Lippincott; 1992.
6. Fugl-Meyer AR, Jaasko L, Leyman I, et al. The post stroke hemiplegic patient: I. A method for evaluation of physical performance. Scand J Rehabil Med 1975;7:13–31.
7. Flansbjer UB, Downham D, Lexell J. Knee muscle strength, gait performance, and perceived participation after stroke. Arch Phys Med Rehabil 2006;87:974–80.
8. Perry J. Classification of walking handicap in the stroke population. Stroke 1995;26:982–9.
9. Pradon D, Roche N, Enette L, et al. Relationship between lower limb muscle strength and 6-minute walk test performance in stroke patients. J Rehabil Med 2013;45:105–8.
10. Taylor-Piliae RE, Latt LD, Hepworth LT, et al. Predictors of gait velocity among community-dwelling stroke survivors. Gait Posture 2011;35:395–9.
11. Tilson JK, Sullivan KJ, Cen SY, et al. Meaningful gait speed improvement during the first 60 days poststroke: minimal clinically important difference. Phys Ther 2010;90:196–208.
12. Bonita R, Beaglehole R. Modification of Rankin scale: recovery of motor function after stroke. Stroke 1988;19:1497–500.

13. Duncan PW, Lai SM, Keighley J. Defining post-stroke recovery: implications for design and interpretation of drug trials. Neuropharmacology 2000;39:835–41.

14. Nesi M, Lucente G, Nencini P, et al. Aphasia predicts unfavorable outcome in mild ischemic stroke patients and prompts throbolytic treatment. J Stroke Cerebrovasc Dis 2014;23:204–8.

15. Tsouli S, Kyritsis AP, Tsagalis G, et al. Significance of aphasia after first-ever acute stroke: impact on early and late outcomes. Neuroepidemiology 2009;33:96–102.

16. Gialanella B. Aphasia assessment and functional outcome prediction in patients with aphasia after stroke. J Neurol 2011;258:343–9.

17. Gonzalez-Fernandez M, Christian AB, Davis C, et al. Role of aphasia in discharge location after stroke. Arch Phys Med Rehabil 2013;94:851–5.

18. Kwakkel G, Kollen BJ. Predicting activities after stroke: what is clinically relevant? Int J Stroke 2013;8:25–32.

19. Cioncoloni D, Martini G, Piu P, et al. Predictors of long-term recovery in complex activities of daily living before discharge from the stroke unit. NeuroRehabilitation 2013;33:217–33.

20. Duerte E, Marco E, Muniesa JM, et al. Early detection of non-ambulatory survivors six months after stroke. NeuroRehabilitation 2010;26:317–23.

21. Khan M, Goddeau RP, Zhang J, et al. Predictors of outcome following stroke due to isolated m2 occlusion. Cerebrovasc Dis Extra 2014;4:52–60.

22. Kwakkel G, Veerbeek JM, Harmeling-van der Wel BC, et al. Diagnostic accuracy of the Barthel index for measuring activities of daily living outcome after ischemic hemispheric stroke: does early post-stroke timing of assessment matter. Stroke 2011;42:342–6.

23. Kwakkel G, Veerbeek JM, van Wegen EE, et al. Predictive value of the NIHSS for ADL outcome after ischemic hemispheric stroke: does timing of early assessment matter? J Neurol Sci 2010;294:57–61.

24. Protopsaltis J, Kokkoris S, Korantzopoulos P, et al. Prediction of long-term functional outcome in patients with acute ischemic non-embolic stroke. Atherosclerosis 2009;203:228–35.

25. Tei H, Uchiyama S, Usui T, et al. Diffusion-weighted aspects as an independent marker for independent outcome. J Neurol 2011;258:559–65.

26. Jongbloed L. Prediction of function after stroke: a critical review. Stroke 1986;17: 765–76.

27. Govan L, Langhorne P, Weir CJ. Categorizing stroke prognosis using different stroke scales. Stroke 2009;40:3396–9.

28. Tilling K, Sterne JA, Rudd AG, et al. A new method for predicting recovery after stoke. Stroke 2001;32:2867–73.

29. Loewen SC, Anderson BA. Predictors of stroke outcome using objective measurement scales. Stroke 1990;21:78–81.

30. Ntaios G, Faouzi M, Ferrari J, et al. An integer-based score to predict functional outcome in acute ischemic stroke. Neurology 2012;78:1916–22.

31. Liu G, Ntaios G, Zheng H, et al. External validation of the astral score to predict 3- and 12-month functional outcome in the China National Stroke Registry. Stroke 2013;44:1443–5.

32. Papavasileiou V, Milionis H, Michel P, et al. Astral score predicts 5-year dependence and mortality in acute ischemic stroke. Stroke 2013;44:1616–20.

33. Schiemanck SK, Kwakkel G, Post MW, et al. Predicting long-term independency in activities of daily living after middle cerebral artery stroke: does information from MRI have added predictive value compared with clinical information. Stroke 2006;37:1050–4.

34. Schiemanck SK, Kwakkel G, Post MW, et al. Predictive value of ischemic lesion volume assessed with magnetic resonance imaging for neurological deficits and functional outcome poststroke: a critical review of the literature. Neurorehabil Neural Repair 2006;20:492–502.
35. Hand PJ, Wardlaw JM, Rivers CS, et al. MR diffusion-weighted imaging and outcome prediction after ischemic stroke. Neurology 2006;66:1159–63.
36. Wardlaw JM, Keir SL, Bastin ME, et al. Is diffusion imaging appearance and independent predictor of outcome after ischemic stroke. Neurology 2002;59:1381–7.
37. Zaidi SF, Aghaebrahim A, Urra X, et al. Final infarct volume is a stronger predictor of outcome than recanalization in patients with proximal middle cerebral artery occlusion treated with endovascular therapy. Stroke 2012;43:3238–44.
38. Puig J, Pedraza S, Blasco G, et al. Acute damage to the posterior limb of the internal capsule on diffusion tensor tractography as an early predictor of motor outcome after stroke. AJNR Am J Neuroradiol 2011;32:857–63.
39. Radlinska B, Ghinani S, Leppert IR, et al. Diffusion tensor imaging, permanent pyramidal tract damage, and outcome in subcortical stroke. Neurology 2010;75:1048–54.
40. Jang SH. The recovery of walking in stroke patients: a review. Int J Rehabil Res 2010;33:285–9.
41. Lord SE, McPherson K, McNaughton HK, et al. Community ambulation after stroke: how important and obtainable is it and what measures appear to be predictive. Arch Phys Med Rehabil 2004;85:234–9.
42. Feigin L, Sharon B, Czaczkes B, et al. Sitting equilibrium 2 weeks after stroke can predict the walking ability after 6 months. Gerontology 1996;42:348–53.
43. Franchignoni FP, Tesio L, Ricupero C, et al. Trunk control test as an early predictor of stroke rehabilitation outcome. Stroke 1997;28:1382–5.
44. Hsieh CL, Sheu CF, Hsueh IP, et al. Trunk control as an early predictor of comprehensive activities of daily living function in stroke patients. Stroke 2002;33:2626–30.
45. Awad LN, Reisman DS, Binder-Macleod SA. Do improvements in balance related to improvements in long-distance walking function after stroke? Stroke Res Treat 2014;2014:6.
46. Reding MJ, Potes E. Rehabilitation outcome following initial unilateral hemispheric stroke: life table analysis. Stroke 1988;19:1354–8.
47. Bijleveld-Uitman M, van de Port IG, Kwakkel G. Is gait speed or walking distance a better predictor for community walking after stroke? J Rehabil Med 2013;45:535–40.
48. Holleran C, Straube DD, Kinnaird CR, et al. Feasibility and potential efficacy of high-intensity stepping training in variable contexts in subacute and chronic stroke. Neurorehabil Neural Repair 2014;28:643–51.
49. Dawes H, Enzinger C, Johansen-Berg H, et al. Walking performance and its recovery in chronic stroke in relation to extent of lesion overlap with the descending motor tract. Exp Brain Res 2008;186:325–33.
50. Kaczmarczyk K, Wit A, Krawczyk M, et al. Associations between gait patterns, brain lesion factors and functional recovery in stroke patients. Gait Posture 2011;35:214–7.
51. Hendricks HT, Pasman JW, van Limbeek J, et al. Motor evoked potentials of the lower extremity in predicting motor recovery and ambulation after stroke: a cohort study. Arch Phys Med Rehabil 2003;84:1373–9.

52. Piron L, Piccione F, Tonin P, et al. Clinical correlation between motor evoked potentials and gait recovery in poststroke patients. Arch Phys Med Rehabil 2005;86: 1874–8.

53. Duncan PW, Goldstein LB, Horner RD, et al. Similar motor recovery of upper and lower extremities after stroke. Stroke 1994;25:1181–8.

54. Higgins J, Mayo NE, Desrosiers J, et al. Upper-limb function and recovery in the acute phase poststroke. J Rehabil Res Dev 2005;42:65–76.

55. Flemming MK, Newham DJ, Roberts-Lewis SF, et al. Self-perceived utilization of the paretic arm in chronic stroke requires high upper limb functional ability. Arch Phys Med Rehabil 2014;95:918–24.

56. Franceschini M, La Porta F, Agosti M, et al. Is health-related-quality of life of stroke patients influenced by neurological impairments at one year after stroke? Eur J Phys Rehabil Med 2010;46:389–99.

57. Morris JH, van Wijck F, Joice S, et al. Predicting health related quality of life 6 months after stroke: the role of anxiety and upper limb dysfunction. Disabil Rehabil 2013;35:291–9.

58. Coupar F, Pollock A, Rowe P, et al. Predictors of upper limb recovery after stroke: a systematic review and meta-analysis. Clin Rehabil 2011;26:291–313.

59. Chen SY, Winstein CJ. A systematic review of voluntary arm recovery in hemiparetic stroke. J Neurol Phys Ther 2009;33:2–13.

60. Collin C, Wade D. Assessing motor impairment after stroke: a pilot reliability study. J Neurol Neurosurg Psychiatry 1990;53:576–9.

61. Kong KH, Chua KS, Lee J. Recovery of upper limb dexterity in patients more than a year after stroke: frequency, clinical correlates and predictors. NeuroRehabilitation 2011;28:105–11.

62. Olsen TS. Arm and leg paresis as outcome predictors in stroke rehabilitation. Stroke 1990;21:247–51.

63. Au-Yeung SS, Hui-Chan CW. Predicting recovery of dextrous hand function in acute stroke. Disabil Rehabil 2009;31:394–401.

64. Kong KH, Lee J. Temporal recovery and predictors of upper limb dexterity in the first year of stroke: a prospective study of patients admitted to a rehabilitation center. NeuroRehabilitation 2013;32:345–50.

65. Wagner JM, Lang CE, Sahrmann SA, et al. Sensorimotor impairments and reaching performance in subjects with poststroke hemiparesis during the first few months of recovery. Phys Ther 2007;87:751–65.

66. Houwink A, Nijland RH, Geurts AC, et al. Functional recovery of the paretic upper limb after stroke: who regains hand capacity. Arch Phys Med Rehabil 2013;94: 839–44.

67. Katrak P, Bowring G, Conroy P, et al. Predicting upper limb recovery after stroke: the place of early shoulder and hand movement. Arch Phys Med Rehabil 1998; 79:758–61.

68. Smania N, Gambarin M, Tinazzi M, et al. Are indexes of arm recovery related to daily life autonomy in patients with stroke? Eur J Phys Rehabil Med 2009;45: 349–54.

69. Smania N, Paolucci S, Tinazzi M, et al. Active finger extension: a simple movement predicting recovery of arm function in patients with acute stroke. Stroke 2007;38:1088–90.

70. Nijland RH, van Wegen EE, Harmeling-van der Wel BC, et al. Presence of finger extension and shoulder abduction within 72 hours after stroke predicts functional recovery- early prediction of functional outcome after stroke: the EPOS cohort study. Stroke 2010;41:745–50.

71. Stinear C, Barber PA, Petoe M, et al. The prep algorithm predicts potential for upper limb recovery after stroke. Brain 2012;135:2527–35.

72. Wolf SL, Binder-Macleod SA. Electromyographic biofeedback applications to the hemiplegic patient. Phys Ther 1983;63:1393–403.

73. Wolf SL, Winstein CJ, Miller JP, et al. Effect of constraint-induced movement therapy on upper extremity function 3 to 9 months after stroke: the excite randomized clinical trial. JAMA 2010;296:2095–104.

74. Fritz SL, Light KE, Patterson TS, et al. Active finger extension predicts outcomes after constraint-induced movement therapy for individuals with hemiparesis after stroke. Stroke 2005;36:1172–7.

75. Lin KC, Huang YH, Hsieh YW, et al. Potential predictors of motor and functional outcomes after distributed constraint-induced therapy for patients with stroke. Neurorehabil Neural Repair 2009;23:336–42.

76. Feys H, De Weerdt W, Nuyens G, et al. Predicting motor recovery of the upper limb after stroke rehabilitation: value of a clinical examination. Physiother Res Int 2000;5:1–18.

77. Prabhakaran S, Zarahn E, Riley C, et al. Inter-individual variability in the capacity for motor recovery after ischemic stroke. Neurorehabil Neural Repair 2008;22: 64–71.

78. Winters C, van Wegen EE, Daffershofer A, et al. Generalizability of the proportional recovery model for the upper extremity after an ischemic stroke. Neurorehabil Neural Repair 2015;29(7):614–22.

79. Schiemanck SK, Kwakkel G, Post MW, et al. Impact of internal capsule lesions on outcome of motor hand function at one year post-stroke. J Rehabil Med 2008;40: 96–101.

80. Shelton F, Reding MJ. Effect of lesion location on upper limb motor recovery after stroke. Stroke 2001;32:107–12.

81. Wenzelburger R, Kopper F, Frenzel A, et al. Hand coordination following capsular stroke. Brain 2005;128:64–74.

82. Schaechter JD, Fricker ZP, Perdue KL, et al. Microstructural status of ipsilesional and contralesional corticospinal tract correlates with motor skill in chronic stroke patients. Hum Brain Mapp 2009;30:3461–74.

83. Lindenberg R, Renga V, Zhu LL, et al. Structural integrity of corticospinal motor fibers predicts motor impairment in chronic stroke. Neurology 2010;74:280–7.

84. Pizzi A, Carrai R, Catuscia F, et al. Prognostic value of motor evoked potentials in motor function recovery of upper limb after stroke. J Rehabil Med 2009;41: 654–60.

85. Hendricks HT, Zwarts MJ, Plat EF, et al. Systematic review for the early prediction of motor and functional outcome after stroke by using motor-evoked potentials. Arch Phys Med Rehabil 2002;83:1303–8.

86. van Kuijk AA, Pasman JW, Hendricks HT, et al. Predicting hand motor recovery in severe stroke: the role of motor evoked potentials in relation to early clinical assessment. Neurorehabil Neural Repair 2009;23:45–51.

87. Hendricks HT, van Limbeek J, Geurts AC, et al. Motor recovery after stroke: a systematic review. Arch Phys Med Rehabil 2002;83:1629–37.

88. Stinear C. Prediction of recovery of motor function after stroke. Lancet Neurol 2010;9:1228–32.

89. Lazar RM, Minzer B, Antoniello D, et al. Improvement in aphasia scores after stroke is well predicted by initial severity. Stroke 2010;41:1485–8.

90. Pedersen PM, Vinter K, Olsen TS. Aphasia after stroke: type, severity and prognosis. The Copenhagen Aphasia Study. Cerebrovasc Dis 2004;17:35–43.

91. Hachioui HE, Lingsma HF, van de Sandt-Koenderman MW, et al. Long-term prognosis of aphasia after stroke. J Neurol Neurosurg Psychiatry 2013;84:310–5.

92. Price CJ, Seghier ML, Leff AP. Predicting language outcome and recovery after stroke: the PLORAS system. Nat Rev Neurol 2010;6:202–10.

93. Saur D, Ronneberger O, Kummerer D, et al. Early functional magnetic resonance imaging activation predicts language outcome after stroke. Brain 2010;133: 1252–64.

94. Payabvash S, Kamalian S, Fung S, et al. Predicting language improvement in acute stroke patients presenting with aphasia: a multivariate logistic model using location-weighted atlas-based analysis of admission CT perfusion scans. AJNR Am J Neuroradiol 2010;31:1661–8.

95. Forkel SJ, de Schotten MT, Dell'Acqua F, et al. Anatomical predictors of aphasia recovery: a tractography study of bilateral perisylvian language networks. Brain 2014;137:2027–39.

96. Kim SH, Lee DG, You H, et al. The clinical application of the arcuate fasciculus for stroke patients with aphasia: a diffusion tensor tractography study. NeuroRehabilitation 2011;29:305–10.

Upper Limb Motor Impairment After Stroke

Preeti Raghavan, MD

KEYWORDS

- Stroke • Arm • Weakness • Hemiparesis • Motor control

KEY POINTS

- Weakness or paresis is the key impairment early on that leads to learned nonuse. Sensory impairment, immobility, and chronic pain may further contribute to learned nonuse.
- Spasticity, spastic cocontraction, and abnormal motor synergies occur as recovery proceeds and may lead to abnormal compensatory movements, which if repeated and reinforced lead to learned bad use.
- Impairment in sensorimotor adaptation can lead to transient retention of new skills despite extensive practice; this is referred to as forgetting.

THE NATURE OF UPPER LIMB MOTOR IMPAIRMENT

According to the International Classification of Functioning, Disability and Health (ICF) model,[1] impairments may be described as (1) impairments of body function such as a significant deviation or loss in neuromusculoskeletal and movement-related function related to joint mobility, muscle power, muscle tone, and/or involuntary movements or (2) impairment of body structures such as a significant deviation in structure of the nervous system or structures related to movement, for example, the arm and/or hand. A stroke may lead to both types of impairments. Upper limb impairments after stroke cause the functional limitations in using the affected upper limb after stroke, therefore a clear understanding of the underlying impairments is necessary for restoration of upper limb function. However, understanding upper limb impairments in any given patient is complex for two reasons. (1) The impairments are not static, that is, as motor recovery proceeds, the type and nature of the impairments may change; therefore the treatment needs to evolve to target the impairment(s) contributing to dysfunction at a given point in time. (2) Multiple impairments may be present simultaneously, that is, a patient may present with weakness of the arm and hand immediately after a

Funding: NIH R01HD071978.
Motor Recovery Research Laboratory, Department of Rehabilitation Medicine, Rusk Rehabilitation, New York University School of Medicine, 240 East 38th Street, 17th Floor, New York, NY 10016, USA
E-mail address: Preeti.Raghavan@nyumc.org

Phys Med Rehabil Clin N Am 26 (2015) 599–610
http://dx.doi.org/10.1016/j.pmr.2015.06.008
1047-9651/15/$ – see front matter © 2015 Elsevier Inc. All rights reserved.

stroke, which may not have resolved when spasticity sets in a few weeks or months later; hence there may be a layering of impairments over time making it difficult to decide what to treat first. It is useful to review the progression of motor recovery as described by Twitchell[2] and Brunnstrom[3] to understand how impairments may be layered over time (**Fig. 1**).

UNDERSTANDING MOTOR IMPAIRMENT FROM A FUNCTIONAL PERSPECTIVE

The most useful way to understand how impairments contribute to upper limb dysfunction may be to examine them from the perspective of their functional consequences. There are three main functional consequences of stroke on the upper limb: (1) learned nonuse, (2) learned bad use, and (3) forgetting as determined by behavioral analysis of a task such as reaching for a food pellet and bringing it to the mouth in animal models of stroke.[4] These consequences are equally valid for human behavior. Each of the functional consequences and the underlying impairments are elaborated in the following sections.

LEARNED NONUSE

Initially after a stroke, individuals may not use their affected upper limb, eventually leading to learned nonuse. Nonuse can result from several impairments. Initially nonuse may occur because of weakness/paralysis or sensory loss. However, as time progresses, nonuse may become habitual and the limb may not be incorporated into functional activities, even though the individual can move it. Now it becomes a learned behavior and is referred to as learned nonuse.

Weakness or paralysis is the predominant impairment that contributes to dysfunction after stroke[5,6]; it is a direct consequence of the lack of signal transmission from the motor cortex, which generates the movement impulse, to the spinal cord, which executes the movement via signals to muscles. This lack of transmission results in delayed initiation and termination of muscle contraction,[7] and slowness in developing force,[8] manifested as an inability to move or move quickly with negative functional consequences. Abnormally increased electromyographic (EMG)-force slopes are

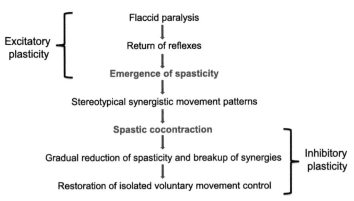

Fig. 1. Sequential progression of motor recovery as described by Twitchell[2] and Brunnstrom.[47,48] Note that while recovery is proceeding from one stage to the next, residual impairment from preceding stages may still be present leading to the layering of impairment. Excitatory and inhibitory plasticity are the presumed underlying physiologic processes that could account for progression of recovery from one stage to the next.

seen on the affected side compared with the contralateral side as well as compared with neurologically intact subjects, suggesting that greater EMG activity is necessary to generate a given force in patients with stroke.[9] This requirement is thought to result from a combination of abnormal firing rate patterns and changes in motor unit control. Weakness may affect all muscle groups of the upper limb, or may be selective, affecting some muscle groups more than the others. Large intersubject differences exist in the pattern of muscle weakness across muscle groups, but research has shown that no consistent proximal to distal gradient or greater extensor relative to flexor weakness exists.[10,11] The absolute strength in any particular muscle group has not been shown to predict function, whereas the rate of change of force development in wrist extensor and handgrip strength[12] are good predictors of upper limb function. Isolated motor deficits in a single arm can occur after a stroke without other cranial or sensory dysfunction; these are rare and easily misdiagnosed, requiring a high index of suspicion and assessment of risk factors for stroke.[13,14] In cases in which trauma accompanies the vascular lesion, the pattern of weakness may need to be examined carefully to rule out spinal cord injury or peripheral nerve injury. Weakness leads to immobility, which can initiate a cascade of problems that can further contribute to motor impairment (**Fig. 2**), as described in the following discussion.

Sensory loss across tactile, proprioceptive, and/or higher-order sensory modalities such as deficits in 2-point discrimination, stereognosis, and graphesthesia are common after stroke and may be associated with the degree of weakness and the degree of stroke severity, as well as mobility, independence in activities of daily living, and recovery.[15] Sensory impairments without motor weakness may also occur from specific lesions in the parietal cortex.[16] In studies that compared the ability of hemiparetic and healthy subjects to produce symmetric forces with both upper limbs, it was found that joint maximum voluntary forces and proprioceptive impairments in the affected limb

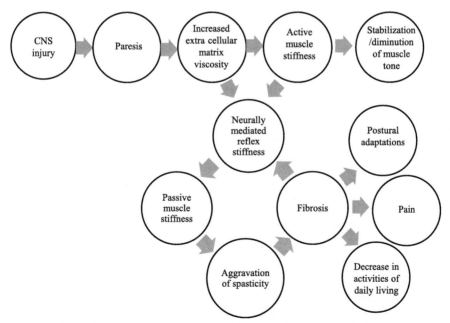

Fig. 2. Model of the contribution of paresis and immobility to the evolution of spasticity. (*From* Stecco A, Stecco C, Raghavan P. Peripheral mechanisms of spasticity and treatment implications. Curr Phys Med Rehabil Rep 2014;2(2):121–7; with permission.)

predicted the errors in force matching.[17] These results suggest that sensory impairments may lead to inaccurate motor output, even though motor capacities were adequate to perform the task. In fact the term learned nonuse was coined from observations in deafferented monkeys that could move but did not do so voluntarily.[18] Chronic loss of sensation may contribute to motor impairment because of inaccurate internal representations of the task and/or inability to control the motor output appropriately owing to lack of feedback about the consequences of the motor action.

Weakness leads to immobility, which can be considered a functional impairment according to the ICF classification.[1] Immobility in turn can begin a vicious circle of problems including peripheral soft tissue changes that reduce tissue compliance, potentiation of reflex mechanisms, and spasticity, eventually leading to muscle fibrosis and contributing to abnormal limb posturing, pain, and decreased function (see **Fig. 2**).[19] Spasticity is now thought to arise as a consequence of contractures rather than being a cause of contractures.[20] Hence early interventions to reduce immobility and preserve range of motion either passively or actively despite paresis, and prevent contractures may be critical to prevent spasticity and its ensuing complications. Passive tissue restraint and agonist weakness, rather than antagonist restraint, have been shown to be the most common contributors to decreased active range of motion.[21] Immobility also leads to changes in bone mineral density with increased risk of developing osteoporosis on the paralyzed side particularly in the upper limbs.[22,23] In fact, fractures are common on the paretic side after stroke.[24] Practitioners need to pay more attention to changes in bone mineral density after stroke and take active measures to prevent problems arising from immobility.

Motor and sensory impairments and immobility are associated with an increased risk for stroke-related pain.[25] Stiffness in the connective tissue of the immobilized limb may stimulate free nerve endings and proprioceptors, such as Pacini and Ruffini corpuscles[26–28] in the tissue producing pain.[29,30] Shoulder pain on the paretic side is common after stroke and is strongly associated with abnormal shoulder joint examination, ipsilateral sensory abnormalities, and arm weakness.[31] Deafferentation and sensory loss may also lead to the development of neuronal hypersensitivity, and eventually, chronic central pain[32–34] which is often difficult to treat. Pain can lead to learned nonuse, which may persist even after the pain has resolved.

LEARNED BAD USE

When the paretic limb is forced to move, weakness, sensory impairments, and pain can prevent normal movement; instead compensatory strategies are used to complete the task or tasks.[35] Furthermore, stiffness and contractures resulting from immobility and the development of spasticity and abnormal motor synergies can contribute to compensatory movements. The use of compensatory strategies has been well described for human reaching and grasping after stroke.[36] Patients with stroke use trunk flexion rather than elbow extension to reach for objects,[37] forearm pronation and wrist flexion rather than neutral forearm position and wrist extension to orient the hand for grasping, and metacarpophalangeal joint flexion rather than proximal interphalangeal joint flexion to grasp objects.[38] Although the use of compensatory strategies may lead to initial success in completing a task, over time success is reduced because of poor accuracy, which increases the probability of failure. Reinforcement of the abnormal strategy by occasional successes can lead to it becoming a bad habit over time,[39] and performance declines despite extended training because the abnormal behavior is repeated and reinforced at the cost of the correct pattern of behavior.[40] Thus in the absence of appropriate feedback and correction of the abnormal motor behavior, learned bad use develops. When the focus of training is to reduce compensatory behaviors, for example, when the trunk is restrained during reach practice, the typical use of a more normal pattern of reaching by extending the elbow is restored along with a reduction in overall impairment.[41,42]

Spasticity and incoordination because of abnormal motor synergies can lead to the development of learned bad use. Spasticity is defined as a motor disorder character- ized by a velocity-dependent increase in muscle tone with exaggerated tendon jerks, resulting from hyperexcitability of the stretch reflex, as one component of the upper motor neuron syndrome.[43] The prevalence of spasticity increases with time since stroke[44] and is related to the secondary effects of weakness and immobility on skel- etal muscles.[25,45,46] Initially, spasticity is considered a positive development because it suggests that the nervous system is beginning to initiate repair mechanisms to restore muscle tone and movement. Indeed, patients who demonstrate spasticity are further along in their recovery than individuals who are more flaccid.[47,48] However, when the threshold for reflex activity continues to reduce because of progressive reor- ganization of the supraspinal descending drive to the spinal cord, peripheral structures of the muscle, muscle spindles, and fascia are further shortened and spasticity evolves into stretch-sensitive forms such as spastic cocontraction.[49] Spastic cocon- traction refers to inappropriate antagonist recruitment triggered by volitional com- mand.[50] Clinically, spastic cocontraction leads to involuntary movement in the opposite direction of the intended voluntary movement and contributes to impairment in active function. The degree of spastic cocontraction has been shown to be positively related to the Fugl-Meyer score,[51,52] suggesting that individuals with spastic cocontraction, although significantly impaired, are further along in their recovery process. Spasticity and spastic cocontraction may, however, lead to learned bad use. Reduction in spasticity with botulinum toxin injections has been shown to improve kinematic parameters such as velocity and smoothness, without significant changes in clinical outcomes such as hand function.[53] It is possible that weakness and atrophy produced by the injections negates the benefit of improvement in the form of the movement, or that functional improvement requires aggressive concurrent therapy.[54]

Abnormal motor synergies have been well described after stroke.[48] For example, during reaching, the shoulder must flex while the elbow extends. However, in patients with stroke, attempts at voluntary forward reaching often result in shoulder abduction and elbow flexion because of the constraining effect of abnormal descending motor commands.[55] The abnormal muscle synergies were not related to proximal weakness or abnormalities in the elbow flexor-extensor strength balance. More recently, it has been found that the common drive to muscles that are functionally coupled during reaching in healthy individuals, for example, the anterior deltoid and triceps brachii, is weakened after stroke likely because of interruption of information flow in the cor- ticospinal pathway.[56] Abnormal muscle synergies have been shown to be indepen- dent of weakness, slowness of muscle activation, excessive cocontraction, and spasticity, and instead reflect a loss of skill in generating spatial and temporal muscle activation patterns that conform with environmental demands.[57] Training strategies that promote movement outside of the abnormal motor patterns may be needed to retrain more normal movement patterns.

FORGETTING

Once a motor skill is attained through training, there is an expectation that it will be retained forever, despite intervals of no training (in the same way that one never forgets how to ride a bicycle). However, rats with motor cortex injury show a decline in performance during intervals of no training and additional training is required to get performance back to pretraining levels.[4] Breaks in rehabilitation similarly lead to forgetting of upper extremity motor skills in humans after stroke.[58,59] Thus new skills, although reasonably stable in healthy individuals, are more transient after stroke. Skill learning requires that at least three independent processes occur across multiple timescales.[60] First, precise task-specific sensorimotor mappings occur through trial-and-error adaptation during practice with appropriate error sensing. Adaptation is a fast learning process,[61] which leads to a rapid reduction in movement error, and typically takes only a few trials;[62] however it is easily forgotten.[63,64] The second process is repetition, which alters movement biases depending on what is repeated. Repetition leads to a slow tuning of directional biases toward the repeated movement.[65] A task can be repeated with or without adaptation to error and does not require error sensing. The third process is reinforcement, whereby movements are rewarded intrinsically or extrinsically and reward leads to faster relearning or savings on subsequent attempts.[66] Although these three processes occur independently, it has been shown that learning is most successful when sensorimotor adaptation is combined effectively with repetition[60] **(Fig. 3)**. For instance, appropriate sensorimotor mappings learned through adaptation must be repeated over time for sustained and appropriate changes in skill to occur.[67] Impaired sensorimotor adaptation and lack of opportunities for long-term practice can lead to unlearning or forgetting after stroke.[68]

Studies from several laboratories have shown that adaptation of reach and grasp are impaired after stroke despite reasonable amounts of repetition with the affected hand.[38,69–71] This finding suggests that patients may be unable to effectively sense the error with their affected hand and/or subsequently update their motor behavior. Adaptation requires specific sensory inputs: kinesthetic sense from muscle forces used to lift objects is required to produce fingertip load forces appropriate for object weight;[72] tactile sensation from touch receptors is required to produce grip forces appropriate for object texture, with higher grip forces needed to hold smoother objects;[73] and visual input about object contours determines how the hand is shaped during reach.[74–76] In reaching experiments, both vision and proprioception provide

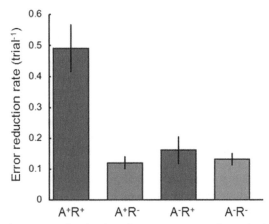

Fig. 3. Error reduction rates, reflecting learning, are greatest when adaptation (A) and repetition (R) combine. (*Adapted from* Huang VS, Haith A, Mazzoni P, et al. Rethinking motor learning and savings in adaptation paradigms: model-free memory for successful actions combines with internal models. Neuron 2011:70(4);793; with permission.)

information about arm configuration, but faulty integration of visual and proprioceptive signals may introduce errors in motor planning;[77–79] this might explain why we close our eyes when we want to enhance feeling. Thus, although multiple sensory contexts may collaborate to maintain task performance,[80] they can also compete and interfere with the acquisition of accurate sensorimotor associations.[77,81,82] In the presence of sensory deficits after a stroke, however, one sensory context may substitute for another to improve the accuracy of sensorimotor maps.[83] Information about how and when sensory substitution should be used is key to the development of effective rehabilitation protocols for the recovery of motor skill. Even mild sensory and/or motor deficits can impair error sensing and affect adaptation of movements and forces with the affected hand after stroke.[38,71] Thus, the first step in overcoming learned bad use and forgetting is to facilitate the formation of sensorimotor mappings or adaptation, which can then be repeated and reinforced for faster relearning during subsequent encounters.

THERAPEUTIC CONSIDERATIONS

A key consideration to determine treatment may be to first examine which impairments are contributing to the present functional status of the patient. If weakness and immobility are predominant and leading to nonuse, then interventions that potentiate excitatory plasticity (see **Fig. 1**) may be warranted. On the other hand, if spasticity, spastic cocontraction, and abnormal motor synergies are predominant and lead to the use of abnormal compensatory strategies to accomplish the task, one might consider interventions that potentiate inhibitory plasticity.[51] As patients with paresis likely evolve to develop some degree of spasticity, the interventions may need to evolve with the stage of recovery.

Furthermore, in patients with chronic stroke, owing to the layering of impairments, it may be important to bear in mind that treatment of one of the impairments might unmask other underlying impairments. For example, spasticity and weakness often coexist. Therefore, treatment of spasticity may unmask the underlying weakness, which might now need specific intervention. It may be necessary to work on several underlying impairments simultaneously for the best results, and the treatment regimen may need to be individualized for each patient.

CLINICAL OUTCOMES

Simple self-report measures used to characterize weakness in the upper limb after stroke, such as the National Institutes of Health Stroke Scale and the Stroke Impact Scale, provide information about the degree of impairment particularly in severely affected individuals but are not sensitive to mild or moderate weakness of the upper limb after stroke.[84]

The Fugl-Meyer scale is based on the observation of sequential recovery of motor function by Twitchell[2] and Brunnstrom.[47,48] This scale is the most widely used quantitative measure of motor recovery after stroke;[85,86] the scores have been shown to correlate with the extent of corticospinal tract damage.[87] The minimal detectable change on the upper extremity component of the Fugl-Meyer scale is found to be approximately 8% of the maximum score of 66 (5.28 points), supporting its utility in clinical settings.[88,89] However, the Fugl-Meyer scale was constructed on the assumptions that recovery proceeds in a proximal to distal manner and from synergistic to isolated movements;[85,90] however, both of these assumptions have been contested recently.[91–93] Furthermore, the Fugl-Meyer scale may show ceiling effects for fine motor skills in higher functioning patients.[94]

Grip strength has been found to be a useful objective measure of motor impairment, particularly the rate of increase in grip force.[12] Task-based kinematic measures such as speed and extent of isolated joint range of motion[38,51] might be useful direct, objective, and reliable measures of movement ability. In fact it has been shown that active range of motion early on predicts function at later time points.[95] However, longitudinal measurements of active range of motion may not show a linear improvement profile as the Fugl-Meyer scale does, especially when spasticity and spastic cocontraction set in. Hence more than one type of measurement and frequent assessment of motor impairment to inform a change in strategy to target the critical impairment(s) may be warranted in the clinical setting.

REFERENCES

1. Geyh S, Cieza A, Schouten J, et al. ICF core sets for stroke. J Rehabil Med 2004; 44(Suppl):135–41.
2. Twitchell TE. The restoration of motor function following hemiplegia in man. Brain 1951;74(4):443–80.
3. Brunnstrom S. Associated reactions of the upper extremity in adult patients with hemiplegia: an approach to training. Phys Ther Rev 1956;36(4):225–36.
4. Whishaw IQ, Alaverdashvili M, Kolb B. The problem of relating plasticity and skilled reaching after motor cortex stroke in the rat. Behav Brain Res 2008; 192(1):124–36.
5. Canning CG, Ada L, Adams R, et al. Loss of strength contributes more to physical disability after stroke than loss of dexterity. Clin Rehabil 2004;18(3):300–8.
6. Wagner JM, Lang CE, Sahrmann SA, et al. Sensorimotor impairments and reaching performance in subjects with poststroke hemiparesis during the first few months of recovery. Phys Ther 2007;87(6):751–65.
7. Chae J, Yang G, Park BK, et al. Delay in initiation and termination of muscle contraction, motor impairment, and physical disability in upper limb hemiparesis. Muscle Nerve 2002;25(4):568–75.
8. Canning CG, Ada L, O'Dwyer N, et al. Slowness to develop force contributes to weakness after stroke. Arch Phys Med Rehabil 1999;80(1):66–70.
9. Suresh NL, Zhou P, Rymer WZ. Abnormal EMG-force slope estimates in the first dorsal interosseous of hemiparetic stroke survivors. Conf Proc IEEE Eng Med Biol Soc 2008;2008:3562–5.
10. Mercier C, Bourbonnais D. Relative shoulder flexor and handgrip strength is related to upper limb function after stroke. Clin Rehabil 2004;18(2):215–21.
11. Tyson SF, Chillala J, Hanley M, et al. Distribution of weakness in the upper and lower limbs post-stroke. Disabil Rehabil 2006;28(11):715–9.
12. Renner CI, Bungert-Kahl P, Hummelsheim H. Change of strength and rate of rise of tension relate to functional arm recovery after stroke. Arch Phys Med Rehabil 2009;90(9):1548–56.
13. Castaldo J, Rodgers J, Rae-Grant A, et al. Diagnosis and neuroimaging of acute stroke producing distal arm monoparesis. J Stroke Cerebrovasc Dis 2003;12(6):253–8.
14. Hiraga A. Pure motor monoparesis due to ischemic stroke. Neurologist 2011; 17(6):301–8.
15. Tyson SF, Hanley M, Chillala J, et al. Sensory loss in hospital-admitted people with stroke: characteristics, associated factors, and relationship with function. Neurorehabil Neural Repair 2008;22(2):166–72.
16. Bassetti C, Bogousslavsky J, Regli F. Sensory syndromes in parietal stroke. Neurology 1993;43(10):1942–9.

17. Mercier C, Bertrand AM, Bourbonnais D. Differences in the magnitude and direction of forces during a submaximal matching task in hemiparetic subjects. Exp Brain Res 2004;157(1):32–42.
18. Taub E, Heitmann RD, Barro G. Alertness, level of activity, and purposive movement following somatosensory deafferentation in monkeys. Ann N Y Acad Sci 1977;290:348–65.
19. Stecco A, Stecco C, Raghavan P. Peripheral mechanisms of spasticity and treatment implications. Curr Phys Med Rehabil Rep 2014;2(2):121–7.
20. Ward AB. A literature review of the pathophysiology and onset of post-stroke spasticity. Eur J Neurol 2012;19(1):21–7.
21. Reinkensmeyer DJ, Schmit BD, Rymer WZ. Mechatronic assessment of arm impairment after chronic brain injury. Technol Health Care 1999;7(6):431–5.
22. Hamdy RC, Krishnaswamy G, Cancellaro V, et al. Changes in bone mineral content and density after stroke. Am J Phys Med Rehabil 1993;72(4):188–91.
23. Hamdy RC, Moore SW, Cancellaro VA, et al. Long-term effects of strokes on bone mass. Am J Phys Med Rehabil 1995;74(5):351–6.
24. Ramnemark A, Nyberg L, Borssén B, et al. Fractures after stroke. Osteoporos Int 1998;8(1):92–5.
25. Lundström E, Terént A, Borg J. Prevalence of disabling spasticity 1 year after first-ever stroke. Eur J Neurol 2008;15(6):533–9.
26. Stecco C, Gagey O, Belloni A, et al. Anatomy of the deep fascia of the upper limb. Second part: study of innervation. Morphologie 2007;91(292):38–43.
27. Tesarz J, Hoheisel U, Wiedenhöfer B, et al. Sensory innervation of the thoracolumbar fascia in rats and humans. Neuroscience 2011;194:302–8.
28. Yahia L, Rhalmi S, Newman N, et al. Sensory innervation of human thoracolumbar fascia. An immunohistochemical study. Acta Orthop Scand 1992;63(2):195–7.
29. Bell J, Holmes M. Model of the dynamics of receptor potential in a mechanoreceptor. Math Biosci 1992;110(2):139–74.
30. Stecco A, Meneghini A, Stern R, et al. Ultrasonography in myofascial neck pain: randomized clinical trial for diagnosis and follow-up. Surg Radiol Anat 2014; 36(3):243–53.
31. Gamble GE, Barberan E, Laasch HU, et al. Poststroke shoulder pain: a prospective study of the association and risk factors in 152 patients from a consecutive cohort of 205 patients presenting with stroke. Eur J Pain 2002; 6(6):467–74.
32. Boivie J, Leijon G, Johansson I. Central post-stroke pain–a study of the mechanisms through analyses of the sensory abnormalities. Pain 1989;37(2):173–85.
33. Klit H, Finnerup NB, Jensen TS. Central post-stroke pain: clinical characteristics, pathophysiology, and management. Lancet Neurol 2009;8(9):857–68.
34. Rausell E, Cusick CG, Taub E, et al. Chronic deafferentation in monkeys differentially affects nociceptive and nonnociceptive pathways distinguished by specific calcium-binding proteins and down-regulates gamma-aminobutyric acid type A receptors at thalamic levels. Proc Natl Acad Sci U S A 1992;89(7): 2571–5.
35. McCrea PH, Eng JJ, Hodgson AJ. Saturated muscle activation contributes to compensatory reaching strategies after stroke. J Neurophysiol 2005;94(5): 2999–3008.
36. Levin MF, Kleim JA, Wolf SL. What do motor recovery and compensation mean in patients following stroke? Neurorehabil Neural Repair 2009;23(4):313–9.
37. Cirstea MC, Levin MF. Compensatory strategies for reaching in stroke. Brain 2000;123(Pt 5):940–53.

38. Raghavan P, Santello M, Gordon AM, et al. Compensatory motor control after stroke: an alternative joint strategy for object-dependent shaping of hand posture. J Neurophysiol 2010;103(6):3034–43.

39. Skinner BF, editor. The behavior of organisms: an experimental analysis. New York: Appleton-Century; 1938.

40. Dickinson A. Actions and habits: the development of behavioral anatomy. Philos Trans R Soc Lond B Biol Sci 1985;308:67–78.

41. Michaelsen SM, Luta A, Roby-Brami A, et al. Effect of trunk restraint on the recovery of reaching movements in hemiparetic patients. Stroke 2001;32(8):1875–83.

42. Woodbury ML, Howland DR, McGuirk TE, et al. Effects of trunk restraint combined with intensive task practice on poststroke upper extremity reach and function: a pilot study. Neurorehabil Neural Repair 2009;23(1):78–91.

43. Lance JW. The control of muscle tone, reflexes, and movement: Robert Wartenberg Lecture. Neurology 1980;30(12):1303–13.

44. Watkins CL, Leathley MJ, Gregson JM, et al. Prevalence of spasticity post stroke. Clin Rehabil 2002;16(5):515–22.

45. Dietz V, Berger W. Cerebral palsy and muscle transformation. Dev Med Child Neurol 1995;37(2):180–4.

46. Hufschmidt A, Mauritz KH. Chronic transformation of muscle in spasticity: a peripheral contribution to increased tone. J Neurol Neurosurg Psychiatry 1985;48(7):676–85.

47. Brunnstrom S. Motor testing procedures in hemiplegia: based on sequential recovery stages. Phys Ther 1966;46(4):357–75.

48. Brunnstrom S. Movement therapy in hemiplegia. A neurophysiological approach. New York: Harper & Row; 1970.

49. Gracies J-M. Pathophysiology of spastic paresis. I: paresis and soft tissue changes. Muscle Nerve 2005;31:535–51.

50. Gracies JM. Pathophysiology of spastic paresis. II: emergence of muscle overactivity. Muscle Nerve 2005;31(5):552–71.

51. Aluru V, Lu Y, Leung A, et al. Effect of auditory constraints on motor performance depends on stage of recovery post-stroke. Front Neurol 2014;5:106.

52. Chae J, Yang G, Park BK, et al. Muscle weakness and cocontraction in upper limb hemiparesis: relationship to motor impairment and physical disability. Neurorehabil Neural Repair 2002;16(3):241–8.

53. Bensmail D, Robertson JV, Fermanian C, et al. Botulinum toxin to treat upper-limb spasticity in hemiparetic patients: analysis of function and kinematics of reaching movements. Neurorehabil Neural Repair 2010;24(3):273–81.

54. Canning CG. Constraint-induced movement therapy after injection of Botulinum toxin improves spasticity and motor function in chronic stroke patients. Aust J Physiother 2009;55(4):286.

55. Beer RF, Ellis MD, Holubar BG, et al. Impact of gravity loading on post-stroke reaching and its relationship to weakness. Muscle Nerve 2007;36(2):242–50.

56. Kisiel-Sajewicz K, Fang Y, Hrovat K, et al. Weakening of synergist muscle coupling during reaching movement in stroke patients. Neurorehabil Neural Repair 2011;25(4):359–68.

57. Canning CG, Ada L, O'Dwyer N. Abnormal muscle activation characteristics associated with loss of dexterity after stroke. J Neurol Sci 2000;176(1):45–56.

58. Krakauer JW. Motor learning: its relevance to stroke recovery and neurorehabilitation. Curr Opin Neurol 2006;19(1):84–90.

59. Takahashi CD, Reinkensmeyer DJ. Hemiparetic stroke impairs anticipatory control of arm movement. Exp Brain Res 2003;149(2):131–40.

60. Huang VS, Haith A, Mazzoni P, et al. Rethinking motor learning and savings in adaptation paradigms: model-free memory for successful actions combines with internal models. Neuron 2011;70(4):787–801.
61. Joiner WM, Smith MA. Long-term retention explained by a model of short-term learning in the adaptive control of reaching. J Neurophysiol 2008;100(5):2948–55.
62. Gordon AM, Westling G, Cole KJ, et al. Memory representations underlying motor commands used during manipulation of common and novel objects. J Neurophysiol 1993;69(6):1789–96.
63. Benson BL, Anguera JA, Seidler RD. A spatial explicit strategy reduces error but interferes with sensorimotor adaptation. J Neurophysiol 2011;105(6):2843–51.
64. Schweighofer N, Lee JY, Goh HT, et al. Mechanisms of the contextual interference effect in individuals poststroke. J Neurophysiol 2011;106(5):2632–41.
65. Galea JM, Celnik P. Brain polarization enhances the formation and retention of motor memories. J Neurophysiol 2009;102(1):294–301.
66. Haith AM, Huberdeau DM, Krakauer JW, et al. The influence of movement preparation time on the expression of visuomotor learning and savings. J Neurosci 2015;35(13):5109–17.
67. Bastian AJ. Understanding sensorimotor adaptation and learning for rehabilitation. Curr Opin Neurol 2008;21(6):628–33.
68. Kitago T, Ryan SL, Mazzoni P, et al. Unlearning versus savings in visuomotor adaptation: comparing effects of washout, passage of time, and removal of errors on motor memory. Front Hum Neurosci 2013;7:307.
69. Hermsdörfer J, Hagl E, Nowak DA, et al. Grip force control during object manipulation in cerebral stroke. Clin Neurophysiol 2003;114(5):915–29.
70. Nowak DA, Hermsdörfer J, Topka H. Deficits of predictive grip force control during object manipulation in acute stroke. J Neurol 2003;250(7):850–60.
71. Raghavan P, Krakauer JW, Gordon AM. Impaired anticipatory control of fingertip forces in patients with a pure motor or sensorimotor lacunar syndrome. Brain 2006;129(Pt 6):1415–25.
72. Johansson RS, Westling G. Coordinated isometric muscle commands adequately and erroneously programmed for the weight during lifting task with precision grip. Exp Brain Res 1988;71(1):59–71.
73. Johansson RS, Westling G. Roles of glabrous skin receptors and sensorimotor memory in automatic control of precision grip when lifting rougher or more slippery objects. Exp Brain Res 1984;56(3):550–64.
74. Marino BF, Stucchi N, Nava E, et al. Distorting the visual size of the hand affects hand pre-shaping during grasping. Exp Brain Res 2010;202(2):499–505.
75. Sakata H, Taira M, Kusunoki M, et al. The TINS Lecture. The parietal association cortex in depth perception and visual control of hand action. Trends Neurosci 1997;20(8):350–7.
76. Santello M, Soechting JF. Gradual molding of the hand to object contours. J Neurophysiol 1998;79(3):1307–20.
77. Gordon AM, Forssberg H, Johansson RS, et al. Visual size cues in the programming of manipulative forces during precision grip. Exp Brain Res 1991;83(3):477–82.
78. Sarlegna FR, Przybyla A, Sainburg RL. The influence of target sensory modality on motor planning may reflect errors in sensori-motor transformations. Neuroscience 2009;164(2):597–610.
79. Scheidt RA, Conditt MA, Secco EL, et al. Interaction of visual and proprioceptive feedback during adaptation of human reaching movements. J Neurophysiol 2005;93(6):3200–13.

80. Holmes NP, Spence C. Visual bias of unseen hand position with a mirror: spatial and temporal factors. Exp Brain Res 2005;166(3–4):489–97.
81. Cole KJ. Lifting a familiar object: visual size analysis, not memory for object weight, scales lift force. Exp Brain Res 2008;188(4):551–7.
82. van Beers RJ, Baraduc P, Wolpert DM. Role of uncertainty in sensorimotor control. Philos Trans R Soc Lond B Biol Sci 2002;357(1424):1137–45.
83. Quaney BM, He J, Timberlake G, et al. Visuomotor training improves stroke-related ipsilesional upper extremity impairments. Neurorehabil Neural Repair 2010;24(1):52–61.
84. Bohannon RW. Adequacy of simple measures for characterizing impairment in upper limb strength following stroke. Percept Mot Skills 2004;99(3 Pt 1):813–7.
85. Gladstone DJ, Danells CJ, Black SE, et al. The Fugl-Meyer assessment of motor recovery after stroke: a critical review of its measurement properties. Neurorehabil Neural Repair 2002;16(3):232–40.
86. van Wijck FM, Pandyan AD, Johnson GR, et al. Assessing motor deficits in neurological rehabilitation: patterns of instrument usage. Neurorehabil Neural Repair 2001;15(1):23–30.
87. Zhu LL, Lindenberg R, Alexander MP, et al. Lesion load of the corticospinal tract predicts motor impairment in chronic stroke. Stroke 2010;41(5):910–5.
88. Lin JH, Hsu MJ, Sheu CF, et al. Psychometric comparisons of 4 measures for assessing upper-extremity function in people with stroke. Phys Ther 2009;89(8):840–50.
89. Rabadi MH, Rabadi FM. Comparison of the action research arm test and the Fugl-Meyer assessment as measures of upper-extremity motor weakness after stroke. Arch Phys Med Rehabil 2006;87(7):962–6.
90. Fugl-Meyer AR, Jääskö L, Leyman I, et al. The post-stroke hemiplegic patient. 1. a method for evaluation of physical performance. Scand J Rehabil Med 1975;7(1):13–31.
91. Beebe JA, Lang CE. Absence of a proximal to distal gradient of motor deficits in the upper extremity early after stroke. Clin Neurophysiol 2008;119(9):2074–85.
92. Crow JL, Harmeling-van der Wel BC. Hierarchical properties of the motor function sections of the Fugl-Meyer assessment scale for people after stroke: a retrospective study. Phys Ther 2008;88(12):1554–67.
93. Woodbury ML, Velozo CA, Richards LG, et al. Dimensionality and construct validity of the Fugl-Meyer Assessment of the upper extremity. Arch Phys Med Rehabil 2007;88(6):715–23.
94. Thompson-Butel AG, Lin G, Shiner CT, et al. Comparison of three tools to measure improvements in upper-limb function with poststroke therapy. Neurorehabil Neural Repair 2015;29(4):341–8.
95. Beebe JA, Lang CE. Active range of motion predicts upper extremity function 3 months after stroke. Stroke 2009;40(5):1772–9.

Hemiparetic Gait

Lynne R. Sheffler, MD[a,b,c,]*, John Chae, MD[a,b,c,d]

KEYWORDS

- Stroke rehabilitation • Gait • Hemiparesis

KEY POINTS

- The most common pattern of walking impairment poststroke is hemiparetic gait.
- Hemiparetic gait is characterized by asymmetry associated with an extensor synergy pattern of hip extension and adduction, knee extension, and ankle plantar flexion and inversion.
- There are characteristic changes in the spatiotemporal, kinematic and kinetic parameters, and dynamic electromyography (EMG) patterns in hemiparesis, which may be assessed most accurately in a motion studies laboratory.
- Increased energy cost of walking is due to the muscle work necessary to lift the body's center of mass (CM) against gravity during the paretic limb swing phase.
- An understanding of normal human gait is necessary to assess the complex interplay of motor, sensory, and proprioceptive loss; spasticity; and/or ataxia on hemiparetic gait.

INTRODUCTION

Seventy-five percent of patients who sustain a stroke have limitations in walking,[1] and the most common pattern of walking impairment poststroke is hemiparetic gait. This review provides a comprehensive overview of the characteristic features and analysis of poststroke hemiparetic gait. An understanding of normal human gait, including basic concepts of the neural control of gait and gait cycle terminology, is a prerequisite for analyzing and treating poststroke patients with hemiparetic gait dysfunction. This article also defines spatiotemporal and kinematic parameters of normal gait as well as key changes in these same parameters in hemiparesis. Although patients with

This work was supported in part by grant K23HD060689 from the National Institute of Child Health and Human Development.
The authors report no relevant commercial or financial conflicts of interest.
[a] Department of Physical Medicine and Rehabilitation, Case Western Reserve University, 2109 Adelbert Road, Cleveland, OH 44106, USA; [b] MetroHealth Rehabilitation Institute of Ohio, MetroHealth System, 4229 Pearl Road, Cleveland, OH 44109, USA; [c] Cleveland Functional Electrical Stimulation Center, 10701 East Boulevard, Cleveland, OH 44106, USA; [d] Department of Biomedical Engineering, Case Western Reserve University, 2109 Adelbert Road, Cleveland, OH 44106, USA
* Corresponding author. Department of Physical Medicine and Rehabilitation, MetroHealth Medical Center, 4229 Pearl Road, Cleveland, OH 44109.
E-mail address: lrsheffler@gmail.com

poststroke hemiparesis may demonstrate classic changes in spatiotemporal, kinematic, and kinetic parameters, they also demonstrate greater gait variability than neurologically intact controls.[2] More advanced assessments of gait, including kinematic, kinetic, and dynamic electromyography (EMG) analyses, can also be done using quantitative gait analysis. The energy cost of normal walking and the increase in energy costs associated with maintaining walking velocity in poststroke hemiparesis are described. Lastly, the authors assert that good clinical care of patients for poststroke hemiparetic gait does not always require the sophisticated analysis provided by a gait laboratory but instead an astute clinician's understanding of the complex interplay of motor strength deficits, variable spasticity, sensory and proprioceptive loss, and/or ataxia on motor control and functional gait performance. Thus, a rubric for the clinician to describe hemiparetic gait in the clinical setting is presented.

NEURAL CONTROL OF NORMAL HUMAN GAIT

The neural control of human gait is dependent on both spinal and supraspinal mechanisms; thus, neurologically based gait impairment results from an interruption at either level. The concept of a locomotor center located at the level of the spinal cord was originally proposed in 1911 by T.G. Brown.[3,4] In his research, Brown noted that cats with transected spinal cords and cut dorsal roots were still capable of producing rhythmic alternating contractions in the ankle flexors and extensors. One century later, the term, *central pattern generator (CPG)*, is now commonly used to describe a spinal locomotor center. CPGs, a term first coined and described in invertebrates and fish, are innate neural networks that are capable of generating self-sustained, rhythmic patterned output, independent of sensory input.[5] Although only indirect evidence exists for human pattern generation, it is generally believed that CPGs, existing within the low thoracic and lumbar regions of the human spinal cord, generate rhythmic patterned outputs largely responsible for control of human locomotion. CPGs are capable of responding to multiple afferent inputs, which modulate human gait patterns, and include a complex interplay of supraspinal afferents originating from the brainstem reticular formation, basal ganglia, premotor and motor cortex, and cerebellum as well as sensory afferents from vestibular, visual, and proprioceptive systems. Information regarding limb positioning and kinesthesia is relayed from proprioceptors within tendons, muscles, ligaments, and joints via the medial leminiscus within the dorsal column of the spinal cord. The convergence of spinal reflex pathways and descending pathways on common spinal interneurons are known to be integrative.[6] In human and other primate gait patterns, however, it is believed that supraspinal input may play a greater role in the regulation of gait than in other species, due to the importance and prominence of the corticospinal tract.[7,8] Supraspinal afferents specifically play a prominent role in the volitional control of gait, such as occurs with change in walking speed, walking direction, or obstacle avoidance. In humans, damage within the central nervous system, secondary to a cerebrovascular accident, ultimately results in an alteration of the normal neural control of gait.

NORMAL HUMAN WALKING

Normal human walking is characterized by a repetitive sequence of limb motion whereby an ipsilateral lower limb alternately provides support for the contralateral lower limb as the body advances forward. Optimal human walking results in the forward translation of the body, using bipedal support, with maximal symmetry, stability, and energy efficiency. Although there is no specific standard for measurement of poststroke gait symmetry, Patterson and colleagues[9] recommend using a symmetry ratio equation, which includes step length, swing time, and stance time as parameters in the equation. Gait stability may be defined as the body's ability to remain safely in an upright posture with minimal susceptibility to perturbations during walking. Stability during walking is determined by a functional balance between the alignment of the body and the muscle activity at each lower limb joint. Gait stability may be influenced by 3 important factors: (1) the generally disproportionate amount of total body weight that relies on the bilateral lower limbs for support, (2) the multisegmented nature of the 2 supporting lower limbs, and (3) the unique mechanical characteristics of each of the lower limb joints. Poststroke gait stability is particularly important due to an increased risk of falls after stroke.[2] Lastly, the efficiency of walking is defined as the ratio of the work accomplished to the energy expended. At a basic level, the cyclic movement of the limbs that characterizes walking requires energy for muscle contraction and thus any disruption to the normal gait cycle, due to alterations in the intensity or pattern of muscle activation, can result in an increase in the energy expenditure of walking.

NORMAL HUMAN GAIT CYCLE
Spatiotemporal Parameters of Gait

The human gait cycle is defined as the temporal sequence of events, which begins at heel strike of an ipsilateral lower limb and ends at the subsequent heel strike of that same limb. The term, *stride*, is used interchangeably with the term, *gait cycle*, and thus the term, *stride length*, refers to the distance to complete 1 gait cycle. The term, *step length*, refers to the distance between heel strike of an ipsilateral limb to heel strike of the contralateral limb. *Cadence* is defined as the number of steps per unit time (minute). *Walking speed*, distance per unit time, is the most important predictor of ambulation status after stroke,[10] and the efficacy of any rehabilitation intervention is most commonly assessed by change in comfortable or self-selected walking speed.

The gait cycle is characterized by alternating *single-support* and *double-support periods*. During a single-support period, only 1 lower limb is in contact with the ground. During a double-support period, both lower limbs are concurrently in contact with the ground. In normal walking, double-support periods occur twice during 1 gait cycle. The first occurs when the ipsilateral limb is at heel-strike and the contralateral limb is at toe off (early gait cycle of ipsilateral limb) and the second occurs when the ipsilateral limb is at toe off and the contralateral limb is at heel strike (midgait cycle of ipsilateral limb). Double-support time decreases as walking speed increases and is eliminated altogether during running. During normal walking, each lower limb spends approximately 80% of the gait cycle in single support and 20% of the gait cycle in double support. More sophisticated gait analysis is required to measure single- and double-support time as well as step width, all of which are parameters indicative of gait symmetry and stability.

The gait cycle is divided into 2 primary phases, called the *stance phase* and the *swing phase*. Stance phase is defined as the period of time during which the ipsilateral lower limb is in direct contact with the ground. During normal walking, the stance phase comprises approximately the first 60% of the gait cycle. Stance phase is further divided into the following periods: (1) initial contact of the limb (heel strike) or early stance, (2) midstance (weight shifting from heel strike anteriorly over a flat foot), (3) terminal stance (weight shifting anteriorly from flat foot to forefoot), and (4) preswing (heel rise to toe off). Swing phase is defined as the period of time that the ipsilateral lower limb is advancing forward while in the air (ie, not bearing weight). The swing phase comprises the latter 40% of the gait cycle and is further divided into the following periods: (1) initial swing (immediately after toe off), (2) midswing, and (3) terminal swing (immediately prior to heel strike). Ankle plantar flexion at preswing, hip flexion, and forward inertia of the tibia are the primary determinants of swing onset. The specific duration of each gait cycle phase has an inverse relationship to walking speed. Thus, when walking speed increases, the durations of both the stance and swing periods of the normal gait cycle decrease. **Fig. 1** demonstrates the normal human gait cycle.

Kinematics and Kinetics of Gait

Although a full discussion of segmental lower limb movement throughout the gait cycle falls outside the scope of this review, a basic understanding of normal pelvis, hip, knee, and ankle joint movements through stance and swing phases is specifically important when considering kinematic and kinetic changes in hemiparetic gait. *Kinematics* provides a description of joint angles and movement without specific consideration to the forces acting at each joint. *Kinetics* describes the forces, moments, and mechanical energy that act on each joint during ambulation. For the purposes of this review, primarily the hip, knee, and ankle joint angles in the sagittal plane are focused on.

Although hip angle is commonly believed to define the relationship between the thigh and the vertical, pelvic tilt significantly influences the arc of hip motion created by displacement of the thigh. At heel strike, the ipsilateral hip is in a flexed position of approximately 20°. The hip then begins a progressive movement arc from flexion to extension as the limb transitions through stance with the normal arc of hip motion in stance being approximately 40°. At preswing, the hip begins a gradual reverse progression of hip extension to reach approximately 25° of flexion by terminal swing. Thus, the hip moves through 2 arcs of motion during 1 gait cycle.

Movement of the knee in the sagittal plane (knee flexion and extension) is essential for lower limb advancement. In normal walking, the knee is generally flexed approximately 5° at heel strike and provides shock absorption at limb loading in early stance. Through midstance, the knee gradually extends until nearly fully extended and provides stability for weight bearing throughout stance. By preswing, the knee flexes to approximately 40° and reaches maximal knee flexion at early swing, which helps facilitate forward advancement of the lower limb and toe clearance. In normal walking, 60° of ipsilateral knee flexion are needed to achieve toe clearance.

At the ankle, there are 2 critical periods of ankle plantar flexion, which occur at early stance after heel strike and at preswing prior to toe off. An important transition at the

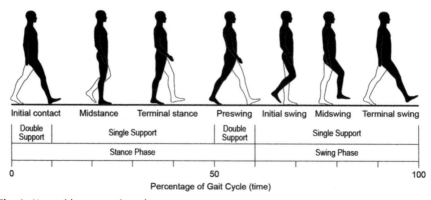

Fig. 1. Normal human gait cycle.

ankle is the gradual dorsiflexion that occurs from midstance to just prior to heel rise. This period of increasing dorsiflexion, during the single-support interval of stance, is a primary determinant of ipsilateral tibial progression. The gastroc-soleus complex stabilizes the ankle at heel rise. During swing, the ankle dorsiflexion muscles contract to realign the ankle to neutral for toe clearance.

MUSCLE ACTIVATION DURING THE GAIT CYCLE

Muscles function to provide stability at the pelvis, hip, knee, and ankle, through coordinated patterns of muscle activation, which are phasic and well described in normal gait. The pattern of contraction of any given muscle may be *concentric* (muscle shortening), *isometric* (muscle contraction without change in length), or *eccentric* (muscle lengthening), depending on the demands of the gait cycle phase. Alterations in the normal activation and termination patterns of muscle fiber activity, including early activation, prolonged duration, delayed activity, curtailed activity, absent activity, and cocontraction of agonist and antagonist muscles groups, are common after a neurologic injury, such as stroke.[11] Dynamic EMG recorded while walking may identify abnormalities in neurologic control and muscle weakness as well as compensatory muscle substitutions.

During stance, hip motion transitions from flexion at heel strike and progresses to extension by heel rise. The hip extensor muscles are responsible for limb deceleration at terminal swing (eccentric contraction) and for restraint of forward momentum as the limb is loaded at heel strike. The primary hip extensors are the gluteus maximus muscle and the 3 hamstring muscles (semimembranosis, biceps femoris, and semitendinosis). The role of the hip abductors (gluteus medius and minimus, tensor fasciae latae) is to counter the contralateral pelvic drop during the cyclic intervals of non–weight bearing throughout ipsilateral stance. The primary hip flexors are the iliopsoas and rectus femoris muscles, both of which contract concentrically at early swing. Although there are 14 specific muscles providing stability at the knee during the gait cycle, the quadriceps complex (vastus medialis longus and oblique, vastus intermedius, and vastus lateralis) is the dominant muscle group for knee extension. Stance stability is also largely reliant on the soleus muscle to control the forward motion of the tibia, iliotibial band tension, and the actions of the rectus femoris, upper portion of the gluteus maximus, and hamstring muscles. Limb deceleration during terminal swing is largely influenced by the balance between the eccentric contraction of the hamstring muscles and the concentric contraction of the quadriceps muscles. The tibialis anterior muscle is the primary ankle dorsiflexor, contracting eccentrically during stance phase (heel strike to foot flat) and concentrically during swing phase. Lastly, the gastroc-soleus complex is the primary ankle plantar flexor, concentrically contracting during terminal stance. **Fig. 2** presents the pattern of lower muscle activation during the normal human gait cycle.

Effect of Center of Gravity on Muscle Activity and Gait

The specific point, within any given body, that is representative of the weight of the body mass, is called the *center of gravity (COG)*. In a typical adult with normal weight distribution, the COG is located just anterior to the 10th thoracic vertebra. During normal walking, the COG moves both vertically and laterally as it is propelled forward. The energy efficiency of any given gait pattern can be assessed by the magnitude of the vertical and lateral displacement of the COG. In a normal adult man, the vertical displacement of the COG within the sagittal plane traces a classic sinusoidal trajectory with amplitude of approximately 2 inches. The COG moves through 2 complete

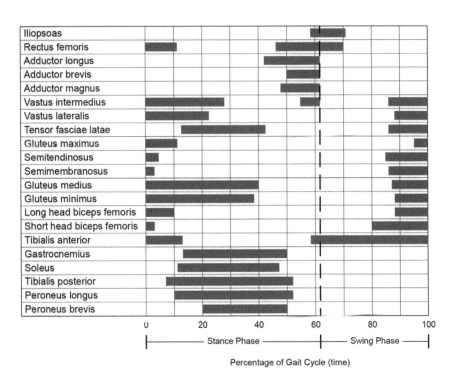

Fig. 2. Pattern of muscle activation of lower limb muscles in normal gait.

oscillations during each cycle so that the sagittal trajectory has 2 peaks and troughs. The COG also oscillates laterally during normal ambulation, tracing a sinusoidal trajectory with amplitude of approximately 2.5 inches. Thus, 1 full lateral sinusoidal oscillation of the COG occurs during each gait cycle. Saunders and colleagues,[12] in 1953, first defined the 6 "determinants of gait" (pelvic rotation, pelvic tilt, knee flexion in midstance, foot and ankle motion, knee motion, and lateral pelvic motion), which, together, minimize vertical and lateral displacement of the COG to maximize energy efficiency in normal walking.

The upper portion of the body (head, trunk, and arms) does not directly contribute to the act of walking yet may contribute up to 70% of total body weight. Alignment of body weight is a critical factor for ambulation and balance of the weight of the upper body is largely dependent on the base of support dictated by lower limb joint alignment and dynamic muscle activity. Muscle action within the trunk and upper spine serves to maintain vertebral alignment. During stance, the effect of body weight on the floor is quantifiable by the resultant *ground reaction force (GFR)*. The GFR is a force generated by the weight-bearing surface, which is of equal magnitude but opposite the direction of force imposed by the body mass on the ground. The *body vector* is a line that represents the location of the GRF at any moment during the stance portion of the gait cycle. By relating the anterior or posterior location of the body vector line (for example, within a sagittal plane), to the individual joint centers (ankle, knee, and hip) at a given moment during stance, the direction of instability at each joint can be known. If the GRF is known, then the muscle and ligamentous forces, which are required to maintain stability at that joint, can also be known. For example, in normal upright standing with both hip and knee extended, if the body vector within the sagittal plane falls posterior to the hip or anterior to the knee, passive stability at those joints can be achieved with only ligamentous tension. Stability at any given joint is thus the result of a balance between the body vector on one side of the joint and ligamentous restraint on the opposite side of that specific joint. In normal upright standing, the body vector falls anterior to the ankle joint, meaning that the human body is inherently unstable in quiet standing. Because the ankle joint does not provide passive stability similar to the knee or hip, isometric contraction of the gastroc-soleus muscle is necessary to maintain standing posture.

Reciprocal flexion and extension of the bilateral upper limbs occurs during walking with ipsilateral arm extension occurring at the same time as ipsilateral lower limb forward propulsion. Thus the arms provide a counterforce to minimize the rotatory displacement of the body associated with lower limb walking mechanics.[13] Arm swing, although involving both passive and active patterns of movement, does not measurably affect the energy cost of walking.[14]

GAIT DEVIATIONS IN HEMIPARESIS

Hemiparetic gait is most commonly characterized by an asymmetric pattern of walking associated with contralateral motor weakness, motor control deficits, sensory and/or proprioceptive loss, and/or ataxia. This review focuses primarily on the effects of motor weakness and motor control deficits on typical hemiparetic gait. The primitive locomotor patterns that emerge early in the poststroke period are described as well as the changes in the spatiotemporal, kinematic, and kinetic parameters, which more commonly characterize hemiparetic walking in the subacute and chronic poststroke periods. Although changes are evident in both the paretic and nonparetic lower limbs, this review focuses primarily on the spatiotemporal, kinematic, and kinetic parameter changes typically seen in the paretic limb only after stroke.

Primitive Locomotor Patterns

In the acute and subacute poststroke period, primitive locomotor patterns emerge that may affect selective motor control, causing an alteration of the normal timing and intensity of muscle contraction of the paretic limb. In the upper limb, a predominant flexor synergy pattern emerges whereas in the lower limb, a predominantly extensor synergy pattern emerges. Loss of selective motor control disrupts the coordinated and fluid sequence of lower limb muscle contraction(s), which characterizes normal walking. In the absence of selective control, a hemiparetic patient can substitute primitive locomotor synergy patterns to increase stance stability and to facilitate walking. Lower limb positioning to achieve stability for weight bearing may be possible due to a *lower limb mass extensor movement pattern*, which is typically marked by hip extension, knee extension, hip adduction, ankle plantar flexion, and ankle inversion. The extensor synergy positioning results, however, in a relative lengthening of the paretic limb compared with the nonparetic limb. The resulting compensation is a tendency to vault over the nonparetic limb, hike the hip on the paretic limb, and circumduct the paretic lower limb at the hip during swing to clear the limb. To minimize these compensations, functional walking is often achieved through the bracing of the ankle (using an ankle foot orthosis) to stabilize the ankle in a neutral position, which is specifically necessary to allow sufficient ipsilateral heel strike, tibial advancement through stance phase, and toe clearance during the swing phase of gait. The prognosis for ambulating at a modified independent level for patients with lower limb extensor synergies is good.

Spatiotemporal Parameters of Hemiparetic Gait

Spatiotemporal parameters of gait refer to walking velocity, step length, stride length, and cadence; these are typically all decreased in hemiparetic walking. Walking velocity is often decreased to maintain an appropriate rate of energy expenditure. Gait asymmetry may be evident in the changes in stance/swing phase durations and single-/double-support durations. Paretic stance duration and paretic single-support duration are both decreased whereas paretic swing duration is increased. Nonparetic limb stance duration[15] and double-support time are both increased. **Table 1** presents the effect of hemiparesis on spatiotemporal gait parameters.

Kinematics of Hemiparetic Gait

Gait kinematics refer to joint angles, velocities, and accelerations during gait. Although gait speed is generally decreased in hemiparesis, a study that evaluated kinematics at variable walking velocities poststroke showed that there is greater variability in poststroke gait kinematics at slower walking speeds.[16] Despite this variability, there are characteristic kinematic changes, which may be observable clinically. At the level of the pelvis, there may be a drop of the pelvis noted on the nonparetic limb side due to weakness of the hip abductors (gluteus medius and minimus) on the paretic side. At the level of the paretic hip, the onset of hip flexion in preswing is delayed[17] and paretic hip flexion at heel strike is typically decreased. Limb instability associated with knee flexion in early stance is more commonly a problem in the early poststroke period and the instability is associated with decreased and/or uncoordinated quadriceps activation. Decreased knee flexion during swing has been commonly described as stiff-knee gait. The combination of decreased paretic hip and knee flexion during the swing phase contributes to decreased ability to clear the paretic lower limb. In chronic hemiparesis, excessive paretic knee extension during mid- to late stance, called *genu recurvatum*, is common. Genu recurvatum may be caused by plantar flexion spasticity, plantar flexion contracture, quadriceps spasticity, hamstring weakness, and/or quadriceps weakness. In a recent study by Cooper and colleagues,[18] a strong association was found between paretic knee hyperextension in midstance and gastroc-soleus weakness. Forward progression of the tibia on the paretic limb is impaired as a result of excessive knee extension during stance, and inadequate plantar flexor power is generated at terminal stance. A recent simulation study[19] suggests that decreased paretic soleus and gastrocnemius contributions to forward propulsion and power generation are the primary impairments, which distinguished a hemiparetic ambulator from a neurologically intact control subject. Lastly, increased

Table 1	
Effect of hemiparesis on spatiotemporal gait parameters	
Walking velocity (m/s)	Decreased
Stride length (m)	Decreased
Step length (m)	Decreased
Cadence (steps/min)	Decreased
Paretic single-stance duration (s)	Decreased
Double-stance duration (s)	Increased
Paretic stance duration (s)	Decreased
Paretic swing duration (s)	Increased

knee extension at terminal stance combined with decreased hip flexion contributes to a shortened step length.

Foot drop may be due to insufficient dorsiflexion strength and/or plantar flexion spasticity and is most noticeable during swing. Dorsiflexion weakness may be the only manifestation of hemiparetic gait in a more mildly impaired patient. In such patients, paretic dorsiflexion weakness may be most clinically evident in midswing with excessive plantar flexion with relatively preserved knee and hip flexion. In more impaired patients, the paretic dorsiflexion angle at heel trike may be decreased such that the positioning of the foot at initial contact is either forefoot first or in a flat foot position. Prolonged gastroc-soleus activation prominently contributes to foot drop associated with inadequate dorsiflexion during swing. Prolonged activation of the posterior and anterior tibialis muscles contribute to inversion positioning of the ankle during swing. Increased ankle inversion results in a shifting of weight bearing to the lateral border of the foot and further instability at the ankle. The term, *equinovarus*, specifically describes foot drop associated with excessive plantar flexion and inversion. Equinovarus deformity occurs when spasticity and primitive locomotor patterns are predominant rather than dorsiflexor muscle weakness. As a result, initial contact occurs with the foot in both a plantar-flexed and inverted position. Equinovarus positioning of the ankle is the most common pathologic limb posture in hemiparesis. **Table 2** presents the typical change in kinematic parameters in hemiparetic gait.

Kinetics of Hemiparetic Gait

Kinetic analysis of gait concerns the forces that produce movement. Quantitative gait analysis laboratories may use either traditional walkways with imbedded force plates or instrumented treadmills to analyze kinetics of gait. Measurement of ground reaction forces to determine joint moments and power may provide insight into the pathogenesis of walking impairment poststroke. In both normal and hemiparetic walking, the primary sources of power generation are the ankle plantar flexors at push off, hip extensors during early stance, and the hip flexors at preswing. In hemiparetic gait, however, the magnitude of power generation at both the hip and ankle are reduced. In a study of the capacity to increase hemiparetic walking velocity, Jonkers and

Table 2 Effect of hemiparesis on kinematic gait parameters	
Pelvis	
Tilt	Increased
Hip	
Flexion at heel strike	Decreased
Flexion at midswing	Decreased
Extension at preswing	Decreased
Knee	
Flexion at heel strike	Decreased
Flexion in swing	Decreased
Extension in stance	Increased
Ankle	
Dorsiflexion at heel strike	Decreased
Plantar flexion in swing	Increased
Inversion in swing	Increased

colleagues[20] found that higher functioning stroke survivors were able to increase walking speed by increasing paretic limb preswing hip flexion power and plantar flexor power at push off. An increase in hip flexion power at preswing alone may compensate for decreased ankle plantar flexion power and facilitate faster walking speeds in patients with greater residual proximal strength.[21] Forward propulsion of gait may be better assessed by measurement of the anteriorly directed GRF (anterior-posterior GRF), a parameter that has been used as a measurement of poststroke recovery over time.

Dynamic Muscle Activation in Hemiparetic Gait

Dynamic EMG can be used to identify abnormalities in timing and/or intensity of EMG signals compared with normal dynamic EMG signals. Clinical correlation between the kinematic gait pattern and dynamic EMG signals is necessary to determine optimal intervention for gait improvement. A recent study suggests that there is compensatory muscle activity of the nonparetic limb muscles that is activated to augment forward propulsion.[22]

ENERGY COSTS OF HEMIPARETIC WALKING

A disruption of the normal gait cycle, as occurs in poststroke hemiparesis, results in an increase in energy expenditure associated with walking.[23] Excessive energy consumption seems mainly due to the extra positive muscle work necessary to lift the body's CM against gravity during the paretic limb swing phase.[24] Thus, the greater metabolic cost of hemiparetic walking is attributed, in part, to compensations required of the nonparetic limb due to the paretic limb not providing adequately timed power at push off. Peterson and colleagues[25] used a 3-D forward dynamics simulation to show that total paretic and nonparetic limb muscle work are increased compared with a control. In 2 simulations that considered effect of walking velocity, the increase in work in hemiparetic gait was related to a decrease in work of the paretic plantar flexors in a lower walking velocity simulation and a decrease in work of the hip abductors and adductors in a higher walking velocity simulation model, with both conditions requiring compensatory work by other muscles. The researchers concluded that hemiparetic walkers expended greater metabolic energy during preswing compared with controls at the same level of mechanical efficiency (matched walking velocity). A recent analysis[26] suggests that the greater metabolic cost of poststroke hemiparetic walking is due to increased work of ambulation, not a decreased gait efficiency.

The higher energy cost of walking has been linked to reduced walking performance, increased deconditioning, and reduced community participation in many stroke survivors.[27] The energy cost of walking can be decreased, however, by either decreasing the walking velocity or performing compensatory gait maneuvers, such as dynamic muscle substitutions, if the patient has sufficient neurologic reserve. The oxygen consumption rate in a hemiparetic subject may be even less than in a healthy control, despite the inefficiency of the gait pattern, if the subject markedly reduces walking velocity. Although comparison between healthy and hemiparetic gait is sometimes carried out when subjects walk overground at preferred speed,[28] most clinical stroke rehabilitation trials attempt to compare gait parameters while controlling for walking velocity.

CLINICAL ASSESSMENT OF HEMIPARETIC GAIT

Many stroke survivors have limitations in walking associated with hemiparesis. The role of the clinician is to improve functional gait, using an individualized approach to therapy interventions, which is largely based on the neurologic examination and observation of gait in an outpatient setting. Quantitative gait analysis, including dynamic EMG, can provide insight into the cause of gait deviation, help determine the best locomotor training strategy, and assess therapeutic options, including orthotics/neuroprosthetics, botulinum toxin, or surgery.[29] A clinician providing care in a typical clinical setting, however, is asked to assess hemiparetic gait and make personalized recommendations for therapy, orthotics, and/or assistive devices without the luxury of quantitative measurements. To successfully do so, the clinician must be able to identify how the gait pattern differs from normal walking and what is the likely cause of the dysfunction. Most studies have found that the within-rater and between-rater reliability of available observational kinematic gait analysis tools is only moderately reliable.[30–32] A recent systematic review of various observational gait analysis tools used in stroke rehabilitation[33] concluded, however, by recommending the Gait Assessment and Intervention Tool[34] for use. Without advocating any specific observational gait analysis tool, the authors propose the following general tenets when evaluating hemiparetic gait in the outpatient setting.

Observational Gait Assessment

The assessment of gait in an outpatient setting should be approached methodically. Observational gait analysis focuses almost entirely on spatiotemporal and kinematics parameters. It is important to fully assess the pattern of walking, preferably as a patient walks down a long hallway or other unencumbered space. The patient should walk with, and then without, any assistive device or orthotic, if deemed safe. Focus first on observations in the frontal and then sagittal planes of gait. A written assessment should include comments on the following elements:

- Identify any assistive device (walker or cane), orthotic (knee or ankle foot orthosis), or neuroprosthetic device (peroneal nerve stimulator) that the patient requires for ambulation.
- Comment on gait speed, symmetry, and stability.
- Comment on posture (head, neck, and trunk) and any unusual patterns of lower limb weight shifting.
- Describe lower limb kinematics starting proximally and proceeding distally.
- Describe alterations in pelvic rotation.
- Describe kinematics at the level of the hip (hip hiking, circumduction, hip extension at push off, and hip flexion in swing).
- Describe kinematics at the knee (knee flexion at heel strike, extension in stance, and knee flexion in swing).
- Described kinematics at the ankle (dorsiflexion at heel strike, plantar flexion at push off, plantar flexion/dorsiflexion/inversion in swing).
- Comment on evidence of spasticity, ataxia, sensory, or proprioceptive deficits evident on neurologic examination, which may be affecting gait performance.

SUMMARY

The most common pattern of walking impairment poststroke is hemiparetic gait. Hemiparetic gait is most commonly characterized by an asymmetric pattern of walking with contralateral motor weakness. Primitive locomotor patterns may emerge poststroke, causing an alteration of the normal timing and intensity of muscle contraction of the paretic limb. In the lower limb, a predominantly extensor synergy pattern marked by hip extension, knee extension, hip adduction, ankle plantar flexion, and ankle inversion emerges, which may provide stance stability and facilitate walking. There are characteristic changes in the spatiotemporal, kinematic, and kinetic parameters of hemiparetic gait, which may be assessed most accurately in the setting of a motion studies laboratory. Additionally, the use of dynamic EMG can provide insight into alterations in normal muscle activation patterns of gait. An increase in the energy costs of walking in hemiparetic gait may be addressed by decreasing walking velocity or by performing compensatory gait maneuvers, if the patient has sufficient neurologic reserve. Knowledge of the neural control and biomechanics of normal human gait is necessary for the clinician to understand the complex interplay of motor strength deficits, variable spasticity, sensory and proprioceptive loss, and/or ataxia on motor control and functional gait performance in hemiparesis.

ACKNOWLEDGMENT

The authors thank medical illustrator Erika Woodrum of the Cleveland Functional Electrical Stimulation Center for her assistance with **Figs. 1** and **2**.

REFERENCES

1. Duncan PW, Zorowitz R, Bates B, et al. Management of adult stroke rehabilitation care: a clinical practice guideline. Stroke 2005;36:e100–43.
2. Kao PC, Dingwell JB, Higginson JS, et al. Dynamic instability during post-stroke hemiparetic walking. Gait Posture 2014;40:457–63.
3. Brown TG. The intrinsic factors in the act of progression in the mammal. Proc Roy Soc Lond 1911;B84:308–19.
4. Brown TG. The factors in rhythmic activity of the nervous system. Proc Roy Soc Lond 1912;B85:278–89.
5. Grillner S. Interaction between sensory signals and the central networks controlling locomotion in lamprey, dogfish, and cat. In: Grillner S, Stein P, Stuart PG, et al, editors. Neurobiology of vertebrate locomotion wenner grem international symposium series. London: MacMillan; 1986. p. 506–12.
6. Dietz V. Proprioception and locomotor disorders. Nat Rev Neurosci 2002;3: 781–90.
7. Armstrong DM. The supraspinal control of mammalian locomotion. J Physiol 1988;405:1–37.
8. Vilensky JA, O'Connor BL. Stepping in nonhuman primates with a complete spinal cord transection: old and new data, and implications for humans. Ann N Y Acad Sci 1998;860:528–30.
9. Patterson KK, Gage WH, Brooks D, et al. Evaluation of gait symmetry after stroke: a comparison of current methods and recommendations for standardization. Gait Posture 2010;31:241–6.
10. Perry J, Garrett M, Gronley JK, et al. Classification of walking handicap in the stroke population. Stroke 1995;26:982–9.
11. Perry J. Dynamic electromyography. In: Perry J, editor. Gait analysis normal and pathological function. New York: McGraw-Hill, Inc; 1992. p. 397.
12. Saunders JB, Inman VT, Eberhart HD. The major determinants in normal and pathological gait. J Bone Joint Surg Am 1953;35-A:543–58.
13. Elftman H. The functions of the arms in walking. Hum Biol 1939;11:529–36.
14. Ralston H. Effect of immobilization of various body segments on the energy cost of human locomotion. Proc. 2nd IEA Conference. Dortmund, 1965. Ergonomics (Supplement) 1965. p. 53–60.
15. Goldie PA, Matyas TA, Evans OM. Gait after stroke: initial deficit and changes in temporal patterns for each gait phase. Arch Phys Med Rehabil 2001;82:1057–65.

16. Oken O, Yavuzer G. Spatio-temporal and kinematic asymmetry ratio in subgroups of patients with stroke. Eur J Phys Rehabil Med 2008;44:127–32.
17. De Quervain IA, Simon SR, Leurgans S, et al. Gait pattern in the early recovery period after stroke. J Bone Joint Surg Am 1996;78:1506–14.
18. Cooper A, Alghamdi GA, Alghamdi MA, et al. The relationship of lower limb muscle strength and knee joint hyperextension during the stance phase of gait in hemiparetic stroke patients. Physiother Res Int 2012;17:150–6.
19. Peterson CL, Hall AL, Kautz SA, et al. Pre-swing deficits in forward propulsion, swing initiation and power generation by individual muscles during hemiparetic walking. J Biomech 2010;43:2348–55.
20. Jonkers I, Delp S, Patten C. Capacity to increase walking speed is limited by impaired hip and ankle power generation in lower functioning persons post-stroke. Gait Posture 2009;29:129–37.
21. Williams G, Morris ME, Schache A, et al. People preferentially increase hip joint power generation to walk faster following traumatic brain injury. Neurorehabil Neural Repair 2010;24:550–8.
22. Raja B, Neptune RR, Kautz SA. Coordination of the non-paretic leg during hemiparetic gait: expected and novel compensatory patterns. Clin Biomech 2012;27:1023–30.
23. Detrembleur C, Dierick F, Stoquart G, et al. Energy cost, mechanical work, and efficiency of hemiparetic walking. Gait Posture 2003;18:47–55.
24. Chen G, Patten C, Kothari DH, et al. Gait differences between individuals with post-stroke hemiparesis and non-disabled controls at matched speeds. Gait Posture 2005;22:51–6.
25. Peterson CL, Kautz SA, Neptune RR. Muscle work is increased in pre-swing during hemiparetic walking. Clin Biomech 2011;26:859–66.
26. Farris DJ, Hampton A, Lewek MD, et al. Revisiting the mechanics and energetics of walking in individuals with chronic hemiparesis following stroke: from individual limbs to lower limb joints. J Neuroeng Rehabil 2015;12:24.
27. Awad LN, Palmer JA, Pohlig RT, et al. Walking speed and step length asymmetry modify the energy cost of walking after stroke. Neurorehabil Neural Repair 2015;29(5):416–23.
28. Rinaldi LA, Monaco V. Spatio-temporal parameters and intralimb coordination patterns describing hemiparetic locomotion at controlled speed. J Neuroeng Rehabil 2013;10:53.
29. Ferrarin M, Rabuffetti M, Bacchini M, et al. Does gait analysis change clinical decision-making in post-stroke patients? Results from a pragmatic prospective observational study. Eur J Phys Rehabil Med 2015;51(2):171–84.
30. Krebs DE, Edelstein JE, Fishman S. Reliability of observational kinematic gait analysis. Phys Ther 1985;65:1027–33.
31. Eastlack ME, Arvidson J, Snyder-Mackler L, et al. Interrater reliability of video-taped observational gait-analysis assessments. Phys Ther 1991;71:465–72.
32. McGinley JL, Goldie PA, Greenwood KM, et al. Accuracy and reliability of observational gait analysis data: judgments of push-off in gait after stroke. Phys Ther 2003;83:146–60.
33. Ferrarello F, Bianchi VA, Baccini M, et al. Tools for observational gait analysis in patients with stroke: a systematic review. Phys Ther 2013;93:1673–85.
34. Daly JJ, Nethery J, McCabe JP, et al. Development and testing of the Gait Assessment and Intervention Tool (G.A.I.T.): a measure of coordinated gait components. J Neurosci Methods 2009;178:334–9.

Spasticity Management After Stroke

Francois Bethoux, MD

KEYWORDS

- Stroke • Spasticity • Symptom management • Outcome measures • Rehabilitation

KEY POINTS

- Spasticity from stroke is classified as cerebral-origin spasticity, characterized by hyperexcitability of monosynaptic pathways, a rapid rise in excitation, and stereotypical postures involving antigravity muscle groups.
- The prevalence of spasticity after stroke can be as high as 46% in the chronic phase (over 3 months).
- Spasticity is most often associated with other neurologic impairments, in particular paresis, which complicate its evaluation and management.
- Treating spasticity after a stroke entails combining nonpharmacological and pharmacologic interventions.
- There is emerging evidence suggesting that some treatments for spasticity improve upper and lower extremity functional performance.

INTRODUCTION

Spasticity is a movement disorder, defined as a velocity-dependent increase in stretch reflexes[1] due to impaired supraspinal inhibitory signals. Recent observations suggest, however, that decreased homosynaptic depression (ie, impaired depletion of the release of excitatory neurotransmitters with repetitive afferent activation), rather than decreased presynaptic inhibition, is associated with poststroke spasticity.[2] In addition, defective supraspinal control of various spinal inhibitory and facilitatory circuits is associated with abnormal muscle contraction during voluntary movement.[3] Finally, changes in the rheologic and contractile properties of musculoskeletal soft tissue are frequently associated with chronic spasticity and in turn have been linked to increased spasticity.[4]

Cerebral-origin spasticity after a stroke differs from spinal-origin spasticity as encountered in spinal cord injury and multiple sclerosis. Cerebral-origin spasticity is characterized by

Mellen Center Rehabilitation Services, The Cleveland Clinic, 9500 Euclid Avenue/Desk U10, Cleveland, OH 44195, USA
E-mail address: BETHOUF@ccf.org

Phys Med Rehabil Clin N Am 26 (2015) 625–639
http://dx.doi.org/10.1016/j.pmr.2015.07.003
pmr.theclinics.com

- Hyperexcitability of monosynaptic pathways
- A rapid rise in excitation
- Stereotypical postures involving antigravity muscle groups. The hemiplegic posture commonly observed after a stroke consists of
  - In the upper extremity: shoulder adduction; forearm pronation; and elbow, wrist, and finger flexion
  - In the lower extremity: hip adduction, knee extension, ankle plantarflexion, and often pes varus

Spasticity is only one component of the upper motor neuron (UMN) syndrome. As a consequence, other features of the UMN syndrome most often accompany spasticity, such as weakness, loss of dexterity, and synkinetic movements. In one study, 100% of patients with spasticity exhibited limb weakness (vs 50% of patients without spasticity) when assessed over 3 months after a stroke.[5] Because other neurologic impairments are commonly seen after a stroke (eg, visual, sensory, and cognitive), it may be difficult to isolate the specific impact of spasticity on functional limitations. It has been stated that the functional limitations experienced by stroke survivors are mostly related to neurologic deficits other than spasticity.[6]

The prevalence of spasticity after stroke is difficult to ascertain in the absence of rigorous population-based studies. In a survey from the National Stroke Association, 57% of 504 stroke survivors reported tight or stiff muscles, suggesting the presence of spasticity.[7] Clinician-based determination of the prevalence of spasticity is most often conducted in hospital stroke units, with sample sizes ranging from 50 to 200 individuals. Prevalence values are between 4% and 27% in the first month after stroke and between 17% and 46% past 3 months.[8,9] Longitudinal studies generally report higher prevalence values at the chronic phase.[5,9,10]

PATIENT EVALUATION OVERVIEW
Identifying Spasticity

The diagnosis of spasticity is based on clinical features, in the context of a central nervous system disorder. Spasticity is usually associated with some or all of the patient complaints presented in **Table 1**. Even though these symptoms are suggestive of spasticity, they are not sufficient to establish the diagnosis. For example, difficulty moving a limb can be described as "stiffness" even when it is due to weakness. Pain can be related to spasticity (particularly if it is associated with spasms or occurs with passive movement), but central neuropathic pain (particularly after a thalamic stroke) or musculoskeletal pain may also be present.

The diagnosis of spasticity is confirmed by clinical examination findings, summarized in **Table 1**. Some of these signs are associated with passive stretch (resistance

Table 1
Patient complaints and examination findings associated with spasticity

Complaints	Clinical Signs
• Muscle stiffness or tightness	• Resistance to passive movement
• Muscle spasms	• Clonus
• Clonus (shaking)	• Spasms
• Pain	• Co-contraction of agonist and antagonist muscles
• Difficulty performing voluntary movement	• Spastic dystonia
	• Decreased passive range of motion
• Limb deformity (cosmetic or functional concern)	• Abnormal posture
	• Limb deformity

to passive movement, clonus); others are observed only with active movement, such as muscle co-contraction and spastic dystonia. Therefore, spasticity needs to be examined at rest and with voluntary movement (whenever possible) to better understand the functional consequences of spasticity. In addition, it is useful to assess spasticity in various positions (standing vs sitting vs supine) because position-dependent variations in spasticity have been reported and are commonly observed in practice.

Other signs of the UMN syndrome are almost always present, in particular paresis and loss of dexterity but also synergistic movement patterns. In addition, other neurologic impairments often increase the complexity of the clinical presentation but are important to document, because they have an impact on goal setting and treatment planning. Strength output is of particular importance, because increased weakness may occur as spasticity is treated. Finally, the presence of partial or total musculoskeletal contractures should be documented, because they have an impact on the treatment plan, whether or not they are directly related to spasticity.

Spasticity needs to be differentiated from other movement disorders associated with increased tone, in particular

- Dystonia, which causes abnormal sustained or intermittent muscle contractions with twisting movements and abnormal postures. Some of the features of dystonia, however, are observed with spasticity (spastic dystonia), as discussed previously.
- Extrapyramidal hypertonia, which is characterized by cogwheeling and rigidity

Velocity-dependent resistance to passive movement is a useful clinical feature to distinguish spasticity from these other movement disorders but may be difficult to assess in the presence of severe hypertonia and ROM limitations. In addition, various movement disorders may coexist, depending on the location of the stroke.

Measuring Spasticity

Once spasticity is identified, it is useful to rate its severity, particularly for monitoring treatment outcomes. **Table 2** gives examples of some of the assessment tools available to clinicians and researchers.

Most of the spasticity severity scales used in the clinic and in clinical trials measure resistance to passive movement (eg, Ashworth Scale and Tardieu Scale), despite the aforementioned limitations of this approach. In addition, patient-reported questionnaires have been used to quantify spasm frequency and, more recently, patients' overall assessment of their spasticity (spasticity numeric rating scale). Instrumented tests measurements (electromyogram [EMG], dynamometry, and pendulum test) are not routinely used in the clinic, due to time and equipment requirements and because they do not always correlate with clinical findings.

Although functional tests and scales are increasingly used in clinical trials of treatments for spasticity, none of them was specifically developed and validated for this application, to the author's knowledge. The appropriateness of a specific functional test depends on the limb(s) targeted for treatment, the treatment goals, the instrument's psychometric properties, and feasibility. Among others, the Frenchay Arm Test, the Disability Assessment Scale have been used to assess upper limb function; timed walking tests to assess lower limb function; and the Barthel Index and Functional Independence Measure for overall functional status have been used in the evaluation of treatments of spasticity after stroke.

Other neurologic impairments need to be documented in the initial evaluation and taken into account for goal setting but may not need to be monitored in a quantitative

Table 2
Assessment tools for spasticity

Name	Clinical Parameter Assessed	Scoring	Comments
Clinical examination scales			
Ashworth Scale (AS) and Modified Ashworth Scale (MAS)[38]	Resistance to passive movement	AS: 1 (no increase in muscle tone) to 5 (affected part[s] rigid in flexion or extension) MAS: 0 (no increase in muscle tone) to 4 (affected part [s] rigid in flexion or extension) Includes 1+ rating (catch followed by minimal resistance throughout the remainder of the range of motion)	Pros: easy to administer; frequently used in clinical trials Cons: lacks sensitivity to change; inter-rater reliability is an issue; resistance to passive movement is not equivalent to spasticity
Tardieu Scale (TS)[39] and Modified Tardieu Scale (MTS)[40]	Resistance to passive movement	TS: resistance to passive movement assessed at 3 speeds: V1 (as slow as possible), V2 (speed of the limb falling under gravity), V3 (as fast as possible) Two angles measured: R1 (first catch to a quick stretch) and R2 (total passive range of motion with slow stretch) R2–R1 = dynamic tone MTS: only 2 speeds (V1 and V3)	Pros: easy to administer; more detailed assessment than AS or MAS Cons: lacks sensitivity to change; inter-rater reliability is an issue
Triple Spasticity Scale[41]	Change in resistance to passive movement between slow and fast speed, clonus, dynamic muscle length	Total score from 0 to 10 Three subscales: increased resistance between a slow stretch and a fast stretch (0–4), clonus (0–2), dynamic muscle length (0–4)	—
Self-report measures			
Spasm Frequency Scale[42]	Spasm frequency	0 (No spasm) to 4 (more than 10 spontaneous spasms per hour)	Pros: easy to use; frequently used in clinical trials Cons: does not take into account fluctuations of spasm frequency; does not assess spasm severity or pain associated with spasms; lacks sensitivity to change

Spasm Frequency Score[43]	Spasm frequency	0 (No spasms) to 10 (10 or more spasms per day, or continuous contraction)	Pros and cons are similar to those cited for the Spasm Frequency Scale. Not as commonly used in clinical trials.
Spasticity numeric rating scale (NRS)[44]	Global severity of spasticity	0 (No spasticity) to 10 (worst possible spasticity)	Pros: easy to use, good test-retest reliability, correlates with other measures of spasticity. Clinically important difference was calculated at 30% change in score (minimal clinically important difference: 18% change). Cons: validated only for multiple sclerosis–related spasticity
Instrumented measurements			
Isokinetic dynamometry[45]	Resistance to passive movement	Torque	Pros: high test-retest reliability; excellent control of stretch velocity and amplitude; quantification of resistance to passive movement. Cons: equipment and time requirements; correlation with traditional clinical measures not always satisfactory
Pendulum test[46]	Lower leg swing in patient sitting	Amplitude of leg swing around the knee (assessed with electrogoniometer), angle difference between start and finish positions	Pros: simple setup; correlates well with clinical measures of spasticity. Cons: requires equipment; only assesses spasticity around the knee joint
EMG[47]	EMG response to stretch, tendon tap (T reflex) and electrical stimulation of the peripheral nerve (H-reflex)	Threshold values H/M ratio (H = H-reflex threshold, M = M-reflex threshold)	Pros: measures reflex activity. Cons: equipment and time requirements. Poor or no correlation with clinical measures
Tonic stretch reflex threshold (TSRT)[48]	Excitability of motoneurons without stretch (0°/s velocity) TSRT computed from angles where the EMG signal increases for a given velocity of stretch	The TSRT is defined as the intercept value of the linear regression line for dynamic stretch reflex thresholds (at various angular velocities) with the angle axis (dependent variable: angle; independent variable: velocity).	Pros: portable device; moderate inter- and intrarater reliability for moderate to high spasticity; tested in poststroke spasticity. Cons: time consuming; did not correlate with MAS scores in preliminary validation study

manner, because they are expected to remain unchanged. The only notable exception is weakness, because it may also be impacted by treatment. The most common way to document strength in the clinic is the manual muscle testing (despite its limitations in the assessment of central paresis), whereas the Evaluation Database to Guide Effectiveness (EDGE) document published by the Neurology Section of the American Physical Therapy Association recommends the use of handheld dynamometry.[11]

Treatment planning requires assessing the consequences of spasticity and defining realistic goals. Although it is a common process in medicine in general, and in the field of rehabilitation in particular, goal setting can be difficult because spasticity is most often not the only cause of the symptoms and functional limitations observed. Potential consequences of spasticity and related treatment goals are described in **Table 3**.

Once goals have been defined, the Goal Attainment Scaling can be used to quantify treatment results.[12]

Before describing in detail treatment options for spasticity, a few general treatment planning rules must be stated:

- Spasticity does not always need to be treated. If no short-term or long-term adverse consequence is expected, no other intervention that self-management with daily stretching may be required. In one study, 4% of stroke survivors exhibited disabling spasticity requiring treatment 1 year after a first stroke.[13] Patients should be advised to seek medical attention if they notice a worsening of spasticity over time.
- Furthermore, treating spasticity may be detrimental to functional performance due to the compensatory effect of hypertonia in weak limbs and to increased weakness from treatment. Other potential beneficial effects of spasticity, which are reported anecdotally but have not been extensively studied, include maintaining muscle bulk and bone density and improving venous circulation by causing involuntary muscle contraction.
- When treatment is needed, nonpharmacologic treatments are systematically used, either prior to or concomitant with pharmacologic or surgical treatments.
- Treatment modalities can be combined to achieve the desired goals.

The Department of Veterans Affairs/Department of Defense Clinical Practice Guideline for the Management of Stroke Rehabilitation includes simple recommendations for the management of spasticity after stroke.[14] Several review articles provide

Table 3	
Consequences of spasticity and potential treatment goals	
Domain Affected by Spasticity	**Examples of Goals**
Comfort	Alleviate discomfort, pain, or sleep disruption associated with hypertonia and/or spasms
Posture	Improve abnormal posture of a limb or of the body and the potential consequences of abnormal posture (eg, cosmetic impact, interference with positioning and care, and abnormal pressure points)
Ease of care (sometimes called "passive function")	Reduce physical caregiver burden by facilitating passive movement and positioning
Active function	Improve the quality of voluntary movement to enhance functional performance and/or facilitate rehabilitation
Prevention of medical complications	Decrease the risk of contractures and pressure ulcers

more detailed recommendations based on evidence review and expert opinion, including treatment algorithms.[15–17]

NONPHARMACOLOGIC TREATMENT OPTIONS

The first step in managing spasticity (or before escalating treatment in the context of abrupt worsening of spasticity) is to identify any noxious stimulus that can increase its severity, such as a decubitus ulcer, a urinary problem (acute urinary retention, bladder stones, or urinary tract infection), or an ingrown toenail. Addressing these issues may lead to a significant improvement, and obviate further symptomatic treatment.

Education of patients, and often of caregivers, is essential in the management of spasticity. An article published in 2013 by Sunnerhagen and Francisco[18] provides a detailed discussion of issues related to patient-provider communication in the management of spasticity.

Referral to a rehabilitation professional is strongly recommended for all patients with clinically significant spasticity, although treatment modalities and goals vary depending on the extent and severity of the spasticity and on a patient's overall functional status. These modalities include

- Stretching, arguably the most commonly used nonpharmacologic treatment in the management of spasticity. After proper training by a physical or occupational therapist, stretching is performed daily by patients themselves or by a caregiver to help increase or preserve the length of the muscles and other musculoskeletal structures.
- Fitting of splints/braces, and sometimes serial casting, to achieve a similar goal as stretching and to facilitate functional tasks (eg, ankle foot orthosis to correct foot drop due to plantarflexor spasticity)
- Physical modalities, such as ultrasound and thermotherapy
- Neuromuscular electrical stimulation (NEMS), when applied to an agonist muscle, was shown to decrease spasticity in the antagonist muscle, although the effect is usually short-lived. It has been suggested that NEMS applied to a muscle after botulinum toxin (BT) injections may help the medication diffuse and amplify its efficacy.[19] Finally, functional electrical stimulation of the upper and lower extremity is increasingly used, particularly to control distal muscles, such as the finger extensors and the ankle dorsiflexors, in patients with spastic paresis.
- Muscle strengthening (in particular strengthening of an agonist to diminish the consequences of spasticity in the antagonist)
- Aerobic training for fitness and endurance and task-specific functional training
- Use of robotics to perform stretching and movement training. The Lokomat device (Hocoma AG, Volketswil, Switzerland), which combines robotic assist with body weight–supported treadmill training, has been the topic of several publications. To the author's knowledge, its superiority to traditional physical therapy (PT) has not been established, but recent evidence suggests that use of the Lokomat combined with traditional PT is more effective than PT alone.[20] Other devices have been developed for the lower extremity[21] and for the upper extremity.[22]

PHARMACOLOGIC TREATMENT OPTIONS

Oral symptomatic medications for spasticity (sometimes called antispasmodics) are well known and generally safe (**Table 4**). They are typically prescribed in divided doses

Table 4
Pharmacologic treatments for spasticity

Name	Dosing	Most Common Side Effects	Comments
Oral medications			
Baclofen	Up to 80 mg daily in divided doses (3–4 times per day). Higher doses have been used for severe spasticity as tolerated.	Sedation, drowsiness, confusion, dizziness, weakness. Risk of withdrawal.	Structural analog of γ-aminobutyric acid (GABA), binds to pre- and postsynaptic GABA-B receptors
Tizanidine	Up to 36 mg daily in divided doses (3–4 times per day)	Sedation, dry mouth, dizziness, hypotension, elevated liver enzymes, and hallucinations. Drug interaction with ciprofloxacine.	Imidazoline derivative, central α_2-adrenergic receptor agonist
Dantrolene	Up to 400 mg/d in up to 4 divided doses	Muscle weakness, sedation, gastrointestinal symptoms, hepatotoxicity	Hydantoin derivative, reduces the action potential-induced release of calcium from the sarcoplasmic reticulum of skeletal muscle fibers
Diazepam	Up to 30 mg/d in 3–4 divided doses	Sedation, confusion, muscle weakness. Risk of overdose (respiratory depression, coma) and withdrawal (anxiety, agitation, seizures)	GABA-A agonist, decreases mono- and polysynaptic reflexes in the spinal cord. Can be helpful to control painful muscle spasms at night. Benzodiazepines may compromise neurologic recovery.

Local injections

Phenol/alcohol neurolysis	Phenol concentration ≥3% Ethyl alcohol concentration ≥50%	Local: injection pain, weakness, dysesthesia, inflammation, tissue sloughing, deep vein thrombosis, ischemia General: central nervous system depression, seizures, cardiovascular compromise	Immediate effect, duration 6 mo or more Low cost Primarily motor nerves are preferred, to decrease the risk of dysesthesia
BT	Intramuscular injections every 3–4 mo. Doses vary depending on the size of the muscles injected, the severity of the spasticity, and the treatment goals. Dosing guidelines have been published.[49]	Local: pain, weakness, muscle atrophy General: fatigue, nausea, "spread of effect" (dissemination of chemodenervation effect beyond the muscle targeted)	BT A and B are available. Injection guidance with EMG, electrical stimulation, and more recently ultrasound, is not mandatory but helpful with smaller and deeper muscles. Higher cost

Intrathecal therapy

ITB	Continuous intrathecal delivery, with a wide range of daily rates expressed in μg/d	Weakness Complications related to the surgery (eg, cerebrospinal fluid leak or infection) or to device malfunction (catheter more frequently than the pump) Risk of baclofen overdose or withdrawal	A screening injection is usually performed before planning surgery. The ITB infusion system consists of a programmable pump implanted subcutaneously in the abdominal area and a catheter between the pump and the intrathecal space.

throughout the day, due to their short duration of effect (usually 4–6 hours), although single dosing at bedtime is an option if controlling night time spasms is the primary treatment goal. Their use is often limited, however, by side effects, in particular sedation and weakness. Baclofen and tizanidine are the most commonly used oral agents, but tizanidine has been recommended over baclofen for patients with chronic stroke. The use of these agents as well as benzodiazepines is discouraged during the post-stroke recovery period due to a potential negative impact on brain plasticity.[14] Antiepileptic drugs, such as gabapentin and pregabalin, are not considered first-line options for spasticity but can be used as adjunct therapies, particularly when central neuropathic pain is present. Cannabis derivatives are approved in some countries to treat spasticity from multiple sclerosis, based on positive results from phase III clinical trials, but not for poststroke spasticity.[23]

Local treatments present several advantages, including the ability to selectively treat specific muscles and the absence of sedation. They are indicated particularly when spasticity is focal but are also helpful when spasticity is diffuse and focal goals are identified.

- Injections of local anesthetics to produce transient neuromuscular blocks are used for treatment planning, mainly to differentiate between contractures and severe spasticity and sometimes to assess whether decreasing spasticity may have negative consequences (particularly functional), but their effect is too short-lived to consider them a treatment modality.
- Injections of phenol or alcohol (chemical neurolysis) are preferably performed on purely or predominantly motor nerves, to decrease the risk of chronic dysesthesia. The most common targets include the musculocutaneous, obturator, and tibial nerves.[24]
- BT, when injected intramuscularly, causes chemodenervation by blocking the release of acetylcholine at the neuromuscular junction. The effect is not as immediate and does not last as long as that of chemical neurolysis, yet BT therapy has become the most widely used local treatment of spasticity, with a large body of evidence supporting its efficacy on poststroke spasticity but more limited data on its functional impact. In 2008, the Therapeutics and Technology Assessment Subcommittee of the American Academy of Neurology published an evidence-based review on the use of BT for upper and lower extremity spasticity. The investigators concluded that BT is effective in reducing tone and improving passive function in adults with spasticity (level A recommendation) and probably effective on active function (level B recommendation, based on one class I study).[25] Recently published literature reviews and meta-analyses on the functional impact of BT for spasticity after stroke found a small (0.044 m/s) but statistically significant improvement in gait velocity after BT injections for spastic equinovarus in a pooled sample of 228 patients[26] and reported a moderate BT treatment effect on various measures of upper extremity function.[27] Several preparations of BT type A and one preparation of BT type B have been used to treat spasticity. There is no fully reliable dosing conversion factor between these preparations.

Intrathecal baclofen (ITB) therapy is a neuromodulation treatment that allows the delivery of baclofen intrathecally, via a programmable pump implanted subcutaneously in the abdominal area and connected to a catheter whose distal end is inserted into the spinal canal. Although the point of entry of the catheter into the spine is usually at the upper lumbar level, the catheter tip can be located at various levels, with higher catheter tip locations considered when upper extremity spasticity relief is sought.

ITB therapy is generally indicated in patients with severe spasticity refractory to other treatments, in particular oral baclofen (insufficient efficacy and/or side effects). Evidence regarding the effectiveness of ITB therapy in poststroke survivors and potential procedure-related or device-related complications were summarized in guidelines published in 2006[28] and in a more recent review.[17] Compared with oral baclofen, ITB therapy is usually more effective on spasticity and less sedative. The absence of adverse effect (weakness) on the nonaffected limbs was demonstrated.[29] Functional improvement in the lower extremity[30] and upper extremity[31] was reported in uncontrolled open-label studies.

SURGICAL TREATMENT OPTIONS

Overall, surgical treatments are not used as frequently as other options in the management of spasticity. They can be classified into orthopedic and neurosurgical procedures.

Orthopedic surgery addresses the consequences of spasticity more than the movement disorder itself and consist mainly of tendon release and tendon transfer procedures, in the setting of fixed contractures and severe deformity with cosmetic, functional, or medical (eg, skin ulcers) consequences.

Neurosurgical interventions include neurotomy and selective dorsal rhizotomy (SDR):

- Neurotomy is mainly considered for distal lower limb spasticity (in particular equinovarus deformity and toe clawing). An open-label study on 34 patients found that tibial nerve neurotomy was more effective than BT therapy on a variety of outcomes, including spasticity, range of motion, and lower extremity function, up to 1 year after the neurotomy procedure.[32]
- SDR consists of severing dorsal lumbar nerve fascicles exhibiting an abnormal response to electrical stimulation, resulting in a diffuse improvement of lower body spasticity. SDR has been mainly used in children with cerebral palsy, although less frequently since the introduction of ITB therapy. A recent literature review of non– cerebral palsy indications for SDR[33] identified 11 relevant care series reporting on a total of 145 patients, but only 2 of those patients were ischemic stroke survivors, who exhibited good results after unilateral SDR (functional improvement in 1 patient and improved pain in the other).[34]

COMBINING INTERVENTIONS

Managing spasticity most often requires combining treatment modalities as is thought appropriate to achieve predefined goals. For example,

- Stretching should be combined with all other treatment modalities.
- Task-specific functional training is needed if the goal is to enhance active function.
- Oral medications to decrease the overall level of spasticity may be combined with local injections of BT to address focal problems related to spasticity.
- When orthopedic procedures, such as tendon release, are contemplated, controlling spasticity with medication is recommended to decrease the risk of recurrence of contractures or orthopedic deformities.

Therefore, interventions are often combined based on an individualized treatment plan. Unfortunately, there is a lack of evidence to demonstrate the outcomes of combined interventions. A recently published Cochrane review of the effects of multidisciplinary rehabilitation after local treatments of poststroke spasticity (including BT therapy) found only low-level evidence supporting the efficacy of rehabilitation on active function and no evidence on passive function.[35]

TREATMENT RESISTANCE/COMPLICATIONS

The main potential side effects and complications of treatments for spasticity are described above (or were described previously).

Long-term loss of efficacy of symptomatic medications for spasticity is observed empirically, but its cause is often unclear. Factors related to the patient may include aging, difficulty taking the prescribed dose due to side effects, the development of comorbidities leading to increased spasticity (eg, decubitus ulcers), and the consequences of chronic immobility (eg, development of contractures). Two drug therapies have been associated with pharmacologic phenomenons that may limit their efficacy:

- The development of a pharmacologic tolerance has been described with oral and intrathecal baclofen, mainly in patients with spinal cord injury and multiple sclerosis, but not systematically investigated. In case series of patients treated with intrathecal baclofen, some investigators have interpreted the stabilization of group average doses on the long-term as evidence of the absence of tolerance.[36]
- BT injections may lead to the development of neutralizing antibodies that are not known to cause harm to the patient but compromise the biological effects of the treatment. The observed incidence of antibodies in clinical trials is generally low; however, the observation period is often short.[37]

SUMMARY

A significant proportion of stroke survivors present with chronic spasticity of cerebral origin. Diagnosis and assessing the consequences of spasticity require thorough clinical examination, including testing at rest in various positions and functional testing. Spasticity can have an impact on comfort, posture, ease of care, and active function and may increase the risk of comorbid complications, such as contractures and skin ulcers. Conversely, spasticity can also help preserve function. Therefore, the treatment plan should be tailored to specific goals and not merely be driven by the presence of spasticity. Stretching, rehabilitation, and the use of orthotics are commonly combined with pharmacologic therapies. A variety of medications are available, administered via different routes (oral, local injections, and intrathecal), and their efficacy, safety profile, and relative indications are documented in a growing body of evidence. Functional outcomes, however, remain to be better characterized and predictors of response need to be identified to guide clinical decision making.

REFERENCES

1. Lance J. Symposium synopsis. In: Feldman RG, Young RR, Koella WP, editors. Spasticity: disordered motor control. Chicago: Year Book Medical Publishers; 1980. p. 485–94.
2. Lamy JC, Wargon I, Mazevet D, et al. Impaired efficacy of spinal presynaptic mechanisms in spastic stroke patients. Brain 2009;132:734–48.
3. Burke D, Wissel J, Donnan GA. Pathophysiology of spasticity in stroke. Neurology 2013;80(3 Suppl 2):S20–6.

4. Dietz V, Sinkjaer T. Spastic movement disorder: impaired reflex function and altered muscle mechanics. Lancet Neurol 2007;6:725–33.
5. Wissel J, Schelosky LD, Scott J, et al. Early development of spasticity following stroke: a prospective, observational trial. J Neurol 2010;257(7):1067–72.
6. Landau WM. Spasticity after stroke: why bother? Stroke 2004;35:1787–8.
7. National Stroke Association Stroke Perceptions Study, June 2006. Available at: http://support.stroke.org/site/DocServer/StrokePerceptions_FinalSurveyResults_2006.pdf?docID=1941, Accessed March 1, 2015.
8. Wissel J, Manack A, Brainin M. Toward an epidemiology of poststroke spasticity. Neurology 2013;80(3 Suppl 2):S13–9.
9. Opheim A, Danielsson A, Alt Murphy M, et al. Upper limb spasticity during the first year after stroke: stroke arm longitudinal study at the University of Gothenburg. Am J Phys Med Rehabil 2014;93:884–96.
10. Welmer AK, Widén Holmqvist L, Sommerfeld DK. Location and severity of spasticity in the first 1-2 weeks and at 3 and 18 months after stroke. Eur J Neurol 2010;17(5):720–5.
11. Available at: http://www.neuropt.org/docs/stroke-sig/strokeedge_taskforce_summary_document.pdf?sfvrsn=2. Accessed March 1, 2015.
12. Turner-Stokes L, Baguley IJ, De Graaff S, et al. Goal attainment scaling in the evaluation of treatment of upper limb spasticity with botulinum toxin: a secondary analysis from a double-blind placebo-controlled randomized clinical trial. J Rehabil Med 2010;42(1):81–9.
13. Lundstrom E, Terent A, Borg J. Prevalence of disabling spasticity 1 year after first-ever stroke. Eur J Neurol 2008;15:533–9.
14. VA/DoD Clinical Practice Guideline for the Management of Stroke Rehabilitation. Version 2.0. October 2010. Available at: http://www.rehab.research.va.gov/jour/10/479/pdf/VADODcliniaclGuidlines479.pdf. Accessed March 1, 2015.
15. Bakheit AM. The pharmacological management of post-stroke muscle spasticity. Drugs Aging 2012;29(12):941–7.
16. Yelnik AP, Simon O, Parratte B, et al. How to clinically assess and treat muscle overactivity in spastic paresis. J Rehabil Med 2010;42(9):801–7.
17. Francisco GE, McGuire JR. Post-stroke spasticity management. Stroke 2012;43:3132–6.
18. Sunnerhagen KS, Francisco GE. Enhancing patient-provider communication for long-term post-stroke spasticity management. Acta Neurol Scand 2013;128(5):305–10.
19. Santus G, Faletti S, Bordanzi I, et al. Effect of short-term electrical stimulation before and after botulinum toxin injection. J Rehabil Med 2011;43(5):420–3.
20. Dundar U, Toktas H, Solak O, et al. A comparative study of conventional physiotherapy versus robotic training combined with physiotherapy in patients with stroke. Top Stroke Rehabil 2014;21(6):453–61.
21. Zhang M, Davies TC, Xie S. Effectiveness of robot-assisted therapy on ankle rehabilitation–a systematic review. J Neuroeng Rehabil 2013;10:30.
22. Fazekas G, Horvath M, Troznai T, et al. Robot-mediated upper limb physiotherapy for patients with spastic hemiparesis: a preliminary study. J Rehabil Med 2007;39(7):580–2.
23. Malfitano AM, Proto MC, Bifulco M. Cannabinoids in the management of spasticity associated with multiple sclerosis. Neuropsychiatr Dis Treat 2008;4(5):847–53.
24. Kocabas H, Salli A, Demir AH, et al. Comparison of phenol and alcohol neurolysis of tibial nerve motor branches to the gastrocnemius muscle for treatment of

spastic foot after stroke: a randomized controlled pilot study. Eur J Phys Rehabil Med 2010;46(1):5–10.

25. Simpson DM, Gracies JM, Graham HK, et al. Assessment: botulinum neurotoxin for the treatment of spasticity (an evidence-based review): report of the Therapeutics and Technology Assessment Subcommittee of the American Academy of Neurology. Neurology 2008;70(19):1691–8.

26. Foley N, Murie-Fernandez M, Speechley M, et al. Does the treatment of spastic equinovarus deformity following stroke with botulinum toxin increase gait velocity? A systematic review and meta-analysis. Eur J Neurol 2010;17(12):1419–27.

27. Foley N, Pereira S, Salter K, et al. Treatment with botulinum toxin improves upper-extremity function post stroke: a systematic review and meta-analysis. Arch Phys Med Rehabil 2013;94(5):977–89.

28. Francisco GE, Yablon SA, Schiess MC, et al. Consensus panel guidelines for the use of intrathecal baclofen therapy in poststroke spastic hypertonia. Top Stroke Rehabil 2006;13(4):74–85.

29. Ivanhoe CB, Francisco GE, McGuire JR, et al. Intrathecal baclofen management of poststroke spastic hypertonia: implications for function and quality of life. Arch Phys Med Rehabil 2006;87:1509–15.

30. Francisco GE, Boake C. Improvement in walking speed in poststroke spastic hemiplegia after intrathecal baclofen therapy: a preliminary study. Arch Phys Med Rehabil 2003;84;1194–9.

31. Schiess MC, Oh IJ, Stimming EF, et al. Prospective 12-month study of intrathecal baclofen therapy for poststroke spastic upper and lower extremity motor control and functional improvement. Neuromodulation 2011;14:38–45.

32. Rousseaux M, Buisset N, Daveluy W, et al. Comparison of botulinum toxin injection and neurotomy in patients with distal lower limb spasticity. Eur J Neurol 2008;15:506–11.

33. Gump WC, Mutchnick IS, Moriarty TM. Selective dorsal rhizotomy for spasticity not associated with cerebral palsy: reconsideration of surgical inclusion criteria. Neurosurg Focus 2013;35(5):E6.

34. Fukuhara T, Kamata I. Selective posterior rhizotomy for painful spasticity in the lower limbs of hemiplegic patients after stroke: report of two cases. Neurosurgery 2004;54:1268–73.

35. Demetrios M, Khan F, Turner-Stokes L, et al. Multidisciplinary rehabilitation following botulinum toxin and other focal intramuscular treatment for post-stroke spasticity. Cochrane Database Syst Rev 2013;(6):CD009689.

36. Draulans N, Vermeersch K, Degraeuwe B, et al. Intrathecal baclofen in multiple sclerosis and spinal cord injury: complications and long-term dosage evolution. Clin Rehabil 2013;27(12):1137–43.

37. Naumann M, Boo LM, Ackerman AH, et al. Immunogenicity of botulinum toxins. J Neural Transm 2013;120(2):275–90.

38. Pandyan AD, Johnson GR, Price CIM, et al. A review of the properties and limitations of the Ashworth and Modified Ashworth Scales as measures of spasticity. Clin Rehabil 1999;13:373–83.

39. Tardieu G, Shentoub S, Delarue R. A la recherche d'une technique de mesure de la spasticite. Rev Neurol 1954;91:143–4.

40. Mehrholz J, Wagner K, Meißner D, et al. Reliability of the Modified Tardieu Scale and the Modified Ashworth Scale in adult patients with severe brain injury: a comparison study. Clin Rehabil 2005;19:751–9.

41. Li F, Wu Y, Xiong L. Reliability of a new scale for measurement of spasticity in stroke patients. J Rehabil Med 2014;46(8):746–53.

42. Penn RD, Savoy SM, Corcos D, et al. Intrathecal baclofen for severe spinal spasticity. N Engl J Med 1989;320:1517–21.

43. Snow BJ, Tsui JKC, Bhatt MH, et al. Treatment of spasticity with botulinum toxin: a double blind study. Ann Neurol 1990;28:512–5.

44. Farrar JT, Troxel AB, Stott C, et al. Validity, reliability, and clinical importance of change in a 0-10 numeric rating scale measure of spasticity: a post hoc analysis of a randomized, double-blind, placebo-controlled trial. Clin Ther 2008;30(5): 974–85.

45. Pisano F, Miscio G, Conte CD, et al. Quantitative measures of spasticity in poststroke patients. Clin Neurophysiol 2000;111:1015–22.

46. Bohannon RW, Harrison S, Kinsella-Shaw J. Reliability and validity of pendulum test measures of spasticity obtained with the Polhemus tracking system from patients with chronic stroke. J Neuroeng Rehabil 2009;6:30.

47. Bakheit AM, Maynard VA, Curnow J, et al. The relation between Ashworth scale scores and the excitability of the alpha motor neurones in patients with poststroke muscle spasticity. J Neurol Neurosurg Psychiatry 2003;74:646–8.

48. Calota A, Levin MF. Tonic stretch reflex threshold as a measure of spasticity: implications for clinical practice. Top Stroke Rehabil 2009;16(3):177–88.

49. Ward AB, Aquilar M, De Beyl Z, et al. Use of botulinum toxin type A in management of adult spasticity—a European consensus statement. J Rehabil Med 2003; 35:98–9.

Hemiplegic Shoulder Pain

Richard D. Wilson, MD*, John Chae, MD

KEYWORDS

- Stroke • Shoulder pain • Diagnosis • Treatment

KEY POINTS

- Hemiplegic shoulder pain (HSP): Shoulder pain is common after stroke, and it interferes with recovery and lowers quality of life. Multiple causes may contribute, with many experiencing multiple concurrent pathologies.
- Diagnosis: Careful history taking, musculoskeletal examination, and neurologic examinations must be performed. Imaging may aid in diagnosing some causes, although asymptomatic anatomic abnormalities may lead to misdiagnosis.
- Treatment: Conservative treatments should be attempted first, with emphasis on improving the biomechanics of the shoulder and function. Pain should be controlled with both non-pharmacologic and pharmacologic approaches. Some may benefit from more invasive treatments.

INTRODUCTION

The prevalence of HSP among stroke survivors is as high as 84%, although estimates vary depending on study methods.[1] Shoulder pain may develop early in the course of recovery, with an estimated prevalence of 17% in the first week, and remains elevated throughout recovery with 20% to 24% experiencing it from 1 to 16 months after stroke.[2,3] The prevalence in rehabilitation settings may be higher because this population has a greater number of associated risk factors for shoulder pain. Early diagnosis and appropriate treatment lead to resolution of symptoms in most patients; however, up to 32% of moderate to severely impaired stroke survivors have shoulder pain many years after their stroke.[4]

Shoulder pain after stroke is not limited to a single pathology, and many will be affected by more than one pathologic condition, creating a multifactorial pain syndrome.[5] The myriad of causes that have been reported includes impingement

The authors have the following disclosures: R.D. Wilson has received research funding from, and is a consultant to, SPR Therapeutics, LLC. J. Chae is a consultant and Chief Medical Advisor to SPR Therapeutics, LLC. Dr J. Chae also owns equity in SPR Therapeutics, LLC. SPR Therapeutics, LLC, has a commercial interest in the device presented in this article.
Physical Medicine and Rehabilitation, MetroHealth Medical Center, MetroHealth Rehabilitation Institute, Case Western Reserve University, 4229 Pearl Rd., Cleveland, OH 44109, USA
* Corresponding author.
E-mail address: rwilson@metrohealth.org

syndrome, rotator cuff dysfunction, tendinopathy, bursitis, adhesive capsulitis, peripheral nerve injuries, complex regional pain syndrome (CRPS), spasticity, central hypersensitivity, and contractures. Similarly, many different risk factors for shoulder pain have also been reported in the literature. The severity of motor impairment is one of the most frequently reported risk factors and also underlies other risks.[2,3,6–9] The literature has also identified the duration of motor impairment,[9] sensory impairment,[3,8] reduced range of motion,[8] spasticity,[10] central sensitization,[11] soft tissue injuries,[12] and comorbidities such as diabetes mellitus as increasing the risk of shoulder pain.[3,8] Shoulder pain is also common among those without neurologic injury, which makes it likely that stroke survivors may experience shoulder pain that is not related to their stroke.

PATIENT EVALUATION OVERVIEW

The approach to evaluation of a painful hemiplegic shoulder should begin with a history and physical examination, including neurologic examination of the central and peripheral nervous system of the upper limbs, active and passive range of motion, scapular motion, and careful palpation of potential anatomic structures that might generate pain. It is important to gather information from the patient or caregiver regarding prior injuries to the shoulder or premorbid symptoms that might have worsened. Salient features of the examination are described in the following sections relative to specific causes. HSP has neither a standard clinical definition nor a validated clinical examination. Providers need to be aware that many with HSP may have multiple underlying pathologies, may have noncontributory anatomic abnormalities, or may have overriding stroke-related symptoms that make precise diagnosis impossible. It may be helpful to consider the following systematic approach to integrating potential underlying pathologies in HSP: (1) impaired motor control, (2) soft tissue lesions, and (3) altered peripheral and central nervous activity (**Box 1**).[13]

Impaired Motor Control and Tone Changes

Glenohumeral subluxation

Glenohumeral subluxation has been reported to occur in up to 81% of stroke survivors.[14] Subluxation can be measured with the patient seated and the arm in a dependent position allowing the weight of the limb to distract the humeral head from the glenoid fossa.[10,14,15] Subluxation can be measured by the number of fingerbreadths between the acromion and humeral head, or by radiographs, computed tomography, ultrasonography, and MRI. The fingerbreadth measurement is adequate in clinical practice because the relationship between subluxation and pain remains controversial. Some studies show an association between subluxation and pain,[1,10] whereas others have demonstrated no association.[6,15,16] It is likely that subluxation predisposes the shoulder to other types of painful pathologies such as CRPS, peripheral neuropathies, and rotator cuff injury.[1,17,18]

Scapular dyskinesis

The impaired strength, unbalanced tone, and lack of control of the hemiplegic shoulder can disrupt the timed and coordinated movements known as scapulohumeral rhythm that can increase the risk for HSP.[19] Aberrant recruitment of the infraspinatus muscle, serratus anterior muscle, and inferior trapezius muscles that stabilize the scapula during humeral movement have been found in those with HSP compared with pain-free stroke survivors, and the aberrant patterns are similar to recruitment patterns seen in nonstroke impingement syndrome of the shoulder.[20] Evidence of impaired shoulder control can be detected with observation of scapular movement,

Box 1
Systemization of pathologies underlying HSP
Impaired motor control and tone changes
Flaccidity
Spasticity
Loss of motor function
Glenohumeral subluxation
Scapular dyskinesis
Spasticity of shoulder muscles
Soft tissue lesions
Impingement syndrome, rotator cuff tendinopathy
Bicipital tendinopathy
Adhesive capsulitis
Myofascial pain
Altered peripheral and central nervous activity
Peripheral nerve entrapment
Complex regional pain syndrome
Central poststroke pain
Central hypersensitivity
Adapted from Kalichman L, Ratmansky M. Underlying pathology and associated factors of hemiplegic shoulder pain. Am J Phys Med Rehabil 2011;90(9):776; with permission.

with comparison with the unaffected shoulder, during a clinical examination and characterized into specific patterns[21] (**Table 1**), although the reliability in stroke survivors is unknown. Further evidence for scapular dyskinesis can be detected with improvement in symptoms during range of motion with the scapular repositioning test[22] and the scapular assistance test.[23]

Table 1	
Classification of scapular dyskinesis	
Inferior angle (type I)	At rest: prominence of inferior medial scapular border During arm motion: dorsal tilt of inferior angle, ventral tilt of acromion Axis of the rotation: horizontal plane
Medial border (type II)	At rest: prominence of entire medial border During arm motion: dorsal tilt of medial scapular border Axis of rotation: vertical in the frontal plane
Superior border (type III)	At rest: elevation of superior border with possible anterior displacement During arm motion: shoulder shrug initiates movement without significant winging Axis of rotation: sagittal plane

Adapted from Kibler WB, Uhl TL, Maddux JW, et al. Qualitative clinical evaluation of scapular dysfunction: a reliability study. J Shoulder Elbow Surg 2002;11(6):551; with permission.

Spastic shoulder muscles

Upper motor neuron lesions can result in a movement disorder characterized by a velocity-dependent resistance to passive stretching known as spasticity. The spasticity affects not only muscles at the shoulder but also the scapular stabilizers. The typical pattern of spasticity of the upper limb after stroke is internal rotation and adduction of the shoulder with flexion at the elbow, the wrist, and the fingers.[24,25] The result is impairment in active and passive movement to varying degrees and impaired control of shoulder motion that can cause injury. The adducted humerus coupled with an increase in tone in the trapezius and rhomboids that impairs scapular elevation increases the risk of shoulder impingement and can lead to pain. Constant pull of adductors can also increase the strain of muscles on their attachment sites to bone, also causing pain.[26] It is common for spasticity to lead to contractures of the shoulder that can be associated with pain during movement, although the pain might also be due to spasticity resulting from stretch.[26]

Clinical evaluation of spasticity can be performed with the use of a descriptive scale. The Modified Ashworth Scale is frequently used and qualitatively describes the increase in resistance encountered during passive stretch.[27] The Modified Ashworth Scale is an efficient, reliable, and simple measurement scale, although it has the downside of not ascribing a reason for any increase in resistance around a joint. For example, the scale does not discern between spasticity and other causes of increased resistance to passive stretch, such as contractures and rigidity.

Soft Tissue Lesions

The evaluation of a patient with shoulder pain should include provocative maneuvers in addition to a standard physical examination that includes range of motion and neurologic evaluation of the upper limb[28–30] (**Table 2**). Many causes of shoulder pain overlap, and imaging or other diagnostic studies may be beneficial.

Impingement syndrome and rotator cuff injury

Impingement syndrome is often thought of as an injury to the supraspinatus muscle or tendon resulting from repetitive compression between the inferior border of the

---

Table 2
Examination for soft tissue lesions in HSP

	Impingement Syndrome/Rotator Cuff Tendinopathy	Bicipital Tendinopathy	Adhesive Capsulitis	Myofascial Pain
Examination	Positive result of abduction test Positive result of drop arm test Presence of Neer sign Positive result of Hawkin test	Positive result of Yergason test Positive result of Speed test	External rotation <15° Early scapular motion	Palpation of shoulder and scapular muscles
Diagnostic test	Subacromial lidocaine injection MRI Ultrasonography	Tendon sheath injection of lidocaine	MRI Arthrogram	None

Adapted from Black-Schaffer RM, Kirsteins AE, Harvey RL. Stroke rehabilitation. 2. Co-morbidities and complications. Arch Phys Med Rehabil 1999;80(5 Suppl 1):S14; with permission.

acromion and the greater tuberosity of the humerus, although it encompasses many injuries of the shoulder including rotator cuff tendinopathy, rotator cuff tears, and bursitis. Although not extensively studied as a cause for HSP, one cross-sectional study has found that half of those with chronic HSP have evidence of impingement syndrome.[16] Biomechanical changes after stroke such as laxity of passive restraints due to subluxation, weakness of muscles that stabilize the joint, abnormal muscle tone, and motor recovery in a proximal to distal gradient may place stroke survivors at greater risk for impingement syndrome and rotator cuff injury.

Imaging studies may be particularly helpful in identifying anatomic abnormality of the shoulder in those with HSP, although the presence of a tear or a tendinopathy is not related to the severity of pain.[31] Recent MRI studies comparing those with shoulder pain with a pain-free group did not find differences in the prevalence of rotator cuff pathology or subacromial bursitis.[32,33] Impingement syndrome and rotator cuff injuries may be common in those with stroke because they are common in the general population and the incidence increases with age.[34] The high prevalence of rotator cuff pathology in asymptomatic patients increases the risk of misdiagnosis in those with shoulder pain after stroke.[34]

Bicipital tendinopathy
The prevalence of bicipital tendinopathy in those with HSP is estimated between 7% and 54%.[31,35] Bicipital tendinopathy is more likely in those with spasticity or movement synergies that result in greater activation of the biceps as an elbow flexor or a forearm supinator. The diagnosis is suggested when there is greater tenderness to palpation of the long head of the biceps at the anterior shoulder compared with the unaffected side.[36] Provocative maneuvers, such as Yergason test that provokes pain at the anterior shoulder with resisted forearm supination, can be useful when the patient is able to participate. Imaging may also identify abnormalities of the long head of the biceps, although the findings may not correlate with pain in the acute phase of recovery in spite of the prevalence approaching 40%.[12] Injection of an anesthetic agent at the point that is most painful over the bicipital groove can also provide evidence of the diagnosis if resulting in pain relief.

Adhesive capsulitis
Adhesive capsulitis is characterized by shoulder pain with gradual loss of range of motion because of shortening and thickening of the glenohumeral joint capsule along with adhesions of the capsule.[37] In addition to shoulder pain with range of motion testing, the primary physical finding is a reduction in external rotation. Unfortunately, pain and reduced range of motion are also found with other pathologies in those with HSP, such as pain with spasticity. The prevalence of thickening and synovial membrane contrast enhancement on MRI is higher in those with HSP than in pain-free controls[32,33]; however, adhesive changes have been found in over 30% of stroke survivors in the contralateral shoulders when evaluated with arthography.[38]

Myofascial pain
Myofascial pain is commonly associated with shoulder pain in those with HSP[11] and nonstroke shoulder pain.[39] Precipitating factors of myofascial pain, such as trauma, poor posture, muscle imbalance, degenerative changes, and stress, are common in those with stroke.[29] Myofascial pain may be secondary to another condition, but the muscles may be pain generators contributing to the overall condition. Typical findings are hyperalgesic muscles around the shoulder, neck, and scapular stabilizers that exhibit taught bands, tender points, and trigger points that may result in referred pain.

Altered Peripheral and Central Nervous Activity

Peripheral nerve entrapment

Brachial plexus injury and other peripheral nerve injuries in HSP are difficult to diagnose because of the overlap with prominent symptoms due to the central nervous system (CNS) damage from the stroke, as well as because of limitations of electrodiagnostic studies in diagnosing proximal lesions. It has been hypothesized that injury to peripheral nerves may occur because of traction caused by inferior subluxation,[18] trauma incurred as a result of hemiplegia,[17,18] or trauma incurred through incorrect transfers.[40] To date, electrophysiologic studies have been mixed in support of peripheral nerve injury as the cause of HSP, although it should be considered if a mechanism for injury is present or with findings of lower motor neuron injury in the setting of shoulder subluxation.

Complex regional pain syndrome

CRPS after stroke generally refers to CRPS type I because it follows CNS injury rather than damage to a peripheral nerve.[41] The prevalence of CRPS type I in hemiplegia ranges from 12.5%[42] to 70%,[43] reflecting differences in study design and inclusion of study cohorts before routine treatment in rehabilitation centers. Risk factors for CRPS type I include motor impairment[44] and trauma related to altered shoulder biomechanics.[45] Other risk factors might exist and are not yet known because the pathophysiology of CRPS type I has not yet been elucidated.[46] The diagnosis of CRPS type I is based on clinical examination and can be aided by standardized criteria (**Box 2**).[47]

Box 2
Clinical diagnostic criteria for CRPS

1. Continuing pain, which is disproportionate to any inciting event

2. Must report at least 1 symptom in 3 of the 4 following categories:

   - Sensory: Reports of hyperalgesia and/or allodynia

   - Vasomotor: Reports of temperature asymmetry, skin color changes, and/or skin color asymmetry

   - Sudomotor/edema: Reports of edema, sweating changes, and/or sweating asymmetry

   - Motor/trophic: Reports of decreased range of motion, motor dysfunction (weakness, tremor, dystonia), and/or trophic changes (hair, nail, skin)

3. Must display at least 1 sign[a] at the time of evaluation in 2 or more of the following categories:

   - Sensory: Evidence of hyperalgesia (to pinprick) and/or allodynia (to light touch, deep somatic pressure, and/or joint movement).

   - Vasomotor: Evidence of temperature asymmetry, skin color changes, and/or asymmetry

   - Sudomotor/edema: Evidence of edema, sweating changes, and/or sweating asymmetry

   - Motor/trophic: Evidence of decreased range of motion, motor dysfunction (weakness, tremor, dystonia), and/or trophic changes (hair, nail, skin)

4. There is no other diagnosis that better explains the signs and symptoms

[a]A sign is counted only if it is observed at the time of diagnosis.
From Harden RN, Oaklander AL, Burton AW, et al. Complex regional pain syndrome: practical diagnostic and treatment guidelines, 4th edition. Pain Med 2013;14(2):184; with permission.

Triple-phase bone scan has been recommended as an adjunct diagnostic tool,[48] although the highest sensitivity may be during the acute phase of CRPS type I.

Central poststroke pain

Formerly known as thalamic pain syndrome, central poststroke pain (CPSP) is a neuropathic pain syndrome that can arise from a stroke within the spinothalamocortical pathway,[49] and most with CPSP have multiple lesions on MRI.[50] The pain may be due to the lesion, although it might also be caused by neuroplasticity that occurs after the stroke.[51] Typically the pain arises gradually, within the first month after stroke, although it may arise many months later.[52] If pain arises more than 12 months after stroke, it might be reasonable to look for a new cause, including a new stroke. The clinical presentation of CPSP can be variable, including multiple sensations within a single individual, making diagnosis difficult. An algorithm to improve the diagnosis has been proposed[53] (**Box 3**), although standard diagnostic criteria for CPSP have not been established.

Central hypersensitivity

There is evidence that alterations in pain perception because of amplifications of neural signaling within the CNS that increases pain sensation,[54] termed central hypersensitivity, contributes to HSP.[8,55] An initial injury may result in tissue damage and acute pain, but maladaptive changes in the brain and spinal cord may allow the pain to persist or worsen beyond the initial injury, even after the initial injury has healed.[56] Central hypersensitivity is characterized by a reduction in pain thresholds, an exaggerated response to noxious stimuli, pain after the end of a stimulus, and a spread of sensitivity to normal tissue.[54] There is no diagnostic test or established criteria for diagnosis. Central hypersensitivity should be considered when a patient exhibits allodynia or hyperalgesia, spread of pain sensitivity to uninvolved areas, alterations of sensation after a stimulus, and the maintenance of pain by stimuli that do not typically evoke any ongoing pain.

Box 3
Diagnostic criteria for CPSP

Mandatory criteria

Pain within an area of the body corresponding to the lesion of the CNS

History suggestive of a stroke and onset of pain at or after stroke onset

Confirmation of a CNS lesion by imaging or negative or positive sensory signs confined to the area of the body corresponding to the lesion

Other causes of pain, such as nociceptive or peripheral neuropathic pain, are excluded or considered highly unlikely

Supportive criteria

No primary relation to movement, inflammation, or other local tissue damage

Descriptors such as burning, painful cold, electric shocks, aching, pressing, stinging, and pins and needles, although all pain descriptors can apply

Allodynia or dysesthesia to touch or cold

From Klit H, Finnerup NB, Jensen TS. Central post-stroke pain: clinical characteristics, pathophysiology, and management. Lancet Neurol 2009;8(9):860; with permission.

TREATMENT OPTIONS
All Causes

Prevention

That HSP is most associated with severity of hemiplegia leads many to think that the weakness in the flaccid stage increases the risk of injury due to malpositioning and improper handling by health care providers[57] and caregivers[6] alike; however, there is little evidence to support specific positioning or handling of the hemiparetic upper limb to prevent the development or worsening of HSP.[58] It is recommended that the patient, caregivers, and providers who work with stroke survivors be educated on proper handling and positioning of the arm to prevent injury.[59,60] A common recommendation on positioning includes protracted shoulder, arm forward, neutral to slightly supinated wrist, and extended fingers.[61] Positions need to change with alterations of posture, activity, and position, and also need to be tailored for individual comfort.

Straps or slings

It is recommended to consider the use of straps or slings to prevent trauma or subluxation,[59,60] although randomized controlled trials (RCTs) of glenohumeral strapping and slings have shown mixed results.[62,63] It is likely that some will benefit from straps or slings, and their use should be encouraged on an individual basis if benefit can be demonstrated.

Exercise

Supervised exercise therapy is a cornerstone of stroke rehabilitation as well as in the prevention and treatment of HSP. Passive range of motion should be started early to reduce soft tissue contractures and complications related to immobility. In particular, external rotation has been shown to be efficacious in maintaining range of motion and preventing harmful positions.[64] Aggressive range of motion programs, and the use of overhead pulleys, should be avoided because of the risk of injury.[65] Active training should be used as it is able to improve biomechanics to reduce the risk of injury, although moderate intensity is encouraged because high-intensity programs can increase the risk of injury.[66]

Specific Causes

Spasticity

In addition to stretching, pharmacologic modalities may be necessary to reduce spasticity at the shoulder that might contribute to pain, although no controlled trials have demonstrated efficacy in reducing shoulder pain. Thermoplastic splints are often used to reduce contracture associated with spasticity, although they may not reduce contracture, spasticity, or pain.[67] There is limited evidence that botulinum toxin is efficacious in reducing HSP in those with spastic hemiplegia,[68] although there is no consensus on which muscles to target or what is the appropriate dose.[69] An algorithm for the approach to pharmacologic management of spasticity that is based on the extent of bodily involvement has been proposed[70] (**Table 3**).

Soft tissue lesions

Therapeutic exercise is the first-line treatment of soft tissue lesions. Oral analgesics may be necessary to reduce discomfort during exercise and at rest. Typical recommendations for oral analgesics apply to stroke survivors with HSP with the exception of more judicious use of nonsteroidal antiinflammatory medications because of risks associated with coadministration with aspirin and the potential to increase the risk of heart attack and stroke.[71]

Table 3
Pharmacologic management of spasticity

Focal	Multifocal	Regional	Generalized
Botulinum toxins	Botulinum toxins	Intrathecal therapy	Intrathecal therapy
Phenol/alcohol neurolysis	Phenol/alcohol neurolysis	Botulinum toxins	Oral medications
	Oral medications	Phenol/alcohol neurolysis	Botulinum toxins[a]
			Phenol/alcohol neurolysis[a]

[a] If focal problem in addition to generalized.

Adapted from Francisco GE, McGuire JR. Poststroke spasticity management. Stroke 2012;43(11):3134; with permission.

Subacromial corticosteroid injections may be helpful in those who are likely affected by impingement syndrome or rotator cuff tendinopathy.[72,73] A peritendinous corticosteroid injection is also recommended for those who have a tendinopathy of the long-head biceps[74(p446)], although it has not been studied in a controlled trial. A corticosteroid injection at the glenohumeral joint for those with adhesive capsulitis also seems to improve symptoms as much as physical therapy,[75] and the combination may provide faster relief than physical therapy alone.[76]

The primary approach to treating isolated myofascial pain, or that co-occurring with another shoulder pathology, is with physical modalities and often supplemented with needling, myofascial release, ischemic compression, laser therapy, and multimodal treatment.[77] The treatments are not well studied in stroke, and reviews of needling[78] and myofascial release,[79] in particular, have not found support in systematic reviews of varying pain syndromes.

Complex regional pain syndrome
There are no definitive treatments for CRPS, although multiple potential treatments have been proposed. The general approach to treatment of CRPS includes reducing edema, treating pain, maintaining joint motion and strength, and functional restoration.[45,80,81] In the absence of a better understanding of the cause of CRPS, and based on the fact that multiple causes may contribute, it has been proposed to choose specific interventions based on prominent symptoms,[46] although this approach has not been evaluated in a clinical trial (**Box 4**).

Central poststroke pain
The treatment of CPSP is typically through pharmacologic means. Two oral medications have been shown to have positive effects in RCTs that included subjects with CPSP. The tricyclic antidepressant amitriptyline, 75 mg/d, significantly reduced pain, although side effects such as fatigue and dry mouth were common.[82] The antiepileptic lamotrigine in doses up to 200 mg/d significantly reduced pain, although with frequent side effects.[83] The efficacy of pregabalin has been mixed in 2 RCTs.[84,85] The use of multidrug regimens has not been studied, although it has been advocated if a single-drug regimen is not effective.[86]

Central hypersensitivity
The contribution of central hypersensitivity in those with HSP is now recognized, although methods for measuring and diagnosing central hypersensitivity are still being developed. Thus, there are no established methods for treating central hypersensitivity. Until more is known about the cause of central hypersensitivity, it is likely that a multimodal treatment approach is best, possibly with alteration based on chronicity and distribution of complaints.[87] Those with more recent and focal complaints at

---

Box 4
Interventions for the treatment of CRPS

Symptoms: sweating, trophic changes, coldness

Sympathetic nerve block at stellate ganglion

Mobilization, strengthening, desensitization, and functional restoration

Symptoms: hyperesthesia, hyperalgesia, allodynia

Desensitization

Antiepileptic medications (gabapentin, carbamazepine)

Heterocyclic antidepressants

NMDA receptor antagonists

Symptoms: impaired tactile discrimination, referred sensation, dystonia

Edema control, mobilization, strengthening

Mirror therapy

Mental imagery

Symptoms: warmth, erythema, edema, pain

Oral corticosteroids

Nonsteroidal antiInflammatory drugs

Others potential interventions

Bisphosphonates

Biofeedback

Abbreviation: NMDA, N-methyl-D-aspartate.
  Data from Chae J. Poststroke complex regional pain syndrome. Top Stroke Rehabil 2010;17(3):151–62.

---

the shoulder may benefit from shoulder joint mobilization manual therapy and specific exercises to improve the shoulder complaint. If the pain is chronic, or affects a larger regional or diffuse area of the body, then it is likely more appropriate to use a physical and cognitive approach to treatment by education focused on functional movements combined with attempts to address myofascial pain along with incorporation of global exercises. Pharmaceutical analgesics may also enhance the multimodal treatment, although they have not been studied.

Emerging Treatment Options

Suprascapular nerve block

The suprascapular nerve is a mixed nerve that innervates the infraspinatus and supraspinatus muscles, large portions of the capsule and ligaments in the shoulder joint, and sympathetic fibers. It has been found to be safe and efficacious in nonstroke shoulder conditions[88] and is now being studied for HSP. A RCT compared suprascapular nerve block of a corticosteroid and a local anesthetic with placebo for subjects with HSP of up to 12 months duration and found a statistically greater reduction in pain for at least 12 weeks after the intervention.[89]

Percutaneous peripheral nerve stimulation

Stimulation of peripheral nerves of the shoulder by wire electrodes placed through the skin and into the underlying muscle of the affected shoulder is safe and has shown promise in providing long-term relief for subjects with chronic HSP with a short-term stimulation paradigm of 3 to 6 weeks. A RCT showed that a treatment that stimulated the trapezius, supraspinatus, middle deltoid, and posterior deltoid muscles for 6 h/d for 6 weeks provided greater pain reduction for at least 12 months when compared with the use of a hemisling.[90] A simpler approach of a single-wire electrode stimulating the axillary nerve to produce contraction of the middle and posterior deltoid muscles for 6 h/d for 3 weeks was compared with physical therapy in an RCT.[91] Peripheral nerve stimulation produced greater pain reduction than physical therapy for at least 12 weeks.

SUMMARY/DISCUSSION

Health care providers who treat stroke survivors need to be knowledgeable about pathologic conditions of the shoulder, proper evaluation, and available treatments. Diagnosis of the cause of HSP can be challenging to providers because of the overlap of signs and symptoms of different pathologies and because of the frequency at which multiple pathologies coexist. Treatments should be chosen based on symptoms and likelihood of underlying pathologies. Emerging treatments of HSP show promise in providing pain relief.

REFERENCES

1. Najenson T, Yacubovich E, Pikielni SS. Rotator cuff injury in shoulder joints of hemiplegic patients. Scand J Rehabil Med 1971;3:131–7.
2. Lindgren I, Jonsson AC, Norrving B, et al. Shoulder pain after stroke: a prospective population-based study. Stroke 2007;38(2):343–8.
3. Ratnasabapathy Y, Broad J, Baskett J, et al. Shoulder pain in people with a stroke: a population-based study. Clin Rehabil 2003;17:304–11.
4. Broeks JG, Lankhorst GJ, Rumping K, et al. The long-term outcome of arm function after stroke: results of a follow-up study. Disabil Rehabil 1999;21(8):357–64.
5. Lo SF, Chen SY, Lin HC, et al. Arthrographic and clinical findings in patients with hemiplegic shoulder pain. Arch Phys Med Rehabil 2003;84(12):1786–91.
6. Wanklyn P, Forster A, Young J. Hemiplegic shoulder pain (HSP): natural history and investigation of associated features. Disabil Rehabil 1996;18(10):497–501.
7. Gamble GE, Barberan E, Laasch HU, et al. Poststroke shoulder pain: a prospective study of the association and risk factors in 152 patients from a consecutive cohort of 205 patients presenting with stroke. Eur J Pain 2002;6(6):467–74.
8. Roosink M, Renzenbrink GJ, Buitenweg JR, et al. Persistent shoulder pain in the first 6 months after stroke: results of a prospective cohort study. Arch Phys Med Rehabil 2011;92(7):1139–45.
9. Karaahmet OZ, Eksioglu E, Gurcay E, et al. Hemiplegic shoulder pain: associated factors and rehabilitation outcomes of hemiplegic patients with and without shoulder pain. Top Stroke Rehabil 2014;21(3):237–45.
10. VanOuwenaller C, Laplace PM, Chantraine A. Painful shoulder in hemiplegia. Arch Phys Med Rehabil 1986;67:23–6.
11. Soo Hoo J, Paul T, Chae J, et al. Central hypersensitivity in chronic hemiplegic shoulder pain. Am J Phys Med Rehabil 2013;92(1):1–9 [quiz: 10–3].
12. Pong YP, Wang LY, Huang YC, et al. Sonography and physical findings in stroke patients with hemiplegic shoulders: a longitudinal study. J Rehabil Med 2012; 44(7):553–7.
13. Kalichman L, Ratmansky M. Underlying pathology and associated factors of hemiplegic shoulder pain. Am J Phys Med Rehabil 2011;90(9):768–80.

14. Najenson T, Pikielny SS. Malalignment of the gleno-humeral joint following hemiplegia. A review of 500 cases. Ann Phys Med 1965;8:96–9.
15. Zorowitz RD, Hughes MB, Idank D, et al. Shoulder pain and subluxation after stroke: correlation or coincidence. Am J Occup Ther 1996;50(3):194–201.
16. Joynt RL. The source of shoulder pain in hemiplegia. Arch Phys Med Rehabil 1992;73(5):409–13.
17. Chino N. Electrophysiological investigation on shoulder subluxation in hemiplegics. Scand J Rehabil Med 1981;13:17–21.
18. Ring H, Leillen B, Server S, et al. Temporal changes in electrophysiological, clinical and radiological parameters in the hemiplegic's shoulder. Scand J Rehabil Med Suppl 1985;12:124–7.
19. Niessen M, Janssen T, Meskers C, et al. Kinematics of the contralateral and ipsilateral shoulder: a possible relationship with post-stroke shoulder pain. J Rehabil Med 2008;40(6):482–6.
20. De Baets L, Jaspers E, Janssens L, et al. Characteristics of neuromuscular control of the scapula after stroke: a first exploration. Front Hum Neurosci 2014;8:933.
21. Kibler WB, Uhl TL, Maddux JW, et al. Qualitative clinical evaluation of scapular dysfunction: a reliability study. J Shoulder Elbow Surg 2002;11(6):550–6.
22. Tate AR, McClure PW, Kareha S, et al. Effect of the scapula reposition test on shoulder impingement symptoms and elevation strength in overhead athletes. J Orthop Sports Phys Ther 2008;38(1):4–11.
23. Rabin A, Irrgang JJ, Fitzgerald GK, et al. The intertester reliability of the scapular assistance test. J Orthop Sports Phys Ther 2006;36(9):653–60.
24. Hefter H, Jost WH, Reissig A, et al. Classification of posture in poststroke upper limb spasticity: a potential decision tool for botulinum toxin A treatment? Int J Rehabil Res 2012;35(3):227–33.
25. Marciniak C. Poststroke hypertonicity: upper limb assessment and treatment. Top Stroke Rehabil 2011;18(3):179–94.
26. Braun RM, West F, Mooney V, et al. Surgical treatment of the painful shoulder contracture in the stroke patient. J Bone Joint Surg Am 1971;53(7):1307–12.
27. Bohannon RW, Smith MB. Interrater reliability of a modified Ashworth scale of muscle spasticity. Phys Ther 1987;67(2):206–7.
28. Black-Schaffer RM, Kirsteins AE, Harvey RL. Stroke rehabilitation. 2. Comorbidities and complications. Arch Phys Med Rehabil 1999;80(5 Suppl 1): S8–16.
29. Yap EC. Myofascial pain–an overview. Ann Acad Med Singapore 2007;36(1):43–8.
30. Vasudevan JM, Browne BJ. Hemiplegic shoulder pain: an approach to diagnosis and management. Phys Med Rehabil Clin N Am 2014;25(2):411–37.
31. Shah R, Haghpanah S, Elovic E, et al. MRI findings in Painful Post-stroke Shoulder. Stroke 2008;39:1803–13.
32. Tavora DG, Gama RL, Bomfim RC, et al. MRI findings in the painful hemiplegic shoulder. Clin Radiol 2010;65(10):789–94.
33. Pompa A, Clemenzi A, Troisi E, et al. Enhanced-MRI and ultrasound evaluation of painful shoulder in patients after stroke: a pilot study. Eur Neurol 2011;66(3): 175–81.
34. Reilly P, Macleod I, Macfarlane R, et al. Dead men and radiologists don't lie: a review of cadaveric and radiological studies of rotator cuff tear prevalence. Ann R Coll Surg Engl 2006;88(2):116–21.
35. Dromerick AW, Edwards DF, Kumar A. Hemiplegic shoulder pain syndrome: frequency and characteristics during inpatient stroke rehabilitation. Arch Phys Med Rehabil 2008;89(8):1589–93.

36. Patton WC, McCluskey GM 3rd. Biceps tendinitis and subluxation. Clin Sports Med 2001;20(3):505–29.
37. Neviaser JS. Adhesive capsulitis of the shoulder. Med Times 1962;90:783.
38. Hakuno A, Sashika H, Ohkawa T, et al. Arthrographic findings in hemiplegic shoulders. Arch Phys Med Rehabil 1984;65(11):706–11.
39. Paul TM, Soo Hoo J, Chae J, et al. Central hypersensitivity in patients with subacromial impingement syndrome. Arch Phys Med Rehabil 2012;93(12):2206–9.
40. Moskowitz E, Porter JI. Peripheral nerve lesions in the upper extremity in hemiplegic patients. N Engl J Med 1963;269:776–8.
41. Stanton-Hicks M, Janig W, Hassenbusch S, et al. Reflex sympathetic dystrophy: changing concepts and taxonomy. Pain 1995;63(1):127–33.
42. Davis SW, Petrillo CR, Eichberg RD, et al. Shoulder-hand syndrome in a hemiplegic population: a 5-year retrospective study. Arch Phys Med Rehabil 1977;58: 353–6.
43. Perrigot M, Bussel B, Pierrot DE. L'epaule de l'hemiplegique. Ann Med Phys 1975;18:176–87.
44. Daviet JC, Preux PM, Salle JY, et al. Clinical factors in the prognosis of complex regional pain syndrome type I after stroke: a prospective study. Am J Phys Med Rehabil 2002;81(1):34–9.
45. Geurts AC, Visschers BA, van Limbeek J, et al. Systematic review of aetiology and treatment of post-stroke hand oedema and shoulder-hand syndrome. Scand J Rehabil Med 2000;32(1):4–10.
46. Chae J. Poststroke complex regional pain syndrome. Top stroke Rehabil 2010; 17(3):151–62.
47. Harden RN, Oaklander AL, Burton AW, et al. Complex regional pain syndrome: practical diagnostic and treatment guidelines, 4th edition. Pain Med 2013; 14(2):180–229.
48. Petchkrua W, Weiss DJ, Patel RR. Reassessment of the Incidence of complex regional pain syndrome type 1 following stroke. Neurorehabil Neural Repair 2000;14(1):59–63.
49. Hong JH, Bai DS, Jeong JY, et al. Injury of the spino-thalamo-cortical pathway is necessary for central post-stroke pain. Eur Neurol 2010;64(3):163–8.
50. Bowsher D, Leijon G, Thuomas KA. Central poststroke pain: correlation of MRI with clinical pain characteristics and sensory abnormalities. Neurology 1998; 51(5):1352–8.
51. Anderson WS, O'Hara S, Lawson HC, et al. Plasticity of pain-related neuronal activity in the human thalamus. Prog Brain Res 2006;157:353–64.
52. Andersen G, Vestergaard K, Ingeman-Nielsen M, et al. Incidence of central post-stroke pain. Pain 1995;61(2):187–93.
53. Klit H, Finnerup NB, Jensen TS. Central post-stroke pain: clinical characteristics, pathophysiology, and management. Lancet Neurol 2009;8(9):857–68.
54. Woolf CJ. Central sensitization: implications for the diagnosis and treatment of pain. Pain 2011;152(3 Suppl):S2–15.
55. Roosink M, Buitenweg JR, Renzenbrink GJ, et al. Altered cortical somatosensory processing in chronic stroke: a relationship with post-stroke shoulder pain. NeuroRehabilitation 2011;28(4):331–44.
56. Latremoliere A, Woolf CJ. Central sensitization: a generator of pain hypersensitivity by central neural plasticity. J Pain 2009;10(9):895–926.
57. Ring H, Feder M, Berchadsky R, et al. Prevalence of pain and malalignment in the hemiplegic's shoulder at admission for rehabilitation: a preventive approach. Eur J Phys Med Rehabil 1993;3:199–203.

58. Teasell RW, Foley NC, Bhogal SK, et al. An evidence-based review of stroke rehabilitation. Top Stroke Rehabil 2003;10(1):29–58.

59. Bates B, Choi JY, Duncan PW, et al. Veterans affairs/department of defense clinical practice guideline for the management of adult stroke rehabilitation care: executive summary. Stroke 2005;36(9):2049–56.

60. Duncan PW, Zorowitz R, Bates B, et al. Management of adult stroke rehabilitation care: a clinical practice guideline. Stroke 2005;36(9):e100–43.

61. Carr EK, Kenney FD. Positioning of the stroke patient: a review of the literature. Int J Nurs Stud 1992;29(4):355–69.

62. Griffin A, Bernhardt J. Strapping the hemiplegic shoulder prevents development of pain during rehabilitation: a randomized controlled trial. Clin Rehabil 2006; 20(4):287–95.

63. Hanger HC, Whitewood P, Brown G, et al. A randomized controlled trial of strapping to prevent post-stroke shoulder pain. Clin Rehabil 2000;14(4): 370–80.

64. Veerbeek JM, van Wegen E, van Peppen R, et al. What is the evidence for physical therapy poststroke? A systematic review and meta-analysis. PLoS One 2014; 9(2):e87987.

65. Kumar R, Metter EJ, Mehta AJ, et al. Shoulder pain in hemiplegia. The role of exercise. Am J Phys Med Rehabil 1990;69(4):205–8.

66. Lynch D, Ferraro M, Krol J, et al. Continuous passive motion improves shoulder joint integrity following stroke. Clin Rehabil 2005;19(6):594–9.

67. Tyson SF, Kent RM. The effect of upper limb orthotics after stroke: a systematic review. NeuroRehabilitation 2011;28(1):29–36.

68. Singh JA, Fitzgerald PM. Botulinum toxin for shoulder pain: a Cochrane systematic review. J Rheumatol 2011;38(3):409–18.

69. Viana R, Pereira S, Mehta S, et al. Evidence for therapeutic interventions for hemiplegic shoulder pain during the chronic stage of stroke: a review. Top stroke Rehabil 2012;19(6):514–22.

70. Francisco GE, McGuire JR. Poststroke spasticity management. Stroke 2012; 43(11):3132–6.

71. Antman EM, Bennett JS, Daugherty A, et al. Use of nonsteroidal antiinflammatory drugs: an update for clinicians: a scientific statement from the American Heart Association. Circulation 2007;115(12):1634–42.

72. Rah UW, Yoon SH, Moon do J, et al. Subacromial corticosteroid injection on poststroke hemiplegic shoulder pain: a randomized, triple-blind, placebo-controlled trial. Arch Phys Med Rehabil 2012;93(6):949–56.

73. Lakse E, Gunduz B, Erhan B, et al. The effect of local injections in hemiplegic shoulder pain: a prospective, randomized, controlled study. Am J Phys Med Rehabil 2009;88(10):805–11 [quiz: 12–4, 51].

74. Stein J, Harvey RL, Winstein CJ, et al. Stroke recovery and rehabilitation. 2nd edition. New York: Demos Medical; 2014.

75. Arslan S, Celiker R. Comparison of the efficacy of local corticosteroid injection and physical therapy for the treatment of adhesive capsulitis. Rheumatol Int 2001;21(1):20–3.

76. Carette S, Moffet H, Tardif J, et al. Intraarticular corticosteroids, supervised physiotherapy, or a combination of the two in the treatment of adhesive capsulitis of the shoulder: a placebo-controlled trial. Arthritis Rheum 2003;48(3): 829–38.

77. Sergienko S, Kalichman L. Myofascial origin of shoulder pain: a literature review. J Bodyw Mov Ther 2015;19(1):91–101.

78. Tough EA, White AR, Cummings TM, et al. Acupuncture and dry needling in the management of myofascial trigger point pain: a systematic review and meta-analysis of randomised controlled trials. Eur J Pain 2009;13(1):3–10.
79. Ajimsha MS, Al-Mudahka NR, Al-Madzhar JA. Effectiveness of myofascial release: systematic review of randomized controlled trials. J Bodyw Mov Ther 2015;19(1):102–12.
80. Ribbers GM, Geurts AC, Stam HJ, et al. Pharmacologic treatment of complex regional pain syndrome I: a conceptual framework. Arch Phys Med Rehabil 2003;84(1):141–6.
81. Pertoldi S, Di Benedetto P. Shoulder-hand syndrome after stroke. A complex regional pain syndrome. Europa medicophysica 2005;41(4):283–92.
82. Leijon G, Boivie J. Central post-stroke pain–a controlled trial of amitriptyline and carbamazepine. Pain 1989;36(1):27–36.
83. Vestergaard K, Andersen G, Gottrup H, et al. Lamotrigine for central poststroke pain: a randomized controlled trial. Neurology 2001;56(2):184–90.
84. Kim JS, Bashford G, Murphy TK, et al. Safety and efficacy of pregabalin in patients with central post-stroke pain. Pain 2011;152(5):1018–23.
85. Vranken JH, Dijkgraaf MG, Kruis MR, et al. Pregabalin in patients with central neuropathic pain: a randomized, double-blind, placebo-controlled trial of a flexible-dose regimen. Pain 2008;136(1–2):150–7.
86. Kim JS. Pharmacological management of central post-stroke pain: a practical guide. CNS drugs 2014;28(9):787–97.
87. Isabel de-la-Llave-Rincon A, Puentedura EJ, Fernandez-de-Las-Penas C. Clinical presentation and manual therapy for upper quadrant musculoskeletal conditions. J Man Manip Ther 2011;19(4):201–11.
88. Shanahan EM, Shanahan KR, Hill CL, et al. Safety and acceptability of suprascapular nerve block in rheumatology patients. Clin Rheumatol 2012;31(1): 145–9.
89. Adey-Wakeling Z, Crotty M, Shanahan EM. Suprascapular nerve block for shoulder pain in the first year after stroke: a randomized controlled trial. Stroke 2013; 44(11):3136–41.
90. Chae J, Yu DT, Walker ME, et al. Intramuscular electrical stimulation for hemiplegic shoulder pain: a 12-month follow-up of a multiple-center, randomized clinical trial. Am J Phys Med Rehabil 2005;84(11):832–42.
91. Wilson RD, Gunzler DD, Bennett ME, et al. Peripheral nerve stimulation compared with usual care for pain relief of hemiplegic shoulder pain: a randomized controlled trial. Am J Phys Med Rehabil 2014;93(1):17–28.

Poststroke Communication Disorders and Dysphagia

Marlís González-Fernández, MD, PhD*, Martin B. Brodsky, PhD, ScM, CCC-SLP, Jeffrey B. Palmer, MD

KEYWORDS

- Communication disorders • Dysphagia • Aphasia • Stroke • Deglutition disorders

KEY POINTS

- Communication and swallowing disorders are very common after stroke.
- Evaluation of communication disorders after stroke requires formal testing of each area of language for accurate diagnosis.
- Swallowing disorders improve for most stroke patients but chronic deficits occur.
- Treatment of swallowing disorders after stroke should focus on the underlying impairment while maintaining the least restrictive diet.

Stroke can significantly affect a person's ability to communicate and swallow effectively. In many cultures, people interact by conversing during meals. When the ability to express oneself and/or understand others is affected, rehabilitation of other impairments becomes more challenging. The overall goals of rehabilitation for impaired swallowing and communication and swallowing deficits may differ based on the specific deficits caused by the stroke but the main goal is always to improve the patient's everyday interpersonal interactions and optimize participation in society. The specific goals vary, in part because of the variety of functional deficits caused by the stroke. In impairments of communication and swallowing, involvement of a speech language pathologist is valuable for assessment and treatment.

COMMUNICATION DISORDERS

Verbal communication is a complex process dependent on intact language, speech, and hearing functions. The focus here is on speech and language because they are most commonly impaired by stroke. A brain lesion can affect (1) the formulation, expression, and/or understanding language (aphasia); (2) planning and/or

The authors have no commercial or financial conflicts of interest to disclose.
Department of Physical Medicine and Rehabilitation, Johns Hopkins University School of Medicine, Baltimore, MD, USA
* Corresponding author.
E-mail address: mgonzal5@jhmi.edu

coordination of articulatory movements and rate/rhythm for speech production (apraxia of speech [AOS]); or (3) motor patterns (dysarthria).

Neural Control

Aphasia

The brain networks that support language function are largely circumscribed to specific areas of the cerebral cortex and the white matter tracts connecting those areas (**Fig. 1**). Traditional language control models identify Broca area (Brodmann area [BA] 44 and BA45) and Wernicke area (BA22) as among the most crucial cortical locations for language control. Other important areas include the angular gyrus (BA39) and the inferior temporal cortex (BA21). The left posterior inferior frontal gyrus or Broca area is related to most language functions including comprehension and production of language.[1] The superior temporal cortex (Wernicke area) has been associated with language reception and processing. Other important areas include BA6, premotor cortex; BA40, supramarginal gyrus; BA37, posterior inferior and middle temporal cortex and fusiform cortex; BA21, inferior temporal cortex; and BA38, anterior temporal cortex.

Dysarthria

Dysarthria occurs when weakness, dyscoordination, and/or sensory loss affect muscle function in one or more of the five subsystems of speech (ie, respiration, articulation, phonation, resonance, and/or prosody [rate/rhythm]).[2] There is abnormal

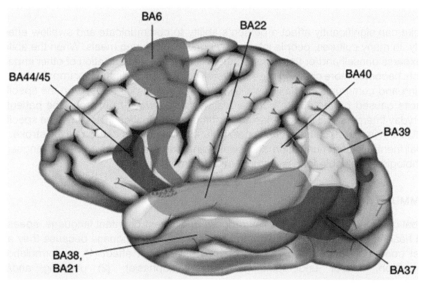

Fig. 1. Network of cortical regions supporting most language tasks. BA44/45: posterior inferior frontal gyrus (Broca area); BA6: premotor cortex; BA22: superior temporal cortex; BA40: supramarginal gyrus; BA39: angular gyrus; BA37: posterior inferior and middle temporal cortex and fusiform cortex; BA38: anterior temporal cortex; BA21: inferior temporal cortex. The white matter tracts that connect these cortical regions are also critical to the language network. Although the entire network may be engaged in the task (if it is sufficiently difficult for the person), lesions to different components of the network cause distinct deficits. BA, Broadmann area. (*From* Gonzalez-Fernandez M, Hillis AE. Speech and language therapy. In: Ovbiagale B, editor. Stroke management and recovery, vol. 1. 1st edition. London: Future Medicine Ltd; 2013. p. 151; with permission.)

neuromuscular control of the structures involved in speech generation. The motor control of the larynx, pharynx, tongue, and lips occurs at the level of the primary motor cortex (M1) through the internal capsule to the brainstem nuclei.[3] Such structures as the basal ganglia, red nucleus, substantia nigra, reticular formation, and cerebellum are also important in speech production as part of the extrapyramidal system.[3] The principal cranial nerve nuclei for the muscles of speech production are the trigeminal, facial, and hypoglossal motor nuclei, and the nucleus ambiguous; they are located in the medulla and pons.

Apraxia of speech

In people who have AOS the high level organization of motor speech is impaired resulting in an inability to plan or coordinate articulatory movements.[4] In this context the person "knows what he or she wants to say and how it should sound" but cannot effect these plans of action into accurate speech.[5] Lesions in the left inferior frontal gyrus (Broca area) have been associated with AOS.[5] Others challenge this notion and have proposed that the left anterior insular cortex is more frequently damaged in AOS.[6] A study contrasting patients with acute stroke with and without insular damage failed to find a significant association between AOS and the insula.[5] Conversely, a strong association was found between AOS and lesions in the left inferior frontal gyrus. Other areas have also been associated with AOS. These include left subcortical structures within the basal ganglia and the left frontal and temporoparietal cortices.[7,8]

Diagnosis

Accurate diagnosis of speech and language deficits requires a systematic approach. Specific language areas and speech in the context of its subsystems have to be tested and deficits clearly described. Treatment efforts are later tailored based on comprehensive testing. A comprehensive speech and language evaluation should include the following:

1. Formal testing within each of the specific language domains.
2. Comprehensive motor speech evaluation to include pitch, loudness, voice quality, duration, contextual speech component integration, and intelligibility and a focused cranial nerve examination.
3. Formal examination of speech samples to characterize phonemic errors and their frequency and pattern.

Aphasia

Important areas in the evaluation of stroke survivors with aphasia include auditory comprehension, reading comprehension, verbal expression, and written expression. Several batteries are available including the Boston Diagnostic Aphasia Examination and the Western Aphasia Battery.[9,10]

Aphasia has been traditionally classified into various syndromes based on clinical deficits (**Table 1**). Classification is based primarily on the identification of deficits in three areas: (1) repetition, (2) auditory comprehension, and (3) fluency. These aphasia syndromes do not have a single underlying cause but tend to co-occur because the brain areas responsible for these functions have shared vascular supply. The co-occurrences of these deficits are important because it can allow clinicians to predict stroke location based on the presence or absence of specific clinical deficits.[11] The use of this classification has been challenged because it has been proposed that classification should be based on theoretically significant groups.[12]

Table 1
Vascular aphasia syndromes

Syndrome	Fluency	Repetition	Comprehension	Content	Naming	Spelling	Reading	Associated Features
Broca	Poor	Poor (nonfluent)	Intact for words/simple sentences	Good	Worse for verbs	Poor	Poor	AOS Right arm weakness
Wernicke	Good	Poor (jargon)	Poor	Poor	Worse for nouns	Poor	Poor	Superior visual field cut
Conduction	Fair-good	Poor	Intact for words/simple sentences	Good	Fair-good	May be spared	May be spared	Poor working memory
Transcortical motor	Poor	Good	Intact for words/simple sentences	Good	Fair-good	May be spared	May be spared	Abulia
Transcortical sensory	Good	Good	Poor	Poor	Poor	Poor	Poor	Right visual field cut
Mixed transcortical	Poor	Good	Poor	Poor	Poor	Poor	Poor	Right hemiplegia
Global	Poor	Poor	Poor	Poor	Poor	Poor	Poor	Right hemiplegia
Anomic	Good	Good	Good	Good	Worse for nouns	May be spared	May be spared	—

Adapted from Hillis AE. Aphasia: progress in the last quarter of a century. Neurology 2007;69:204; with permission.

Dysarthria

Evaluation of the patient with dysarthria includes evaluation of neuromuscular function and speech characteristics. Evaluation should include assessment of prosody (rate and the rhythm, stress, and intonation of speech), articulation (intelligibility), velophayngeal function and resonance (sound quality), phonation (voice qualities, such as pitch variability), and respiratory function (coordination and loudness).[2,13] Based on these characteristics, dysarthria may be classified into the following groups: ataxic, hyperkinetic, hypokinetic, spastic, flaccid, unilateral upper motor neuron, or mixed.[2] Ataxic dysarthria is associated with cerebellar lesions resulting in speech that is dyscoordinated. Disorders affecting the basal ganglia result in hyperkinetic dysarthria. Lesions in the substantia nigra are associated with hypokinetic dysarthria. Spastic dysarthria, characterized by speech slowness and reduced range of motion of articulators, is associated with lesions of the corticopontine or corticobulbar pyramidal tracts. Flaccid dysarthria often presents with varying degrees of slow, labored, and imprecise articulation; a hypernasal resonance; and a hoarse voice, most often related to conditions commonly associated with brainstem impairments. Unilateral upper motor neuron dysarthria is characterized by imprecise articulation and slowed rate and a monotone quality voice and is linked to unilateral upper motor neuron lesions in the central nervous system bulbar or pseudobulbar syndromes.[14]

Apraxia of speech

The apraxia battery for adults is the most commonly used test for AOS evaluation.[15] Other tests available include the Quick Assessment of Apraxia for Speech[16] and the Motor Speech Evaluation.[7] Deficits seen in AOS are difficult to differentiate from those seen in other speech-language disorders. As such, the evaluation of patients by an experienced speech-language pathologist is of paramount importance.

Treatment

Aphasia

Treatments of aphasia can be broadly classified as behavioral or biologic. Behavioral language therapy uses various approaches including stimulation, facilitation, modality model, nondominant hemisphere approach, neurolinguistic, functional communication or pragmatic, or information processing.[17] These treatment approaches are summarized in **Table 2**.

Biologic approaches aim to restore lost neuromuscular function. They are primarily considered adjuvant to traditional aphasia rehabilitation approaches. These may include such medications as bromocriptine, dextroamphetamines, donepezil, and piracetam.[18–22] Drugs with opposite effects on neutotransmitters (ie, cholaminergic and GABAergic effects) should be avoided. Cortical stimulation (including transcranial direct current stimulation and transcranial magnetic stimulation) is thought to facilitate recovery by fostering brain plasticity.[23] For a summary of the evidence on therapeutic interventions for aphasia see the review by Allen and colleagues.[24]

In severe cases, alternative means of communication may be necessary. These include the use of writing, drawing, communication books, or electronic communication devices. Applications have been developed for this purpose for use with smartphones or tablet computers.

Apraxia of speech

The main goal of treatment in AOS is to improve functional communication. Affected features of speech, such as articulatory accuracy, rate, timing, or rhythm, should be targeted specifically. Spared systems can be used to facilitate speech production.

Table 2
Behavioral language therapy approaches

Approach	Treatment Characteristics and Techniques
Stimulation-facilitation	Targets access to language and not complete loss of language to improve language processing Treatment involves intensive auditory stimuli and repetition Errors are not corrected – followed by additional stimulation
Modality model	Language is multimodal thus aphasia is modality specific Performance in strong performing modalities is used to improve performance of weak modalities
Information processing	Based on the cognitive models developed for the specific tasks that are part of language: reading, spelling, naming, semantics, sentence production, auditory discrimination/recognition Treatment focuses on the specific process impaired When treatment of impaired processes is not successful compensation using intact processes is used
Nondominant hemisphere	Based on the hypothesis that nondominant hemisphere capabilities may facilitate communication Visual-spatial, paralinguistic, or musical skills are used to facilitate language
Neurolinguistic	Based on the premise that a specialized rule system applies to the organization of language Treatment focuses on improving disrupted rule-systems (phonologic, semantic, or lexical) by targeting the specific linguistic impairment
Functional communication (pragmatic)	This technique focuses on improving the person's ability to communicate instead of the linguistic accuracy of the message Environmental modifications to facilitate communication may also be part of this treatment approach

Singing or intonation therapies are techniques designed to engage the undamaged contralateral hemisphere to facilitate speech production.[25] The evidence summarized in a recent systematic review suggests a strong effect of articulatory/kinematic and rate/rhythm approaches for the treatment of AOS.[26]

Dysarthria
Treatment of dysarthria focuses on improving control for breathing related to speech, phonation, resonance, articulation, and prosody.[27] Exercises can improve muscle tone, strength, coordination, and precision of speech. Biofeedback can also be helpful.

Specific therapeutic approaches for the treatment of dysarthria are described in **Table 3**.[28–31] In severe cases, augmentative communication techniques may be necessary to allow for functional communication.

DYSPHAGIA

Dysphagia (swallowing impairment) is a common problem after stroke affecting more than 50% of stroke survivors (to various degrees of severity).[32] For most people affected, swallowing impairments improve quickly, with only 11% to 13% of patients having dysfunction at 6 months.[33,34] Long-standing problems can present challenges to hydration, nutrition, respiratory function, and quality of life.

Table 3
Therapy approaches for dysarthria

Approach	Characteristics
Lee Silverman Voice Treatment	Focused on increasing respiratory drive and vocal fold adduction
Behavioral communication interventions	Targets management of respiratory/phonation dysfunction Biofeedback Strategies to increase volume, reduce speed of speech, and improve intelligibility Orofacial and articulation exercises
Speech supplementation strategies	Gestures Alphabet supplementation Semantic/topic supplementation Syntactic supplementation
Systems approach	Targets components, such as breathing, phonation, nasal resonance, articulation, and intonation

Neural Control

The control of swallowing depends on multiple structures at the level of the medulla and cortical and subcortical structures. It is well known that the central pattern generator for swallowing is located in the rostral medulla.[35–37] Damage to this area can result in severe and persistent swallowing dysfunction among other deficits.

Several supratentorial structures are also critical for swallowing. In contrast to language, for which the left cortical hemisphere is dominant in most individuals, no consistent hemispheric dominance has been described. Some studies suggest that swallowing function is lateralized in each individual but that the side varies from person to person.[38,39] Bilateral hemispheric strokes are commonly associated with dysphagia.[40]

Multiple supratentorial structures, including the internal capsule and insula, have been associated with swallowing function (**Table 4**).[41] The specific role of these structures in swallowing is not completely clear, but for most, specific roles have been hypothesized. It is also uncertain which brain structures are critical and what pattern of damage results in persistent dysphagia after stroke.

Diagnosis

The prompt evaluation of dysphagia after stroke is critical to reducing morbidity and mortality. Dysphagia after stroke can result in malnutrition, dehydration, and aspiration pneumonia. The best practice in dysphagia evaluation after stroke should include early screening followed by evaluation by a speech-language pathologist and instrumental evaluation of swallowing when indicated.

Multiple tools exist for early screening for dysphagia after stroke. Some tools have been developed for use by physicians in the emergency room.[42] Others have been developed for use in specialized units, to be administered by nurses.[43] Most of these screening tests depend on a brief history or clinical evaluation followed by a water swallowing test to assess aspiration risk.[44–46]

The sensitivity and specificity of these screening tests is highly variable. The false-negative rate, depending on the test, can be high; thus clinical staff in stroke units should have a high level of suspicion and escalate evaluation even when screening failed to identify increased aspiration risk or the possibility of significant dysphagia.

Table 4	
Brain regions associated with swallowing function	
ROI	**Hypothesized Role in Swallowing Function**
Primary somatosensory, motor and motor supplementary cortices (BA1, BA2, BA3, BA4, and BA6)	Cortical processing of swallowing, including motor regulation and execution and sensorimotor control
Anterior cingulate (BA24 and BA32)	Higher-order motor processing: swallowing movement planning and execution Cognitive perceptual processes, such as attention and response selection
Orbitofrontal cortex (BA10, BA11, BA12, BA44, BA45, and BA47)	Unclear
Parieto-occipital cortex (BA7, BA17, BA18, and BA40)	Sensory processing of swallowing Task-cue processing not swallowing per se Movement planning and execution
Temporopolar cortex (BA22 and BA38)	Unclear
Insular cortex	Processing of gustatory input and intraoral sensory modulation
Internal capsule	Functional connection of the cortical and brain stem nuclei via the corticobulbar tracts
Thalamus	Sensory and motor input processing via thalamocortical and thalamostriatal pathways
Putamen, caudate, basal ganglia	Gating of sensory input
Cerebral peduncle	Unclear
Brainstem	Central pattern generator, swallowing regulation
Cerebellum	Regulation of adaptive coordination, sequencing, timing, learning, and memory of motion

Adapted from Gonzalez-Fernandez M, Kleinman J, Ky P, et al. Supratentorial regions of acute ischemia associated with clinically important swallowing disorders: a pilot study. Stroke 2008;39:3024; with permission.

A speech-language pathologist should formally evaluate people who have a positive screening test or are suspected of having dysphagia on clinical grounds. The protocol used for evaluation of dysphagia after stroke is highly variable by clinician and institution but usually includes a clinical swallow evaluation (bedside) followed by, as deemed necessary, an instrumental evaluation of swallowing that includes videofluoroscopy, fiberoptic endoscopic evaluation of swallowing (FEES), or both.

Several tools have been developed for clinical, noninstrumental evaluation of dysphagia and/or aspiration risk after stroke. Most include a cranial nerve function evaluation followed by an oral-motor assessment, pharyngeal assessment, and swallowing trials. Several validated tools have been published.[47–49] Most are checklists that assign weights to different aspects of swallowing and provide an assessment of the risk of dysphagia and tracheal aspiration. In stroke, the possibility of silent aspiration (aspiration without detectable signs) is a major concern because it cannot be identified with a clinical bedside evaluation; recognition of silent aspiration requires an instrumental examination.

Instrumental evaluation of swallowing can be performed using videofluoroscopy or FEES. Each of these has advantages and disadvantages that are relevant when choosing the appropriate test for a specific patient (**Table 5**).

Table 5		
Comparison of videofluoroscopy and FEES for the evaluation of dysphagia		
	Advantages	**Disadvantages**
Videofluoroscopy	Direct assessment of oral, pharyngeal, and esophageal stages Evaluate bolus flow, temporal and spatial structural measurements Determine the effects of compensatory strategies Direct assessment of UES opening and closing	Radiation exposure limits the length of the examination Difficulty with patient positioning, especially patients with hemiplegia or contractures Nonnatural environment may exacerbate cognitive problems Use of barium as opposed to real food
Videoendoscopy	Completed at bedside Use of real food No time constraints No radiation exposure Direct visualization of the larynx Evaluation of secretions	No visualization of the oral stage No visualization of the actual swallow because of "whiteout"; thus, details of oral and pharyngeal motility must be inferred No ability to assess esophageal functioning Limited to no ability to evaluate bolus flow and analyze structural movement

Abbreviation: UES, upper esophageal sphincter.
From Gonzalez-Fernandez M, Hillis AE. Speech and language therapy. In: Ovbiagale B, editor. Stroke management and recovery, vol. 1. 1st edition. London: Future Medicine Ltd; 2013. p. 160; with permission.

The videofluoroscopic swallowing study (VFSS) is a test in which various liquids and foods combined with barium are consumed while swallowing is visualized in real time and recorded as a movie using pulsed fluoroscopy (x-ray). Oral contrast, typically barium sulfate, is necessary. Several barium consistencies are commercially available in the United States ranging from thin liquid to pudding. The use of solid food requires coating with barium for visualization. Efforts have been made to improve palatability of barium preparations but for some patients this is still a deterrent for participation in the test. VFSS allows the evaluation of full swallowing sequences (from the lips to the stomach). Radiation exposure during a VFSS may be a concern; however, radiation exposure during a VFSS is 50% less than the exposure during a midday flight from New York City to Washington, DC (0.0033 mSv for the flight vs 0.0015 for a VFSS).[50] The VFSS can be performed in the lateral or anterior-posterior projection. One of the most important advantages of the VFSS is that function of the oral cavity, pharynx, larynx, esophagus, and the upper and lower esophageal sphincters can all be directly visualized. Therapeutic and compensatory modifications or maneuvers are tested in real time to determine their efficacy. A standardized tool to systematically evaluate swallowing impairments during videofluoroscopy has been developed.[51]

FEES is the preferred method when radiation exposure is a major concern. It is also useful when transporting the patient to the fluoroscopy suite is not possible, but it should be readily recognized that VFSS and FEES are complementary instrumental assessments.[52] Often, the most weight given to choosing VFSS or FEES is relative to the clinical concern (see **Table 5**). Pharyngeal residue is most easily visualized using FEES. There is no need to use contrast agents for FEES; thus, taste is not changed and foods can be trialed without alteration. FEES also has significant limitations: it does not permit evaluation of the oral or esophageal stages of the swallow. A "white out" occurs at the time of the swallow, only allowing for limited visualization of the pharyngeal

Table 6
Dysphagia treatment interventions and the physiologic impairments they target

Interventions	Physiologic Impairments[a]															
	Oral						Pharyngeal								Es	
	Lip Closure	Hold Position and Tongue Control	Bolus Preparation and Mastication	Bolus Transport and Lingual Motion	Oral Residue	Initiation of Pharyngeal Swallow	Soft Palate Elevation	Laryngeal Elevation	Anterior Hyolaryngeal Excursion	Epiglottic Inversion	Laryngeal Vestibular Closure	Pharyngeal Stripping Wave	PE Segment Opening	Pharyngeal Contraction	Tongue Base Retraction	Esophageal Clearance (Upright)
Compensatory																
Chin tuck						■									■	
Head rotation											■[b]		■			
Head tilt				■												
Compensatory and exercise																
Supraglottic						■			■	■	■				■	
Super-supraglottic						■			■	■	■				■	■
Effortful swallow							■		■	■	■				■	
Mendelsohn								■	■				■		■	
Exercises																
Tongue hold (Masako)														■	■	
Shaker exercises								■	■				■			

Abbreviations: Es, esophageal; PE, pharyngoesophageal.

[a] As part of the MBSImP by Martin-Harris et al. Pharyngeal residue was not included in the table because it is not considered part of the overall impairment score.

[b] Unilateral.

From Vose A, Nonnenmacher J, Singer ML, et al. Dysphagia management in acute and sub-acute stroke. Curr Phys Med Rehabil Rep 2014;2:200; with permission.

swallow to the periods immediately before and after (but not during) the swallow, per se. Evaluations of tongue base retraction, hyoid excursion, pharyngeal and laryngeal elevation, direct observation of airway closure, pharyngeal contraction, and cricopharyngeal opening are not possible during FEES.

Treatment

Treatment of dysphagia after stroke relies on a combination of compensatory maneuvers, diet modifications, and direct dysphagia therapy.[53] Most patients benefit from a carefully designed dysphagia rehabilitation program provided by a speech-language pathologist. A basic tenet of dysphagia rehabilitation is that swallowing is the best therapy for swallowing, and expression of specificity of training. The clinician is challenged to identify the least restrictive diet that the patient can safely consume while reducing the number of changes to a patient's diet and the maneuvers used during consumption of food and drink as needed.

Diet modifications may include the use of thickened liquids or modified food textures. Thickened liquids, particularly honey or pudding consistencies, should be used with caution because of palatability issues; these may lead patients to limit volumes of liquids consumed resulting in inadequate hydration. The texture of solid food may be altered based on the patient's ability to chew, transport food to the pharynx, or to prevent oral food pocketing, and when there is significant impairment of pharyngeal clearance in swallowing.

Dysphagia treatment interventions and the impairments targeted are listed in **Table 6**.[54] The use of compensatory maneuvers after stroke may be hampered by cognitive deficits. Patients may be able to use a simple maneuver, such as the chin tuck, consistently but a more complicated maneuver, such as the Mendelsohn maneuver, may be unable to be trained, let alone abandoned or forgotten. In these cases, alternatives for rehabilitation should be identified.

Stroke-related weakness may be one of the reasons for swallowing dysfunction in this population. In this case, strengthening exercises may prove useful. Exercises targeting tongue, suprahyoid, and vocal fold adductor muscle weakness (among others) have been described.[55,56]

The use of neuromuscular electrical stimulation for dysphagia rehabilitation remains controversial despite considerable study; there is evidence for and against its use. Most agree that it is not a primary mode of treatment and should be used only as an adjunct to other therapies. Neuromuscular electrical stimulation in some situations can produce hyolaryngeal depression rather than elevation.[57] This effect can be used as a resistive exercise to strengthen the muscles of elevation. However, there is an increased risk of aspiration in patients with severe dysphagia when they are unable to overcome such resistance.[58]

A dysphagia rehabilitation program should also promote effective oral hygiene. The mouth is the primary source of bacteria (including anaerobes) that, if aspirated, may result in pneumonia. Intensified oral hygiene programs have been associated with decreased rates of pneumonia after stroke.[59]

SUMMARY

Communication and swallowing disorders are common after stroke. Targeted surveillance followed by prompt evaluation and treatment is of paramount importance. Fortunately, therapeutic or compensatory interventions can decrease the effects that communication and swallowing deficits have on the quality of life of stroke survivors.

ACKNOWLEDGMENTS

This manuscript was supported in part by the National Institutes of Health, grant numbers 5K23DC011056 (MGF) and 5K23DC013569 (MBB).

REFERENCES

1. Gonzalez-Fernandez M, Hillis AE. Speech and language therapy. In: Ovbiagale B, editor. Stroke Management and Recovery. Future Medicine Ltd; 2013. p. 148–64.
2. Darley FL, Aronson AE, Brown JR. Differential diagnostic patterns of dysarthria. J Speech Hear Res 1969;12(2):246–69.
3. Ludlow CL, Hoit J, Kent R, et al. Translating principles of neural plasticity into research on speech motor control recovery and rehabilitation. J Speech Lang Hear Res 2008;51(1):S240–58.
4. Ziegler W, Aichert I, Staiger A. Apraxia of speech: concepts and controversies. J Speech Lang Hear Res 2012;55(5):S1485–501.
5. Hillis AE, Work M, Barker PB, et al. Re-examining the brain regions crucial for orchestrating speech articulation. Brain 2004;127(Pt 7):1479–87.
6. Dronkers NF. A new brain region for coordinating speech articulation. Nature 1996;384(6605):159–61.
7. Wertz RT, LaPointe LL, Rosenbek JC. Apraxia of speech: the disorder and its management. New York: Grune and Stratton; 1984.
8. Ogar J, Slama H, Dronkers N, et al. Apraxia of speech: an overview. Neurocase 2005;11(6):427–32.
9. Goodglass H, Kaplan E. Boston Diagnostic Aphasia Examination. Austin, TX: Pro-Ed; 2001.
10. Kertesz A, editor. Western Aphasia Battery: revised. San Antonio (TX): PsychCorp; 2007.
11. Hillis AE. Aphasia: progress in the last quarter of a century. Neurology 2007;69(2):200–13.
12. Badecker W, Caramazza A. On considerations of method and theory governing the use of clinical categories in neurolinguistics and cognitive neuropsychology: the case against agrammatism. Cognition 1985;20(2):97–125.
13. Darley FL, Aronson AE, Brown JR. Clusters of deviant speech dimensions in the dysarthrias. J Speech Hear Res 1969;12(3):462–96.
14. Hartman DE, Abbs JH. Dysarthria associated with focal unilateral upper motor neuron lesion. Eur J Disord Commun 1992;27(3):187–96.
15. Dabul BL, editor. The apraxia battery for adults. Austin (TX): Pro-Ed; 2000.
16. Tanner D, Culbertson W. Quick assessment for apraxia of speech. Oceanside, CA: Academic Communication Associates; 1999.
17. Cherney LR, Small SA. Aphasia, apraxia of speech and dysarthria. In: Stein J, Harvey RL, Macko RF, et al, editors. Stroke recovery and rehabilitation. New York: Demos Medical; 2009. p. 155–81.
18. Raymer AM, Bandy D, Adair JC, et al. Effects of bromocriptine in a patient with crossed nonfluent aphasia: a case report. Arch Phys Med Rehabil 2001;82(1):139–44.
19. Walker-Batson D, Curtis S, Natarajan R, et al. A double-blind, placebo-controlled study of the use of amphetamine in the treatment of aphasia. Stroke 2001;32(9):2093–8.
20. Martinsson L, Hardemark HG, Wahlgren NG. Amphetamines for improving stroke recovery: a systematic Cochrane review. Stroke 2003;34(11):2766.

21. Berthier ML, Green C, Higueras C, et al. A randomized, placebo-controlled study of donepezil in poststroke aphasia. Neurology 2006;67(9):1687–9.
22. Kessler J, Thiel A, Karbe H, et al. Piracetam improves activated blood flow and facilitates rehabilitation of poststroke aphasic patients. Stroke 2000;31(9):2112–6.
23. Hamilton RH, Chrysikou EG, Coslett B. Mechanisms of aphasia recovery after stroke and the role of noninvasive brain stimulation. Brain Lang 2011;118(1–2): 40–50.
24. Allen L, Mehta S, McClure JA, et al. Therapeutic interventions for aphasia initiated more than six months post stroke: a review of the evidence. Top Stroke Rehabil 2012;19(6):523–35.
25. Albert ML, Sparks RW, Helm NA. Melodic intonation therapy for aphasia. Arch Neurol 1973;29(2):130–1.
26. Ballard KJ, Wambaugh JL, Duffy JR, et al. Treatment for acquired apraxia of speech: a systematic review of intervention research between 2004 and 2012. Am J Speech Lang Pathol 2015;24:316–37.
27. Enderby P. Disorders of communication: dysarthria. Handb Clin Neurol 2013;110: 273–81.
28. Deane KH, Whurr R, Playford ED, et al. Speech and language therapy for dysarthria in Parkinson's disease. Cochrane Database Syst Rev 2001;(2):CD002812.
29. Deane KH, Whurr R, Playford ED, et al. A comparison of speech and language therapy techniques for dysarthria in Parkinson's disease. Cochrane Database Syst Rev 2001;(2):CD002814.
30. Hustad KC, Jones T, Dailey S. Implementing speech supplementation strategies: effects on intelligibility and speech rate of individuals with chronic severe dysarthria. J Speech Lang Hear Res 2003;46(2):462–74.
31. Pennington L, Miller N, Robson S, et al. Intensive speech and language therapy for older children with cerebral palsy: a systems approach. Dev Med Child Neurol 2010;52(4):337–44.
32. Martino R, Foley N, Bhogal S, et al. Dysphagia after stroke: incidence, diagnosis, and pulmonary complications. Stroke 2005;36(12):2756–63.
33. Smithard DG, O'Neill PA, England RE, et al. The natural history of dysphagia following a stroke. Dysphagia 1997;12(4):188–93.
34. Mann G, Hankey GJ, Cameron D. Swallowing function after stroke: prognosis and prognostic factors at 6 months. Stroke 1999;30(4):744–8.
35. Jean A. Brainstem organization of the swallowing network. Brain Behav Evol 1984;25(2–3):109–16.
36. Jean A. Brain stem control of swallowing: neuronal network and cellular mechanisms. Physiol Rev 2001;81(2):929–69.
37. Miller AJ. The search for the central swallowing pathway: the quest for clarity. Dysphagia 1993;8(3):185–94.
38. Hamdy S, Aziz Q, Rothwell JC, et al. Recovery of swallowing after dysphagic stroke relates to functional reorganization in the intact motor cortex. Gastroenterology 1998;115(5):1104–12.
39. Hamdy S, Aziz Q, Rothwell JC, et al. The cortical topography of human swallowing musculature in health and disease. Nat Med 1996;2(11):1217–24.
40. Horner J, Massey EW, Brazer SR. Aspiration in bilateral stroke patients. Neurology 1990;40(11):1686–8.
41. Gonzalez-Fernandez M, Kleinman J, Ky P, et al. Supratentorial regions of acute ischemia associated with clinically important swallowing disorders: a pilot study. Stroke 2008;39(11):3022–8.

42. Antonios N, Carnaby-Mann G, Crary M, et al. Analysis of a physician tool for evaluating dysphagia on an inpatient stroke unit: the modified Mann assessment of swallowing ability. J Stroke Cerebrovasc Dis 2010;19(1):49–57.

43. Martino R, Silver F, Teasell R, et al. The Toronto Bedside Swallowing Screening Test (TOR-BSST): development and validation of a dysphagia screening tool for patients with stroke. Stroke 2009;40(2):555–61.

44. Suiter DM, Leder SB. Clinical utility of the 3-ounce water swallow test. Dysphagia 2008;23(3):244–50.

45. Trapl M, Enderle P, Nowotny M, et al. Dysphagia bedside screening for acute-stroke patients: the Gugging Swallowing Screen. Stroke 2007;38(11):2948–52.

46. Wu MC, Chang YC, Wang TG, et al. Evaluating swallowing dysfunction using a 100-ml water swallowing test. Dysphagia 2004;19(1):43–7.

47. Splaingard ML, Hutchins B, Sulton LD, et al. Aspiration in rehabilitation patients: videofluoroscopy vs bedside clinical assessment. Arch Phys Med Rehabil 1988; 69(8):637–40.

48. Smithard DG, O'Neill PA, Park C, et al. Can bedside assessment reliably exclude aspiration following acute stroke? Age Ageing 1998;27(2):99–106.

49. Mann G. MASA: the Mann assessment of swallowing ability. New York: Singular; 2002.

50. Institut de Radioprotection et de Surete Nucleaire. Calculation of dose: cosmic radiation. 2015. Available at: https://www.sievert-system.org/. Accessed May, 2015.

51. Martin-Harris B, Brodsky MB, Michel Y, et al. MBS measurement tool for swallow impairment–MBSImp: establishing a standard. Dysphagia 2008;23(4):392–405.

52. Langmore SE. Evaluation of oropharyngeal dysphagia: which diagnostic tool is superior? Curr Opin Otolaryngol Head Neck Surg 2003;11:485–9.

53. Huckabee M, Pelletier C. Management of adult neurogenic dysphagia. San Diego (CA): Singular Publishing Group; 1999.

54. Vose A, Nonnenmacher J, Singer ML, et al. Dysphagia management in acute and sub-acute stroke. Curr Phys Med Rehabil Rep 2014;2(4):197–206.

55. Martin BJ, Logemann JA, Shaker R, et al. Normal laryngeal valving patterns during three breath-hold maneuvers: a pilot investigation. Dysphagia 1993;8(1): 11–20.

56. Robbins J, Kays SA, Gangnon RE, et al. The effects of lingual exercise in stroke patients with dysphagia. Arch Phys Med Rehabil 2007;88(2):150–8.

57. Ludlow CL, Humbert I, Saxon K, et al. Effects of surface electrical stimulation both at rest and during swallowing in chronic pharyngeal dysphagia. Dysphagia 2007; 22(1):1–10.

58. Ludlow CL. Electrical neuromuscular stimulation in dysphagia: current status. Curr Opin Otolaryngol Head Neck Surg 2010;18(3):159–64.

59. Sorensen RT, Rasmussen RS, Overgaard K, et al. Dysphagia screening and intensified oral hygiene reduce pneumonia after stroke. J Neurosci Nurs 2013; 45(3):139–46.

Neuropharmacology of Poststroke Motor and Speech Recovery

Zafer Keser, MD[a], Gerard E. Francisco, MD[b],*

KEYWORDS

- Stroke • Recovery • Motor • Speech • Neuropharmacology

KEY POINTS

- Stroke is a common and serious condition.
- The main focus of the article is pharmacologic agents used for motor and speech recovery after stroke.
- Amphetamine, levodopa, selective serotonin reuptake inhibitors, and piracetam were the most commonly used drugs in enhancing motor and speech recovery after stroke.
- Adding drug therapy to conventional rehabilitation seems beneficial in poststroke motor and speech recovery.
- Adequately powered, randomized, double-blind clinical trials are needed to explore pharmacologic enhancement of stroke recovery.

INTRODUCTION

Approximately 6.8 million Americans more than 20 years of age have had a stroke. On average, every 40 seconds, someone in the United States has a stroke. Motor and speech deficits are common results of stroke. Fifty percent of patients have some hemiparesis after stroke and 19% have aphasia.[1] Although physical, occupational, and speech therapies are the most widely used treatment in the rehabilitation of stroke

Conflict of Interest: None declared.

Funding Support: Partial support came from grants from Mission Connect, a project of TIRR Foundation; TIRR Memorial Hermann; and the Department of Physical Medicine and Rehabilitation, UTHealth.

[a] Department of Physical Medicine and Rehabilitation, University of Texas Health Science Center (UTHealth), The NeuroRecovery Research Center Houston, TIRR Memorial Hermann, Houston, 1333B Moursund Street, Room 126, Houston, TX 77030, USA; [b] Department of Physical Medicine and Rehabilitation, University of Texas Health Science Center (UTHealth), The Neuro-Recovery Research Center Houston, TIRR Memorial Hermann, Houston, 1333 Moursund Street, Suite E-108, Houston, TX 77030, USA

* Corresponding author.

E-mail address: Gerard.E.Francisco@uth.tmc.edu

Phys Med Rehabil Clin N Am 26 (2015) 671–689

http://dx.doi.org/10.1016/j.pmr.2015.06.009

survivors, their therapeutic effects are generally modest. There is a growing need for more effective treatment options as add-ons to conventional therapy. For several decades, pharmacologic agents have been used as potential approaches for enhancing motor and speech recovery.

This article summarizes published literature in motor (**Table 1**) and speech (**Table 2**) recovery after stroke. The clinical trials investigating primarily recovery from poststroke depression, poststroke spasticity, cognitive impairment, activities of daily living (ADLs), neuropathic pain, and seizures have not been included. However, if the improvements in these deficits were reported secondarily to motor or speech recovery, they are mentioned. Experimental studies with animals and healthy controls, and case reports, were not included either because of the large number of clinical trials in the past.

Details about adverse events are not included because this is not the scope of the article. Only serious adverse events related to the drug are mentioned. Engelter[46] provides more specific information about adverse events.

PHARMACOLOGIC AGENTS IN MOTOR AND SPEECH RECOVERY
Central Nervous System Stimulators (Amphetamines and Methylphenidate)

Crisostomo and colleagues[3] conducted a small double-blinded and placebo-controlled study with 8 subjects (4 in active and 4 in placebo groups) to see whether dextroamphetamine (D-amphetamine) helps with the motor recovery of patients up to 10 days after ischemic stroke. A single dose of 10 mg of D-amphetamine was combined with 45 minutes of physiotherapy (PT) within 3 hours after drug administration. Fugl-Meyer (FM) was used as an outcome measures and it was shown that patients who were treated with D-amphetamine obtained greater increments in motor scores than the controls.

Another proof of concept study came from Walker-Batson and colleagues,[31] this time focusing more on speech recovery after stroke. They administered 10 doses of 10 mg of D-amphetamine at intervals of 3 to 4 days along with 1 hour of speech therapy 30 minutes after treatment in 6 patients after acute (10–30 days after the injury) non-hemorrhagic stroke. All 6 subjects received active drug and the assessments were performed at baseline, 1 week, 3 months, 6 months, 9 months, and 1 year after starting the therapy. They used the Porch Index of Communicative Ability (PICA) as an outcome assessment. The results were promising and, at 3 months, 5 of 6 subjects had achieved more than 100% of the 6-month predicted scores.

Reding and colleagues[6] studied amphetamine effects on recovery with larger sample sizes. Administration of 10 mg/d of D-amphetamine for 14 days then 5 mg/d for 3 days along with standard inpatient therapy was performed in 21 patients 7 to 45 days after acute ischemic stroke. Nine of the subjects were in the active treatment group and assessments were done at baseline, day 2, and weekly for 4 weeks. FM, Barthel Index (BI), and Zung Self-rating Depression Scale (ZDS) were used to screen the motor, functional, and mood improvement results respectively. The investigators concluded that amphetamine use did not improve motor recovery, functional outcome, or depression scores in acute/subacute stroke.

Contrary to Reding and colleagues,[6] Walker-Batson and colleagues[5] reported encouraging results in the same year. With a similar protocol to their aphasia study 3 years earlier, 10 doses of 10 mg of D-amphetamine at 3-day to 4-day intervals were administered together with 1 hour of PT in 10 patients after acute (16–30 days after) ischemic stroke but this time they had a control group (5 of 10 subjects) to monitor the effects of amphetamine in a more robust fashion. The participants were assessed at baseline, within each session, and at 1 week, 3 months, 6 months, and 12 months after therapy with FM. The investigators observed a 40 point of difference in FM between the active and control groups by the end of 1 year.[5]

Grade and colleagues[8] investigated more general effects of methylphenidate (MP) in patients after acute (14–21 days) stroke with a randomized and placebo-controlled study. They administered 3 weeks of MP, which was started at 5 mg and increased gradually to 30 mg along with routine inpatient rehabilitation. There were 21 patients (10 in the active and 11 in the placebo groups) and their follow-up was limited to the time of inpatient stay. Motor functioning was assessed using the FM and a modified version of the Functional Independence Measure (M-FIM). Mood assessment was performed with Hamilton Depression Rating Scale (HAM-D) and ZDS. Cognitive status was evaluated using the Mini-Mental State Examination. Patients receiving MP treatment scored lower on the HAM-D and ZDS but significantly higher on the M-FIM and higher on the FM than patients receiving placebo.

Sonde and colleagues[11] used a similar study protocol to Walker-Batson and colleagues[5] (the same 10 doses of 10 mg D-amphetamine at intervals of 3–4 days) with larger sample size (39 patients; 12 active/19 placebo) to investigate amphetamine effects on motor recovery in patients with acute (5–10 days) ischemic/hemorrhagic stroke. They assessed motor and functional recovery with FM and BI and they reported that amphetamine-treated patients did not show any increase in motor function or ADL compared with the control group.

Walker-Batson and colleagues[37] published another encouraging study of the effects of amphetamine on the speech recovery of 21 patients (12 active/9 placebo) 16 to 45 days after acute/subacute ischemic stroke. Using the 10 doses of 10 mg of D-amphetamine at intervals of 3 to 4 days along with 1 hour of speech therapy, they showed significantly greater gain in the D-amphetamine group in 1 week and 6 months compared with placebo according to the PICA.[37]

Another study came from Martinsson and Wahlgren[12] 2 years later assessed the effects of different doses of amphetamine on motor and functional recovery. They had 3 groups of 15 patients (10 active/5 placebo) with different drug doses of 2.5, 5, and 10 mg of D-amphetamine for 5 consecutive days in 45 patients with very acute (up to 72 hours) ischemic stroke. The group treated with D-amphetamine had significantly better improvement during the treatment period, as assessed with the Lindmark Motor Assessment Chart (LMAC) motor function score, Scandinavian Stroke Scale (SSS), activity index (AI) motor score, and BI. At the day 7 follow-up, all members of the D-amphetamine group had significantly better improvement with the LMAC motor function score, SSS, and AI motor score. There were no statistically significant differences at 1 or 3 months. No other outcome measure, including the 10-m walking test, was statistically significant at any time point.[12]

Treig and colleagues[13] performed a randomized, placebo-controlled study to assess the effects of amphetamine on the recovery of the motor function and ADLs of 24 patients (12 active/12 control) with acute/subacute (<6 weeks) ischemic stroke with moderate to severe impairment. Ten sessions with 10 mg of D-amphetamine (or placebo) every fourth day in a time period of 36 days were combined with 45 minutes of PT (5 times/wk) within 60 minutes after drug intake. The comparison between groups did not reveal any difference at any time; amphetamine-treated patients did not show any increase in motor function (assessed by Rivermead Motor Assessment [RMA]) or ADL (assessed by BI) compared with the control group.

An experimental study was performed by Tardy and colleagues,[16] who hypothesized that a single dose of MP would modulate cerebral motor activation and behavior in 8 patients with acute (17 days after) subcortical stroke on the corticospinal tract

Table 1
Summary of pharmacologic studies for motor recovery after stroke

Reference	Type of Stroke	Type of Drug Used	Number of Patients (Active/Placebo)	Time Postinjury at Enrollment	Treatment Protocol	Motor Outcome Assessment	Final Follow-up After Enrollment
Hazama et al,[2] 1980	Ischemic/hemorrhagic	Citicoline	55/56/54[a]	>3 mo	High-dose citicoline (1 g/d/8 w), or low-dose citicoline (250 mg/d/8 w) + functional rehabilitation program	Hemiplegia Function Test	8 wk
Crisostomo et al,[3] 1988	Ischemic	D-AMP	8 (4/4)	<10 d	Single dose of 10 mg of D-AMP + 45 min PT	FM	3 d
Ueda et al,[4] 1994	Ischemic/hemorrhagic	Citicoline	248 (124/124)	4 wk–1 y	1 g/8 wk + specific rehabilitation	Hemiplegia Function Test	8 wk
Walker-Batson et al,[5] 1995	Ischemic	D-AMP	6 (5/5)	10–30 d	10 doses of 10 mg D-AMP at 3–4 d interval + 1 h PT	FM	4 wk
Reding et al,[6] 1995	Ischemic	D-AMP	21 (9/12)	7–45 d	10 mg/d D-AMP for 14 d then 5 mg/d for 3 d + standard inpatient rehabilitation	FM	4 wk
Dam et al,[7] 1996	Ischemic	MPT and FLU	46 (14/16/14)[b]	1–6 mo	150 mg/d MPT, 20 mg/d FLU for 3 mo + 1–2 h/d of PT, 2 h of OT, and 1 h of ST if needed 5 d/w	Graded Neurologic Scale	3 mo
Grade et al,[8] 1998	Ischemic/hemorrhagic	MPH	21 (10/11)	14–21 d	3 w of MPH was started at 5 mg and increased gradually to 30 mg for 3 w + standard inpatient rehabilitation	FM	3 wk
Pariente et al,[9] 2001	Ischemic	FLU	8 (8/8)	14 d	1 dose of 20 mg FLU	NHPT, finger tapping	1 d

Study	Stroke type	Drug	N	Time after stroke	Intervention	Outcome	Follow-up
Scheidtmann et al,[10] 2001	Ischemic/hemorrhagic	L-Dopa	53 (26/27)	3 wk–6 mo	100 mg/d of L-dopa for 3 mo + PT	RMA	6 wk
Sonde et al,[11] 2001	Ischemic/hemorrhagic	D-AMP	31 (12/19)	5–10 d	10 doses of 10 mg D-AMP at 3–4 d interval + 30 min PT	FM	3 mo
Martinsson & Wahlgren,[12] 2003	Ischemic	D-AMP	45 (30/15)	<3 d	2.5-5-10 mg of D-AMP for 5 consecutive days	Lindmark Scale	3 mo
Treig et al,[13] 2003	Ischemic	D-AMP	24 (12/12)	<6 wk	10 doses with 10 mg D-AMP every 4th day in 36 d combined with 45 min of PT (5 times/wk)	RMA	1 y
Nadeau et al,[14] 2004	Ischemic/hemorrhagic	DON	20 (10/10)	>1 y	6 wk 10 mg/d DON + 10 times of 6 h CIT of upper limb (at last 2 wk)	BBT, WMFT, FM, MAL, finger tapping	6 mo
Floel et al,[15] 2005	Ischemic	L-Dopa	9 (9/9)	>12 mo	Single dose of 100 mg of L-dopa + motor memory training	TMS-evoked thumb movements	1 d
Tardy et al,[16] 2006	Ischemic/hemorrhagic	MPH	8 (8/8)	17 d	Single dose of 20 mg MPH	Hand grip strength, finger tapping and speed during a target pursuit task, fMRI	1 d
Gladstone et al,[17] 2006	Ischemic/hemorrhagic	D-AMP	71 (34/37)	5–10 d	10 sessions of D-AMP	FM	3 mo
Sonde & Lokk,[18] 2007	Ischemic/hemorrhagic	D-AMP and L-dopa	25 (7/4/7/7)[c]	5–10 d	10 sessions with 20 mg of D-AMP, 100 mg of L-dopa, or 10 mg of D-AMP + 50 mg of L-dopa or placebo	FM	3 mo

(continued on next page)

Table 1
(continued)

Reference	Type of Stroke	Type of Drug Used	Number of Patients (Active/Placebo)	Time Postinjury at Enrollment	Treatment Protocol	Motor Outcome Assessment	Final Follow-up After Enrollment
Sprigg et al,[19] 2007	Ischemic	D-AMP	33 (17/16)	3–30 d	5 mg initially, then 10 mg D-AMP for 10 subsequent doses with 3-d or 4-d separations + inpatient rehabilitation	FM	3 mo
Zittel et al,[20] 2007	Ischemic/hemorrhagic	RBX	10 (10/10)	>6 mo	Single dose of 6 mg of RBX + 1 h of PT	Tapping speed, grip strength, NHPT, and TMS MEPs	1 d
Restemeyer et al,[21] 2007	Ischemic	L-Dopa	10 (10/10)	>6 mo	Single dose of 100 mg L-dopa + 1 h of PT	NHPT, grip strength, and ARAT and TMS cortical excitability	Right after PT
Zittel et al,[22] 2008	Ischemic/hemorrhagic	CIT	8 (8/8)	>6 mo	Single dose of CIT + 1 h of PT	NHPT, hand grip strength	2 h
Iranmanesh & Vakilian,[23] 2008	Hemorrhagic	Citicoline	32 (16/16)	<6 h	250 mg/d citicoline for 14 d	Muscular strength	3 mo
Acler et al,[24] 2009	Ischemic/hemorrhagic	CIT	20 (10/10)	<10 d	10 mg/d CIT for 4 mo + PT	Lindmark Scale	4 mo

Study	Stroke type	Drug	N (groups)	Time since stroke	Treatment	Outcome measures	Follow-up
Cramer et al,[25] 2009	Ischemic/hemorrhagic	RPR	33 (17/16)	1–12 mo	9 w of RPR (0.25–4 mg/d, titrated daily) + 90 min PT	Gait velocity, gait endurance, FM	3 mo
Wang et al,[26] 2011	Ischemic/hemorrhagic	RBX	11 (11/11)	1–12 mo	Single dose of 6 mg RBX	ARAT, hand grip strength, finger tapping, rapid tapping, and fMRI	1 d
Chollet et al,[27] 2011	Ischemic	FLU	113 (57/56)	5–10 d	20 mg/d FLU for 3 mo + PT	FM	3 mo
Kakuda et al,[28] 2011	Ischemic/hemorrhagic	L-Dopa	5 (5/0)	>12 mo	100 mg/d L-dopa for 7 wk + rTMS and OT	FM, WMFT	4 wk
Schuster et al,[29] 2011	Ischemic	D-AMP	16 (7/9)	<2 mo	10 times 10 mg D-AMP over 5 wk + standard inpatient rehabilitation	Chedoke-McMaster Stroke Assessment	1 y
Mohammadianinejad et al,[30] 2014	Ischemic	Lithium	66 (32/34)	<2 d	300 mg twice daily for 1 mo + inpatient therapy	FM	1 mo

Abbreviations: ARAT, Action Research Arm Test; BBT, Box and Block Test; CIT, citalopram; D-AMP, d-amphetamine; DON, donepezil; FLU, fluoxetine; FM, Fugl-Meyer; fMRI, functional MRI; MAL, motor activity log; MEPs, motor evoked potentials; MPH, methylphenidate; MPT, maprotiline; NHPT, Nine-hole Peg Test; OT, occupational therapy; PT, physical therapy; RBX, reboxetine; RMA, rivermead motor assessment; RPR, ropinirole; rTMS, repetitive transcranial magnetic stimulation; ST, speech therapy; TMS, transcranial magnetic stimulation; WMFT, Wolf-Motor Function Test.

[a] 55/56/54 is high dose, low dose, and placebo respectively.
[b] 14/16/14 is maprotiline, fluoxetine, and placebo respectively.
[c] 7/4/7/7 is 20 mg of D-AMP, 100 mg of L-dopa, 10 mg of D-amphetamine, plus 50 mg of L-dopa or placebo respectively.

Table 2
Summary of pharmacologic studies for speech recovery after stroke

Reference	Type of Stroke	Type of Drug Used	Number of Patients (Active/Placebo)	Time Postinjury	Treatment Protocol	Language Outcome Assessment	Final Follow-up
Walker-Batson et al,[31] 1992	Ischemic	D-AMP	6 (6/0)	10–30 d	10 doses of 10 mg D-AMP at 3–4 d interval + 60 min ST	PICA	1 y
Enderby et al,[32] 1994	Ischemic	Piracetam	67 (30/37)	6–9 wk after	12 wk 4.8 g/d piracetam + standard inpatient rehabilitation	Aachen Aphasia Test	24 wk
De Deyn et al,[33] 1997	Ischemic	Piracetam	373 (180/193)	<12 h	Piracetam 12 g in bolus intravenously within 12 h after stroke onset, followed by piracetam 12 g/d IV until fourth d. Thereafter 12 g/d until 4 w, then 4.8 g/d for 8 wk	Frenchay Aphasia Screening Test	12 wk
Bragoni et al,[34] 2000	Ischemic/hemorrhagic	BR	11 (11/0)	>1 y	Phase 1: placebo plus domperidon (30 mg tid) + ST (2 individual sessions weekly) (day 90). Phase 2: BR (started at 2.5 mg up to 30 mg tid, for a 4-wk period) plus domperidon, and ST (day 150). Phase 4. BR (30 mg tid) plus domperidon	Standardized Italian language test, token test, visual naming test	9 mo
Kessler et al,[35] 2000	Ischemic	Piracetam	24 (12/12)	14 d	6 wk of 2400 mg piracetam twice daily + 5 times/w 60 min ST	Aachen Aphasia Test	6 wk
Szelies et al,[36] 2001	Ischemic	Piracetam	24	14 d	6 wk of 2400 mg piracetam twice daily + 5 times/w 60 min ST	Aphasia Test	6 wk
Walker-Batson et al,[37] 2001	Ischemic	D-AMP	21 (12/9)	16–45 d	10 doses of 10 mg D-AMP at 3–4 d intervals + 1 h ST	PICA	6 mo

Study	Stroke type	Drug	N (M/F)	Time since stroke	Dosage/regimen	Outcome measure	Duration
Berthier et al,[38] 2003	Ischemic/hemorrhagic	Donepezil	10 (10/0)	>6 mo	5 mg/d donepezil for first 4 wk, followed by 10 mg/d for 12 wk + ST	WAB and PALPA	20 wk
Laska et al,[39] 2005	Ischemic/hemorrhagic	Moclobemide	66 (34/31)	3 wk	Started with 300 mg moclobemide and escalated to 600 mg in 1 mo for 6 mo + routine inpatient rehabilitation	Reinvang Grunntest for afasi + ANELT	6 mo
Berthier et al,[40] 2006	Ischemic/hemorrhagic	Donepezil	26 (13/13)	>1 y	5 mg/d donepezil for first 4 wk, followed by 10 mg/d for 12 wk + ST	WAB, CAL, and PALPA	20 wk
Ashtary et al,[41] 2006	Ischemic/hemorrhagic	BR	38 (19/19)	Acute (undefined)	Bromocriptine in 2.5-mg/d increments for 4 w to 10 mg/d for a total of 4 mo	Persian Language Test	16 wk
Seniów et al,[42] 2009	Ischemic/hemorrhagic	L-Dopa	39 (20/19)	2–8 wk	100 mg/d L-dopa + ST 5 times/wk for 3 wk	BDAE	3 wk
Berthier et al,[43] 2009	Ischemic/hemorrhagic	Memantine	27 (14/13)	1 y	20 mg/d memantine only for 16 w, followed by memantine + CIAT (weeks 16–18), memantine alone again (weeks 18–20), and washout (weeks 20–24), and then an open-label extension phase of memantine (weeks 24–48)	WAB and CAL	48 wk
Gungor et al,[44] 2011	Ischemic	Piracetam	30 (15/15)	2–32 d	4.8 g piracetam/d for 6 mo	GAT	24 wk
Breitenstein et al,[45] 2015	Ischemic/hemorrhagic	L-Dopa	10 (10/10)	>1 y	100/25 mg of L-dopa/carbidopa or placebo daily + 4 h of ST for 2 wk	Naming Performance and Verbal Communication	6 mo

Abbreviations: ANELT, Amsterdam-Nijmegen Everyday Language Test; BDAE, Boston Diagnostic Aphasia Examination; BR, bromocriptine; CAL, communicative activity log; CIAT, Constrained-Induced Aphasia Training; GAT, Gulhane Aphasia Test; IV, intravenous; PALPA, Psycholinguistic Assessment of Language Processing in Aphasia; PICA, Porch Index of Communicative Ability; tid, 3 times a day; WAB, Western Aphasia Battery.

resulting in a pure motor hemiparesis. On 2 different occasions, patients received 20 mg of MP or placebo and were assessed by functional MRI (fMRI) and hand grip strength, finger tapping test, and speed during a target pursuit task. MP compared with placebo elicited a significant improvement in motor performance of the affected hand at the finger tapping test. fMRI also showed a hyperactivation of the ipsilesional primary sensorimotor cortex, including the motor hand and face areas, and of the contralesional premotor cortex in the MP group.

A large placebo-controlled clinical trial was performed by Gladstone and colleagues[17] in which 71 subjects (34 in active and 37 in placebo groups) with acute stroke (5–10 days after) causing hemiparesis/hemiplegia underwent 10 sessions of PT coupled with either 10 mg of D-amphetamine or placebo and were assessed by FM. Motor scores improved during treatment in both groups. No significant difference was observed in recovery between the treatment groups for the entire cohort or for subgroups with a severe hemiparesis, moderate hemiparesis, or cortically based stroke.

After failing to show any improvements related to amphetamine-only treatment earlier in 2001, Sonde and Lokk[18] investigated combination with L-dopa with higher amphetamine doses. They had 10 sessions with either 20 mg of D-amphetamine plus 100 mg of L-dopa or 10 mg of D-amphetamine plus 50 mg of L-dopa or placebo during a 2-week period along with PT in 25 patients with acute (5–10 days) ischemic/hemorrhagic stroke. All patients improved significantly over the intervention period. Drug-treated patients did not show any additional increase in motor function (assessed by FM) or ADL (assessed by BI).

In the same year another clinical trial failed to show positive results of motor recovery with amphetamine. Thirty-three subjects (17 active/16 placebo) with acute (3–30 days) ischemic stroke received D-amphetamine (5 mg initially, then 10 mg for 10 subsequent doses with 3-day or 4-day separations) or placebo coupled with inpatient PT. Recovery was assessed by motor scale (FM), functional scale (BI), and Modified Rankin Scale (mRS). D-Amphetamine did not improve motor and functional outcomes at 90 days. Also, peripheral and central systolic blood pressure and heart rate were significantly higher (11.2 mm Hg, 9.5 mm Hg, and 7 beats per minute respectively) in the amphetamine group.[19]

Schuster and colleagues[29] investigated motor and functional recovery improvement with amphetamine. They administered 10 mg of D-amphetamine 10 times over 5 weeks along with multidisciplinary inpatient rehabilitation in 16 patients (7 active/9 placebo) with acute/subacute (less than 2 months after) ischemic stroke. Subjects were assessed twice during baseline, every week during the 5-week treatment period, and at follow-up at 1 week, 6 months, and 12 months after intervention with the Chedoke-McMaster Stroke Assessment for motor function and gross motor and walking index for ADLs. There was significant improvement of ADL and arm motor function in favor of the active drug group.

Overall, the information from the 15 studies discussed earlier suggests that amphetamines were somewhat beneficial for motor recovery, with most utility when combined with therapies, but evidence is mixed across studies and limited by differences in design and outcome measures.

Dopaminergic Agonists

Bragoni and colleagues[34] investigated the effects of bromocriptine (BR) on the speech recovery of 11 subjects with chronic (>1 year) nonfluent aphasia with a double-blind study with a high dosage of BR, prescribed according to a dose-escalating protocol. Domperidone (30 mg 3 times a day) was used to prevent BR's side effects and subjects underwent several different treatment phases: speech therapy (ST) only, BR (started at 2.5 mg up to 30 mg 3 times a day over a 4-week period) combined with ST, and then BR only (30 mg 3 times a day). ST only improved dictation; combination therapy improved dictation, reading aloud, repetition, reading comprehension, and verbal latency; and BR only improved reading comprehension and verbal latency (assessed by Italian language and token tests). Final assessment revealed improvement in reading comprehension. Atrial fibrillation, visual hallucinations, and epileptic seizures were observed in several patients and only 5 patients completed the study. Although the results are promising, side effects of high-dose BR are worrying.

Scheidtmann and colleagues[10] conducted a prospective, randomized, placebo-controlled, double-blind study in which they enrolled 53 patients (26 active/27 placebo) with acute/subacute (3 weeks–6 months after) ischemic/hemorrhagic stroke to investigate the effects of levodopa (L-dopa) on motor recovery. For the first 3 weeks patients received single doses of L-dopa 100 mg or placebo daily in combination with standard PT. For the second 3 weeks patients had only PT. Motor recovery, assessed by RMA was significantly improved after 3 weeks of drug intervention in patients on L-dopa and the result was independent of initial degree of impairment. The advantage of the L-dopa group was maintained at study end point 3 weeks after L-dopa was stopped.

Floel and colleagues[15] designed an experimental, crossover, and placebo-controlled study to test L-dopa on motor recovery. On 2 different occasions either single doses of L-dopa (100 mg) and carbidopa (25 mg) or placebo were administered along with motor memory training in 9 patients with chronic (>12 months) ischemic stroke. The investigators concluded that a single oral dose of L-dopa significantly enhanced the ability to encode motor memory (assessed by transcranial magnetic stimulation (TMS) evoked thumb movements) relative to placebo, because transcranial magnetic stimulation (TMS) evoked thumb movements.

Six years later than Bragoni and colleagues,[34] a randomized, double-blind, placebo-controlled study from Ashtary and colleagues[41] with a simple design and low-dose BR (2.5-mg/d increments over 4 weeks to 10 mg/d for a total of 4 months) but larger sample size (38; 19 active/19 placebo) failed to replicate the initial findings. At 4 months, verbal fluency, gesture to command, naming, single-word response repetition, automatic speech, prosody, and global score had significantly improved for both intervention (BR plus standard ST) and placebo (only standard ST) groups (assessed by standardized Persian language test). However, no difference between active and sham groups was observed and this dose seemed to be safer because all patients tolerated the dose-escalation protocol without major side effects.

Two year later, Restemeyer and colleagues[21] designed a similar study to that of Floel and colleagues.[15] On 2 different occasions, 10 subjects with ischemic chronic stroke (>6 months) received either 100 mg of L-dopa or placebo in a randomized order. After drug intake, they participated in 1 hour of PT designed to improve dexterity. Motor functions were tested by application of the Nine-hole Peg Test (NHPT), a dynamometer measuring grip strength, and the Action Research Arm Test (ARAT). In addition, TMS was applied to study intracortical excitability. TMS studies and motor function measurements were performed before drug intake, 45 minutes after drug ingestion, and after the PT. Compared with placebo, L-dopa neither improved motor functions nor changed motor excitability as tested by TMS.

Cramer and colleagues[25] investigated the effects of ropinirole on motor recovery after acute/chronic stroke (1–12 months after) with a large sample size (33; 16 active and 17 placebo). The study protocol was 9 weeks of immediate-release ropinirole or placebo, each with PT, and subjects were followed up for 3 additional weeks. Drug dose (0.25–4 mg once daily) was titrated weekly. For the first 4 weeks, and for weeks

6 to 9, PT was introduced, twice weekly, for 90 minutes per session. Each PT session began 60 minutes after pill ingestion and had 60 minutes focused on gait therapy and 30 minutes on arm therapy. Gait velocity, gait endurance, FM and BI were used in the assessment. At the doses achieved in this trial, increased dopaminergic tone via ropinirole plus PT was generally well tolerated but did not show any improvement beyond the effects of PT alone.[25]

A randomized, placebo-controlled, double-blinded study with 39 patients (20 active/19 placebo) with acute/subacute (2–8 weeks after) and ischemic/hemorrhagic stroke investigating improvement in speech recovery was performed by Seniów and colleagues[42] in the same year. Treatment protocol was either 100 mg of L-dopa or placebo 30 minutes before ST sessions conducted for 45 minutes every morning from Monday to Friday for 3 weeks. The Boston Diagnostic Aphasia Examination showed that patients receiving L-dopa experienced greater language improvement in verbal fluency and repetition, compared with patients receiving placebo. Improvement was particularly distinct in patients with anterior lesions.

A study combining L-dopa with repetitive transcranial magnetic stimulation (rTMS) and occupational therapy (OT) was published in the same year by Kakuda and colleagues.[28] It was a proof of concept study in which 5 chronic subjects (>1 years) received 100 mg/d for 7 weeks (1 week before the admission, 2 weeks during the inpatient stay, 4 weeks after discharge) along with 40 minutes of low-frequency rTMS and 4 hours for 2 weeks at the hospital. All patients showed an increased FM score over that time and the increase was maintained until 4 weeks after discharge in 4 patients. In addition, the sum of performance times for 15 tasks in the Wolf-Motor Function Test (WMFT) shortened over the treatment period and remained that way after the treatment in all the patients. The total WMFT score also increased in all the patients. Three patients showed a decrease in the Modified Ashworth Scale score with the treatment.

The most recent stroke study for this drug class came from Breitenstein and colleagues.[45] They designed a prospective, randomized, placebo-controlled and crossover study in which 10 subjects with chronic (>1 year) stroke received either 100/25 mg of L-dopa/carbidopa or placebo daily combined with 4 hours of language training for 2 weeks. Naming performance and verbal communication improved significantly and persistently for at least 6 months in every patient, but L-dopa had no incremental effect on intensive training.

In summary, mixed results are reported in the studies using dopaminergic agents to increase the effects of behavioral therapy. L-Dopa was the most used agent in these studies. Because of the side effect profile of these agents, some dose-escalation studies attempted to decrease possible side effects related to dopaminergic stimulation by adjusting the dose.

Selective Serotonergic/Noradrenergic Reuptake Inhibitors

A placebo-controlled experiment with crossover design was performed with 8 patients with pure motor hemiparesis caused by acute (2 weeks after) ischemic lacunar stroke. They received either 20 mg of fluoxetine (FLU) or placebo on 2 different occasions. A single dose of FLU was enough to modulate cerebral sensory-motor activation in patients. This redistribution of activation toward the motor cortex output activation was associated with an enhancement of motor performance. Significant improvement in grip strength and finger tapping was observed, but there was no significant difference in NHPT. fMRI showed that primary motor cortex activation enhanced with FLU but remained the same with placebo.[9]

Another experimental study with placebo-controlled and crossover design was performed by Zittel and colleagues[20] for reboxetine (RBX) on motor improvement in 10 patients with ischemic/hemorrhagic chronic stroke. Patients received a single dose of RBX (6 mg) or placebo with PT on 2 different occasions and were assessed by finger tapping speed, grip strength, NHPT, and TMS motor evoked potentials (MEPs). Compared with placebo, RBX ingestion was followed by an increase of tapping speed and grip strength in the paretic hand. Other than that, there was no difference between the two experiments.[20] The same group investigated the effects of citalopram on motor improvement in the same patient population (8 subjects were enrolled) with the same study protocol as in the RBX study. Compared with placebo, citalopram intake significantly improved performance of the NHPT for the paretic hand but not for the unaffected hand. Hand grip strength remained unchanged.[22]

Acler and colleagues[24] performed a placebo-controlled randomized clinical trial in which 20 subjects with acute (<10 days after) ischemic/hemorrhagic stroke were given 10 mg/d of citalopram or placebo coupled with PT for 4 months and assessed by National Institutes of Health Stroke Scale (NIHSS); BI for functional recovery, Lindmark Scale (LS) for hand and arm functionality; hamilton depression scale (HDS), Beck Depression Inventory for depressive symptoms; and TMS-derived values such as motor threshold, MEP amplitudes, and intracortical inhibition. Subjects taking citalopram showed a decrease of excitability compared with the unaffected hemisphere and better clinical improvement without notable side effects. After 1 month, both groups improved their motor performance significantly, but the treated group showed more improvement.

Three years later, Wang and colleagues[26] confirmed Zittel and colleagues'[20] positive findings concerning the effects of RBX on motor performance. They designed a similar experimental crossover study with 11 subjects having subacute/chronic (1–12 months) stroke with mild to moderate hand paresis. Subjects received a single oral dose of 6 mg of RBX or placebo in 2 different experiments and were assessed by ARAT, hand grip strength, finger tapping, rapid pointing movements, and fMRI. RBX administration significantly increased maximum grip power and index finger tapping frequency of the paretic hand. Enhanced motor performance was associated with a reduction of cortical hyperactivity toward physiologic levels as observed in healthy control subjects.[26]

A French group reported the results of their large, multicenter placebo-controlled 1:1 randomized clinical trial (FLAME trial), which enrolled 118 subjects with acute (5–10 days after) ischemic stroke with hemiplegia/hemiparesis undergoing 20 mg FLU or placebo combined with normal PT for 3 months, and assessed by FM, NIHSS, mRS, and Montgomery Asberg Depression Scale (MADRS). FM score at day 90 was significantly greater in the FLU group, but NIHSS, mRS, and MADRS did not differ between the 2 groups. Two of the adverse events in the active group were serious (1 hyponatremia and 1 partial epileptic seizure) and 2 patients died (1 in each group).[27]

Reports from studies with selective serotonin reuptake inhibitors and serotonin-norepinephrine reuptake inhibitors show consistent beneficial results on motor recovery after stroke. However, heterogeneity of outcome measures and lack of standardization of behavioral therapy were the main limiting factors that prevented a definite conclusion.

Acetylcholinesterase Inhibitors (Galantamine/Donepezil/Memantine)

Nadeau and colleagues[14] tested donepezil as an adjuvant to constraint-induced therapy (CIT) for upper-limb recovery with a placebo-controlled, parallel-design clinical trial in which 20 subjects with chronic (>1 year) stroke received 10 mg/d of donepezil or placebo with CIT of upper limb (6 hours 10 times throughout last 2 weeks of 6 weeks of medication therapy). Participants were assessed with various motor and functional tests, such as the Box and Block Test, WMFT, FM Upper Extremity, motor activity log, finger tapping test, Stroke Impact Scale, and Caregiver Strain Index. Subjects in the donepezil group showed greater improvements in WMFT scores but the results of other tests were inconclusive.

Berthier and colleagues[38] performed 2 separate clinical trials in 2003 and 2006 to assess donepezil's effects on poststroke aphasia. The first study was a 20-week open-label pilot study in which 10 subjects with chronic poststroke aphasia received donepezil (5 mg/d for the first 4 weeks, followed by 10 mg/d for 12 weeks, and then a 4-week washout period). Donepezil improved the aphasia quotient (AQ) score of the Western Aphasia Battery (WAB) and Psycholinguistic Assessment of Language Processing in Aphasia (PALPA) scores in 6 of the 9 domains (phonemic discrimination of nonwords, repetition of words, repetition of nonwords, oral word-picture match, naming by frequency, and oral sentence-picture match). There were no differences in performance on AQ-WAB and PALPA between 5-mg and 10-mg daily doses. The second study was 1:1 randomized and placebo controlled, and 26 participants with chronic poststroke aphasia underwent donepezil (with the same 20-week dose-escalation treatment) or placebo along with ST (2 hours/wk for 20 weeks). The severity of aphasia (AQ of the WAB) and the picture-naming subtest of PALPA improved more in the donepezil group than in the placebo group at week 16. Other subsets of PALPA and communicative activity log (CAL) showed no difference between groups.[40]

Berthier and colleagues[43] studied another acetylcholinesterase inhibitor, memantine, in chronic poststroke aphasia 3 years later. Twenty-seven patients were randomized to memantine (20 mg/d) or placebo only during 16 weeks, followed by memantine coupled with constraint-induced aphasia therapy (CIAT) (weeks 16–18), memantine alone again (weeks 18–20), washout (weeks 20–24), and then an open-label extension phase of memantine (weeks 24–48). The memantine group showed significantly better improvement on AQ-WAB and CAL compared with the placebo group during treatment and washout periods. CIAT treatment resulted in significant improvement in both groups, which was even greater in the memantine group. Beneficial effects of memantine were maintained in the long-term follow-up evaluation, and the same effects were seen in patients who switched to memantine from placebo.[43]

Hong and colleagues[47] performed a randomized placebo-controlled study in 45 patients with chronic (>1 year) poststroke aphasia who received galantamine (8 mg/d for 4 weeks, and 16 mg/d for the following 12 weeks) or placebo. AQ score of WAB showed significant improvement in the galantamine group but not in the control group. Subcortical dominant lesion was found to be the independent determinant for galantamine responsiveness.

Studies with acetylcholinesterase inhibitors in poststroke speech recovery showed consistently beneficial effects.[14] However, more studies from different centers around the world are needed to confirm that these agents are helpful in poststroke speech recovery.

Piracetam

Enderby and colleagues[32] investigated piracetam's effects on speech and functional recovery in the subacute period (6–9 weeks after) of cerebral infarction in the carotid artery territory. Sixty-seven aphasic patients received piracetam (4.8 g/d) or placebo for 12 weeks together with standard inpatient rehabilitation and were assessed by BI and Kuriansky Test for ADLs and Aachen Aphasia Test (AAT) for the subset of patients with aphasia. AAT subtest scores revealed a significant overall improvement compared with baseline in favor of piracetam immediately after treatment. There was no significant difference in improvement of ADLs between the two groups.

Another large-scale, randomized, placebo-controlled clinical trial was performed by De Deyn and colleagues[33] 3 years later in 927 patients with very acute ischemic stroke (<12 hours). These patients were recruited from 55 hospitals in 10 European countries, of whom 373 were aphasic and were analyzed separately from the others (placebo group, n = 193; treatment group, n = 180). The active group received piracetam 12 g in a bolus intravenously within 12 hours after stroke onset, followed by piracetam 12 g per day intravenously until the fourth day, then 12 g of piracetam per day orally until 4 weeks, and then 4.8 g per day for 8 weeks. The Frenchay Aphasia Screening Test (FAST) was used for aphasia and BI for ADLs. A statistically significant difference was found in favor of the treated aphasic group on the FAST test at day 84. In a pre-defined subgroup analysis of a group who were aphasic and treated within 7 hours of the stroke, there were statistically significant differences in language function on aphasia testing, and in other parameters of functioning at the end of the study period, in favor of the treated group.

Kessler and colleagues[35] performed a randomized (1:1) placebo-controlled clinical trial in 24 patients with acute ischemic stroke (14 days after) who received 6 weeks of 2400 mg of piracetam twice daily coupled with 30 sessions of ST 5 times a week for 60 minutes. The patients were assessed by AAT, PET, and neuropsychological battery that included a verbal fluency task, Corsi block span test, a modified laterally score after Oldfield, tests for apraxia, progressive matrices of Raven, and the Benton test. Both groups showed significant reduction in the token test error rate. Although the placebo group showed improvement in written language and in comprehension, the piracetam group showed significant improvement not only in the subtests for written language, naming on confrontation, and comprehension but also in spontaneous speech, especially in communicative verbal behavior, and in the semantic and syntactic structure of their speech. In the piracetam group, increase of activation effect was significantly higher in the left transverse temporal gyrus, left triangular part of inferior frontal gyrus, and left posterior superior temporal gyrus. However, the placebo group showed an increase of activation effect only in the left vocalization area.

A year later, another group from Germany confirmed Kessler and colleagues'[35] findings with the same 6-week treatment protocol with the same outcome measures[35] but using electroencephalography (EEG) instead of PET. Both groups improved significantly in most of the assessments but improvement in the syntactic structure of spontaneous speech and reduction in the error rate were in favor of the piracetam group. In the piracetam group, EEG revealed a significant shift in the alpha rhythm from frontal to occipital regions, which can be interpreted as the improvement of the recovery.[36]

Likewise, Gungor and colleagues[44] investigated the effects of piracetam on speech and general recovery in acute ischemic stroke but with a longer treatment protocol. Thirty patients received 4.8 g of piracetam daily or placebo (1:1 design); treatment of 6 months; and assessment by Gulhane Aphasia Test (GAT; includes spontaneous speech, reading fluency, auditory comprehension, reading comprehension, repetition, naming, and writing), mRS, BI, and NIHSS. Other than the auditory comprehension subtest of the GAT, no significant difference was noted in favor of piracetam treatment.

Piracetam was mainly used in speech recovery after stroke. Except for the work of Gungor and colleagues,[44] beneficial effects of earlier studies were not tested by more recent investigations. Another interesting finding is that, to our knowledge, there have been no studies performed with English-speaking subjects.

Citicoline

The first study investigating the effects of citicoline on motor recovery after stroke came from Hazama and colleagues[2] in 1980 in 165 participants with subacute/chronic

(>3 months) stroke and who received a high dose of citicoline (1 g/d/8 weeks; n = 55), low-dose citicoline (250 mg/d/8 weeks; n = 56), or placebo (n = 54) coupled with a functional rehabilitation program. A 12-grade scale (Hemiplegia Function Test) showed that improvements by 1 or more grades in the fourth and eighth weeks were seen in 44.4% and 53.3% of the high-dose patients, in 29.3% and 54.8% of the low-dose treated patients, respectively. These rates of improvement were higher than the 29.3% and 31.8% rates in the placebo group. The difference reached statistical significance at week 8. More than a decade later, the same group performed another placebo-controlled clinical trial to confirm the results of the previous trial but with no low-dose group and limiting the chronicity of stroke by 1 year. The same 8-week design with high-dose and placebo groups going through the same Hemiplegia Function Test was performed with 248 patients. The rates of improvement by 1 or more grades in upper-extremity function were 67.8% in the citicoline group and 55.4% in the placebo group ($P = .047$), with no safety concerns. After 2 trials, it was concluded that citicoline improves motor function in patients with poststroke hemiplegic under rehabilitation programs.[4]

Iranmanesh and Vakilian[23] focused on the efficiency of citicoline to increase muscular strength in patients with nontraumatic very acute (<6 hours) hemorrhagic stroke. Thirty-two patients with supratentorial cerebral infarction received citicoline (250 mg intravenously twice a day) or placebo for 14 days, and their muscular strength was measured through physical examination before treatment and then 3 months later. The mean muscular strength in both groups before intervention was 2.5 out of 5 in manual muscle testing. Muscular strength in patients with cerebral hemorrhage receiving citicoline increased, and this suggests that citicoline may be effective in the treatment of patients with cerebral hemorrhage.[23]

Citicoline, an agent used mainly for overall recovery after ischemic stroke, was also investigated for poststroke motor recovery. Although the positive results in Hazama and Ueda's early large clinical trials were supported by another group with a smaller trial,[23] more studies are needed to reach an agreement on the beneficial effects of the agent.

Moclobemide: Monoamine Oxidase Inhibitor

Moclobemide was studied for acute poststroke aphasia by Laska and colleagues.[39] Sixty-five patients with acute ischemic/hemorrhagic stroke (<3 weeks) received moclobemide (started with 300 mg and escalated to 600 mg in a month) or placebo for 6 months along with routine inpatient rehabilitation. The Reinvang Grunntest for afasi and the Amsterdam-Nijmegen Everyday Language Test were used for assessment and the degree of aphasia decreased significantly at 6 months, with no difference between the moclobemide-treated and the placebo-treated groups. Results of this single study have not been replicated by others.

Lithium

An interesting clinical trial that studied the efficacy of the drug mainly used for bipolar disease, lithium, on the motor and general recovery after very acute (<48 hours) ischemic stroke came from Mohammadianinejad and colleagues[30] in 2014. For 1 month, 66 participants received 300 mg of lithium or placebo twice daily along with inpatient therapy based on the patient's situation, such as splint and orthosis, exercises for strengthening, positioning, stretching, and initials of occupational therapy (OT). Modified NIHSS (mNIHSS) and upper-limb FM were performed the fifth day and at the end of therapy. There were no significant differences in the improvement in mNIHSS and FM after 30 days. However, a subgroup analysis showed that patients with cortical strokes in the lithium group had significantly better improvement in both mNIHSS and FM compared with the placebo group. Despite a narrow therapeutic range and concerns for toxicity, this agent might find a place in poststroke recovery in the future if more studies from different centers confirm the beneficial effects.

SUMMARY

This article summarizes the main past clinical trials with various pharmacologic agents used to enhance motor (see **Table 1**) and speech (see **Table 2**) recovery after stroke. Pharmacologic augmentation of conventional therapies to enhance stroke motor and speech recovery seems beneficial. However, most of the clinical trials have been small, with narrow eligibility criteria, and the results of some are ambiguous. Timing and dose of medication have been variable between studies, as has the type of PT/OT or ST performed. These issues need to be systematically explored in adequately powered, randomized, double-blind clinical trials. Although promising results have been reported, at this point, the use of these pharmacologic agents is not supported by class I evidence.

ACKNOWLEDGMENTS

The authors thank Nikola Dragojlovic, DO, from Physical Medicine and Rehabilitation at University of Texas Health Science Center, Houston for help in the article preparation.

REFERENCES

1. Go AS, Mozaffarian D, Roger VL, et al. Heart disease and stroke statistics–2014 update: a report from the American Heart Association. Circulation 2014;129(3): 399–410.
2. Hazama T, Hasegawa T, Ueda S, et al. Evaluation of the effect of CDP-choline on post-stroke hemiplegia employing a double-blind controlled trial. Int J Neurosci 1980;11:211–25.
3. Crisostomo EA, Duncan PW, Propst M, et al. Evidence that amphetamine with physical therapy promotes recovery of motor function in stroke patients. Ann Neurol 1988;23(1):94–7.
4. Ueda S, Hasegawa T, Ando K, et al. Evaluation of the pharmacological effect of CDP-choline injection in post-stroke hemiplegia. Strides of Medicine 1994;170: 297–314.
5. Walker-Batson D, Smith P, Curtis S, et al. Amphetamine paired with physical therapy accelerates motor recovery after stroke: further evidence. Stroke 1995; 26(12):2254–9.
6. Reding MJ, Solomon B, Borucki S. Effect of D-amphetamine on motor recovery after stroke. Neurology 1995;45(4):A222.
7. Dam M, Tonin P, De Boni A, et al. Effects of fluoxetine and maprotiline on functional recovery in poststroke hemiplegic patients undergoing rehabilitation therapy. Stroke 1996;27(7):1211–4.
8. Grade C, Redford B, Chrostowski J, et al. Methylphenidate in early poststroke recovery: a double-blind, placebo-controlled study. Arch Phys Med Rehabil 1998; 79(9):1047–50.
9. Pariente J, Loubinoux I, Carel C, et al. Fluoxetine modulates motor performance and cerebral activation of patients recovering from stroke. Ann Neurol 2001; 50(6):718–29.

10. Scheidtmann K, Fries W, Muller F, et al. Effect of levodopa in combination with physiotherapy on functional motor recovery after stroke: a prospective, randomized, double-blind study. Lancet 2001;358(9284):787–90.

11. Sonde L, Nordstrom M, Nilsson CG, et al. A double-blind placebo-controlled study of the effects of amphetamine and physiotherapy after stroke. Cerebrovasc Dis 2001;12(3):253–7.

12. Martinsson L, Wahlgren NG. Safety of D-amphetamine in acute ischemic stroke: a randomized, double-blind, controlled dose-escalation trial. Stroke 2003;34(2):475–81.

13. Treig T, Werner C, Sachse M, et al. No benefit from D-amphetamine when added to physiotherapy after stroke: a randomized, placebo-controlled study. Clin Rehabil 2003;17(6):590–9.

14. Nadeau SE, Behrman AL, Davis SE, et al. Donepezil as an adjuvant to constraint-induced therapy for upper-limb dysfunction after stroke: an exploratory randomized clinical trial. J Rehabil Res Dev 2004;41(4):525–34.

15. Floel A, Hummel F, Breitenstein C, et al. Dopaminergic effects on encoding of a motor memory in chronic stroke. Neurology 2005;65(3):472–4.

16. Tardy J, Pariente J, Leger A, et al. Methylphenidate modulates cerebral post-stroke reorganization. Neuroimage 2006;33(3):913–22.

17. Gladstone DJ, Danells CJ, Armesto A, et al. Physiotherapy coupled with dextroamphetamine for rehabilitation after hemiparetic stroke: a randomized, double-blind, placebo-controlled trial. Stroke 2006;37(1):179–85.

18. Sonde L, Lokk J. Effects of amphetamine and/or L-dopa and physiotherapy after stroke? A blinded randomized study. Acta Neurol Scand 2007;115(1):55–9.

19. Sprigg N, Willmot MR, Gray LJ, et al. Amphetamine increases blood pressure and heart rate but has no effect on motor recovery or cerebral hemodynamics in ischemic stroke: a randomized controlled trial (ISRCTN 36285333). J Hum Hypertens 2007;21(8):616–24.

20. Zittel S, Weiller C, Liepert J. Reboxetine improves motor function in chronic stroke. J Neurol 2007;254(2):197–201.

21. Restemeyer C, Weiller C, Liepert J. No effect of a levodopa single dose on motor performance and motor excitability in chronic stroke. A double-blind placebo-controlled cross-over pilot study. Restor Neurol Neurosci 2007;25(2):143–50.

22. Zittel S, Weiller C, Liepert J. Citalopram improves dexterity in chronic stroke patients. Neurorehabil Neural Repair 2008;22(3):311–4.

23. Iranmanesh F, Vakilian A. Efficiency of citicoline in increasing muscular strength of patients with nontraumatic cerebral hemorrhage: a double-blind randomized clinical trial. J Stroke Cerebrovasc Dis 2008;17(3):153–5.

24. Acler E, Robol E, Fiaschi A, et al. A double blind placebo RCT to investigate the effects of serotonergic modulation on brain excitability and motor recovery in stroke patients. J Neurol 2009;256(7):1152–8.

25. Cramer SC, Dobkin BH, Noser EA. Randomized, placebo-controlled, double-blind study of ropinirole in chronic stroke. Stroke 2009;40(9):3034–8.

26. Wang LE, Fink GR, Diekhoff S, et al. Noradrenergic enhancement improves motor network connectivity in stroke patients. Ann Neurol 2011;69(2):375–88.

27. Chollet F, Tardy J, Albucher JF, et al. Fluoxetine for motor recovery after acute ischemic stroke (FLAME): a randomized placebo-controlled trial. Lancet Neurol 2011;10(2):123–30.

28. Kakuda W, Abo M, Kobayashi K, et al. Combination treatment of low-frequency rTMS and occupational therapy with levodopa administration: an intensive

neurorehabilitative approach for upper limb hemiparesis after stroke. Int J Neurosci 2011;121(7):373–8.

29. Schuster C, Maunz G, Lutz K, et al. D-amphetamine improves upper extremity outcome during rehabilitation after stroke: a pilot randomized controlled trial. Neurorehabil Neural Repair 2011;25(8):749–55.

30. Mohammadianinejad SE, Majdinasab N, Sajedi SA, et al. The effect of lithium in post-stroke motor recovery. Clin Neuropharmacol 2014;37(3):73–8.

31. Walker-Batson D, Unwin H, Curtis S, et al. Use of amphetamine in the treatment of aphasia. Restor Neurol Neurosci 1992;4(1):47–50.

32. Enderby P, Broeckx J, Hospers H, et al. Effect of piracetam on recovery and rehabilitation after stroke: a double-blind, placebo-controlled study. Clin Neuropharmacol 1994;17(4):320–31.

33. De Deyn PP, Reuck JD, Deberdt W, et al. Treatment of acute ischemic stroke with piracetam. Stroke 1997;28(12):2347–52.

34. Bragoni M, Altieri M, Di Piero V, et al. Bromocriptine and speech therapy in non-fluent chronic aphasia after stroke. Neurol Sci 2000;21(1):19–22.

35. Kessler J, Thiel A, Karbe H, et al. Piracetam improves activated blood flow and facilitates rehabilitation of poststroke aphasic patients. Stroke 2000;31(9):2112–6.

36. Szelies B, Mielke R, Kessler J, et al. Restitution of alpha-topography by piracetam in post-stroke aphasia. Int J Clin Pharmacol Ther 2001;39(4):152–7.

37. Walker-Batson D, Curtis S, Natarajan R, et al. A double-blind, placebo-controlled study of the use of amphetamine in the treatment of aphasia. Stroke 2001;32(9): 2093–8.

38. Berthier ML, Marcelo L, Hinojosa J, et al. Open-label study of donepezil in chronic poststroke aphasia. Neurology 2003;60(7):1218–9.

39. Laska AC, von Arbin M, Kahan T, et al. Long-term antidepressant treatment with moclobemide for aphasia in acute stroke patients: a randomized, double-blind, placebo-controlled study. Cerebrovasc Dis 2005;19(2):125–32.

40. Berthier ML, Green C, Higueras C, et al. A randomized, placebo-controlled study of donepezil in poststroke aphasia. Neurology 2006;67(9):1687–9.

41. Ashtary F, Janghorbani M, Chitsaz A, et al. A randomized, double-blind trial of bromocriptine efficacy in nonfluent aphasia after stroke. Neurology 2006;66(6): 914–6.

42. Seniów J, Litwin M, Litwin T, et al. New approach to the rehabilitation of post-stroke focal cognitive syndrome: effect of levodopa combined with speech and language therapy on functional recovery from aphasia. J Neurol Sci 2009; 283(1–2):214–8.

43. Berthier ML, Green C, Lara JP, et al. Memantine and constraint-induced aphasia therapy in chronic poststroke aphasia. Ann Neurol 2009;65(5):577–85.

44. Gungor L, Terzi M, Onar MK. Does long term use of piracetam improve speech disturbances due to ischemic cerebrovascular diseases? Brain Lang 2011; 117(1):23–7.

45. Breitenstein C, Korsukewitz C, Baumgärtner A, et al. L-dopa does not add to the success of high-intensity language training in aphasia. Restor Neurol Neurosci 2015;33(2):115–20.

46. Engelter ST. Safety in pharmacological enhancement of stroke rehabilitation. Eur J Phys Rehabil Med 2013;49(2):261–7.

47. Hong JM, Shin DH, Lim TS, et al. Galantamine administration in chronic post-stroke aphasia. J Neurol Neurosurg Psychiatry 2012;83(7):675–80.

Robotic Therapy and the Paradox of the Diminishing Number of Degrees of Freedom

Hermano Igo Krebs, PhD[a,b,c,d,e,*], Eiichi Saitoh, MD[c],
Neville Hogan, PhD[a,f]

KEYWORDS

- Robotic therapy • Rehabilitation robotics • Stroke • Impairment-based therapy
- Functional-based therapy • Degrees of freedom

KEY POINTS

- Robot-assisted therapy for the upper extremity has already achieved class I, level of evidence A for stroke care in the outpatient setting and care in chronic care settings.
- At least in the US Department of Veterans Affairs (VA) health care system, robot-assisted therapy for the upper extremity has not increased the total health care utilization cost.
- Functionally based robotic training did not demonstrate any advantage over impairment-based robotic training.
- The paradox of diminishing number of degrees of freedom (DOFs) suggests an approach to tailor therapy to a particular patient's needs.

INTRODUCTION: DISRUPTIVE TECHNOLOGY

Three years ago, the authors discussed the concept of disruptive technology and rehabilitation robotics (parts of this review have been published elsewhere).[1] As

---

Disclosures: This work was supported in part by grants from the NIH R01 HD069776 to H.I. Krebs and the Eric P. and Evelyn E. Newman Fund. H.I. Krebs and N. Hogan are co-inventors of several Massachusetts Institute of Technology (MIT)–held patents for the robotic technology. They hold equity positions in Interactive Motion Technologies (Watertown, Massachusetts, US) the company that manufactures this type of technology under license to MIT.
[a] Department of Mechanical Engineering, Massachusetts Institute of Technology, 77 Massachusetts Avenue, Cambridge, MA 02139, USA; [b] Department of Neurology, University of Maryland, School of Medicine, 620 W Lexington St, Baltimore, MD 21201, USA; [c] Department of Rehabilitation Medicine I, School of Medicine, Fujita Health University, 1-98 Dengakugakubo, Kutsukake, Toyoake, Aichi, 470-1192, Japan; [d] Institute of Neuroscience, Newcastle University, Framlington Place, Newcastle upon Tyne, NE2 4HH, UK; [e] Department of Mechanical Engineering, Osaka University, 2-1 Yamadaoka, Suita, Osaka 565-0871, Japan; [f] Department of Brain and Cognitive Sciences, Massachusetts Institute of Technology, 77 Massachusetts Avenue, Cambridge, MA 02139, USA
* Corresponding author.
E-mail address: hikrebs@mit.edu

Phys Med Rehabil Clin N Am 26 (2015) 691–702
http://dx.doi.org/10.1016/j.pmr.2015.06.003
1047-9651/15/$ – see front matter © 2015 Elsevier Inc. All rights reserved.

described then and replicated in this article, disruptive technology is a term coined to characterize an innovation that disrupts an existing market or way of doing things and creates a new value network. The concept was introduced by Christensen and colleagues, who described the concept in 1996 as "Generally, disruptive innovations were technologically straightforward, consisting of off-the-shelf components put together in a product architecture that was often simpler than prior approaches.[2,3] They offered less of what customers in established markets wanted and so could rarely be initially employed there. They offered a different package of attributes valued only in emerging markets remote from, and unimportant to, the mainstream." Eventually with improvement, borrowing from Malcolm Gladwell, the moment of critical mass (the threshold or the boiling point) is reached and the old practices and existing value network abandoned in favor of the new one, also referred to "the tipping point."[4]

UPPER EXTREMITY ROBOTIC THERAPY: THE TIPPING POINT

Since the publication of the first controlled study with stroke inpatients,[5] several studies have been completed with both stroke inpatients and outpatients demonstrating the potential of robotic therapy for the upper extremity. These results were discussed in different meta-analyses (for example, in Refs.[6–8]) and led to the 2010 American Heart Association (AHA) guidelines for stroke care: "Robot-assisted therapy offers the amount of motor practice needed to relearn motor skills with less therapist assistance... Most trials of robot-assisted motor rehabilitation concern the upper extremity (UE), with robotics for the lower extremity (LE) still in its infancy... Robot-assisted UE therapy, however, can improve motor function during the inpatient period after stroke." AHA suggested that robot-assisted therapy for the upper extremity has already achieved class I, level of evidence A for stroke care in the outpatient setting and care in chronic care settings. It suggested that robot-assisted therapy for upper extremity has achieved class IIa, level of evidence A for stroke care in the inpatient setting. Class I is defined as "Benefit >>> Risk. Procedure/Treatment SHOULD be performed/administered" (where >>> indicates that "much larger than"); class IIa is defined as "Benefit >> Risk, IT IS REASONABLE to perform procedure/administer treatment" (where >> indicates "larger than"); and level A is defined as "Multiple populations evaluated: Data derived from multiple randomized controlled trials (RCTs) or meta-analysis."[9]

The 2010 VA/Department of Defense (DOD) guidelines for stroke care came to the same conclusion endorsing the use of rehabilitation robots for the upper extremity but went further to recommend against the use of robotics for the lower extremity. More specifically, the VA/DOD 2010 guidelines for stroke care "Recommend robot-assisted movement therapy as an adjunct to conventional therapy in patients with deficits in arm function to improve motor skill at the joints trained." More needs to be done, however, particularly for the lower extremity, as stated in the VA/DOD guidelines: "There is no sufficient evidence supporting use of robotic devices during gait training in patients post stroke" and "Recommendation is made against routinely providing the intervention to asymptomatic patients. At least fair evidence was found that the intervention is ineffective or that harms outweigh benefits."[10]

Currently the largest single study of upper extremity robotics confirms these endorsements for the upper extremity. The multisite, independently run, VA trial CSP-558 (Robotic Assisted Upper-Limb Neurorehabilitation in Stroke Patients [VA ROBOTICS]), on upper extremity rehabilitation robotics, using the commercial version of the MIT-Manus robot for shoulder and elbow therapy together with corresponding antigravity, wrist, and hand robots,[11] included 127 veterans with chronic stroke at least 6 months post–index stroke with an impairment level characterized by very severe to moderate (Fugl-Meyer assessment between 7 and 38 of 66 points for the upper extremity). Veterans with multiple strokes were included in this study that lasted for 36 weeks: a 12-week intervention followed by a follow-up period lasting 6 months. Veterans were randomly assigned to the robotic therapy group (RT), N = 49; the intensity-matched comparison group (ICT), N = 50; and the usual care group (UC), N = 28. VA ROBOTICS compared the efficacy of RT to UC and ICT. Usual care was not dictated or prescribed by the protocol. The treatment was allowed to vary per therapy targeting specifically the upper extremity, which consisted of an average of 3 sessions per week from therapists delivering treatment they deemed clinically appropriate for the upper extremity. The RT received 3 sessions per week of robotic training for the shoulder and elbow, wrist, and hand that delivered 1024 movements per session. The ICT received 3 sessions per week of a therapy created to have a therapist deliver comparable movement intensity and repetition to the RT during the same period. Contrary to other rehabilitation studies that used a control intervention expected to have little effect on the primary outcome,[12–14] VA ROBOTICS was unique in that it included an active control treatment group. The study was based on the hypothesis that RT would experience greater improvement in motor impairment at 12 weeks compared with UC and ICT, as measured by the upper extremity component of the Fugl-Meyer scale. The ICT intervention is not conventional therapy. It uses manual techniques but would likely be impractical to implement as clinical therapy. It is unlikely that therapists could consistently assist the paretic arm during standard clinical care for approximately 1000 movements per session as done for the ICT (instead of the typical 45 movements per session in usual care for chronic stroke patients[15]). The authors created this control treatment specifically to afford an objective cost analysis.[16]

RESULTS

The first and perhaps most understated finding of the VA ROBOTICS was that usual care did not reduce impairment or disability or improve quality of life in chronic stroke survivors. The usual care intervention had no measurable impact and, to conserve financial resources, it was discontinued as futile midway through the study.

The comparison between the RT and UC included (1) the comparison between the RT and UC subjects, which involved approximately only the first half of the RT when the UC was not discontinued, and (2) whether the changes were robust and long lasting. On this score, robot therapy was statistically superior to usual care in Stroke Impact Scale (quality of life) at the completion of the intervention and in the Fugl-Meyer Assessment (impairment) and Wolf Motor Function Test (function) 6 months after the completion of the intervention.

The results are far more impressive if the whole RT is compared with the UC and not just the analysis that focused on the first half of the study. Although the results at 12 weeks showed that the difference between the first half of the RT and UC was more than 2 Fugl-Meyer points, the difference between the complete RT and UC was 5 points in the Fugl-Meyer assessment, which corresponds to a minimum clinically important difference (MCID) in chronic stroke (**Fig. 1**[17–19]).

The reason(s) for the smaller clinical effects of the robotic intervention in the first stage of the study compared with the second stage of the study have not been established. The authors think this discrepancy is most likely due to the omission of a phase-in stage in this study.[20] When testing a new therapy, it is common practice to treat a predetermined number of subjects during the initial phase of the trial with the new therapy at each site before beginning data collection for the actual controlled trial to gain familiarity and expertise with the novel treatment and streamline the

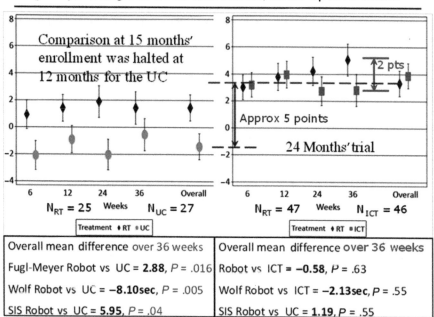

Fig. 1. VA ROBOTICS outcomes. The left column shows the comparison of the first half of the RT (Robot) with the UC. The right column shows the comparison of the RT and ICT. Note the added arrows to the figure: they indicate the advantage of the complete RT and the UC, which achieved the MCID threshold of 5 points in the Fugl-Meyer and the comparison between RT and the ICT after 6 months' follow-up.

process. Nevertheless, even without a phase-in stage, VA ROBOTICS demonstrates the robustness of the results: even when therapists are learning how to use the novel tools and cannot deliver the complete protocol in the prescribed period, the results are better than usual care.

The comparison between the RT and ICT did not show any difference.[16] Also patients in the RT continued to improve even after the intervention was completed at 12 weeks. Thus, the continued and persistent improvement at the 6-month follow-up evaluation suggests improved robustness and perhaps an incremental advantage that prompted further improvement even without intervention. For example, an improvement of approximately 3 points in the Fugl-Meyer scale might enable a severe patient to start to raise his/her arm and to bathe independently or to start to stretch the formerly paralyzed arm so that independent dressing could take place. It might enable a more moderate stroke patient to start to tuck in the shirt or to hike the pants independently or to start to reach overhead and actively grasp an object.

This continued improvement after completion of the intervention is remarkable because VA ROBOTICS included patients with chronic stroke disability in the moderate to severe range and more than 30% had multiple strokes. As such, the majority of this group represented a spectrum of disability burden that many studies have avoided. Moreover, 65% of the volunteers interviewed were enrolled. Together these observations suggest that robotic therapy for the upper extremity offers an opportunity to a broad spectrum of stroke patients.

COST OUTCOMES

In this era of cost containment, an important and unexpected result arose from the recently completed cost-benefit analysis.[21] The purchase cost of the 4 InMotion robotic modules (shoulder and elbow, wrist, antigravity, and hand [Interactive Motion Technologies, Watertown, Massachusetts] **Fig. 2**) was $230,750; the interest rate on borrowing to purchase these robots was estimated at 6.015% with 33% facility overhead on top of the purchase value and a $5000 annual maintenance fee per robot. Yet, the additional costs of delivering RT or ICT were $5152 and $7382, respectively, and the difference was statistically significant (P<.001). Although the active interventions (RT and ICT) added cost, when total cost was compared, which includes the clinical care needed to take care of these veterans for the 36 weeks of the trial (12 weeks of intervention and 6 months without any active intervention), there were no differences between active intervention and usual care. The total cost for the VA was approximately the same: $17,831 for RT; $19,746 for ICT; and $19,098 for UC. The UC used the rest of the health care system more often than the active intervention groups. For 36 weeks of care, the RT cost the VA $5152 for robotic therapy and $12,679 for clinical care. For 36 weeks of care, the UC cost the VA approximately $19,098.

The authors initially speculated that perhaps the surprising decreases in health care cost were due to a placebo or Hawthorne effect; the active groups (RT and ICT) received extra attention during the 36 weeks' trial duration. To determine whether that was the case, the VA health economists (VA Palo Alto Health Care System, Palo Alto, California) continued to collect cost data on these patients. If a placebo or Hawthorne effect accounted for a significant component of the observed cost reductions, costs would be expected to drift upward after trial completion. On the contrary, they did not for the RT. The health care costs until the end of September 2009 (after the 36 weeks of the trial) averaged $7777 for the RT and $14,513 for the ICT;

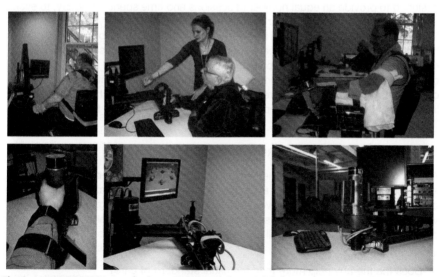

Fig. 2. VA ROBOTICS gym of robots. Top row (*left to right*) shows respectively the antigravity module, the shoulder and elbow robot, and the wrist robot. Bottom row (*left to right*) shows the hand module, the wrist module mounted at the tip of the shoulder and elbow robot, and the hand module mounted at the end-effector of the shoulder and elbow robot.

this difference was statistically significant ($P<.04$). In a nutshell, at least in the VA system, these results suggest better care for the same total cost.

LOWER EXTREMITY ROBOTIC THERAPY: IN ITS INFANCY

The 2 most common lower extremity robotic rehabilitation devices are the Lokomat (Hocoma, Zurich, Switzerland) and the AutoAmbulator (HealthSouth/Motorika, Caesarea, Israel). There are already more than 500 Lokomats and 100 AutoAmbulators in clinical settings, yet the negative perception of lower extremity robotic rehabilitation is not without merit. Although the installed robotic base is reasonably large, there are few published RCTs supporting their use. Some of the large studies using the Lokomat showed statistically significantly inferior results compared with those produced by usual care as practiced in the United States for both chronic and for subacute stroke patients.[22,23] The characteristics and intensity of usual care might vary according to the country; hence, it is important to acknowledge that these results are primarily valid for the United States. Nevertheless, these discouraging results demand explanation.

There are many plausible reasons for these results and the apparent immaturity of lower extremity robotic therapy. Given the success of upper extremity robotic therapy, it seems unlikely that the difficulties can be attributed to the use of technology. Instead, the authors think an important factor is that better understanding of the difference between best practices and tested practices is needed. Clinicians and technologists assumed that body weight–supported treadmill training (BWSTT) delivered by 2 or 3 therapists was an effective and superior form of therapy compared with usual care; thus, automating BWSTT seemed a logical approach. A National Institutes of Health–sponsored RCT demonstrated, however, that, contrary to the hypothesis of its clinical proponents, BWSTT administered by 2 or 3 therapists for 20 to 30 minutes followed by 20 to 30 minutes of overground carryover training did not lead to superior results compared with a home program of strength training and balance (Locomotor Experience Applied Post-Stroke [LEAPS] study[13]). The comparison treatment was designed to provide an equal number of sessions and time spent in therapy, to evoke a cardiovascular response similar to BWSTT, and to be sufficiently credible that participants considered themselves involved in meaningful therapy but "...expected to have little or no effect on the primary outcome, gait speed."[24] These are landmark results that must be seriously acknowledged by both roboticists and clinicians: the goal of rehabilitation robotics is to optimize care and augment the potential of individual recovery. It is not to automate current rehabilitation practices, which for the most part lack a scientific evidential basis, primarily due to the lack of tools to properly assess the practices themselves.[25]

DEFINING SUCCESS IN ROBOTIC REHABILITATION

A benchmark to determine whether a disruptive technology has gone beyond emerging markets and passed a tipping point to enter the mainstream must be defined.[4] To satisfy all perspectives and users without generating too much controversy, the authors think that the success of a therapeutic neurorehabilitation can be defined by positive answers to all of the following questions:

1. Does the therapy help?
2. Does the therapy help more than the usual standard of care?
3. Does the therapy help more than the usual standard of care at the same or lower cost?

   OR, if higher cost, does it present a positive cost/benefit ratio?

Take the example of VA ROBOTICS: the researchers compared 3 sets of chronic stroke patients: RT, ICT, and UC in the VA system.

Although the RT and ICT improved, the UC did not satisfy the first criterion: it did not lead to any measureable improvement in chronic stroke.

The RT and ICT also satisfied the second criterion: RT and ICT improved more than usual care.

When the authors benchmark these groups against each other in terms of cost, RT was considerably cheaper than the ICT and it led to slightly lower overall health care cost (intervention plus all the health care utilization costs) than both UC and ICT, thereby satisfying the third benchmark at least in the VA system, and whether the same is true in the United Kingdom will soon be learned (https://research.ncl.ac.uk/ratuls/).

In view of these 3 positive answers to the benchmarks, it can be argued that upper extremity interactive robotic rehabilitation has reached the tipping point,[4] moving it into mainstream rehabilitation services.

BEYOND THE TIPPING POINT: FUNCTIONAL REHABILITATION

Despite the evidence of success, there is little doubt that further progress is sorely needed (parts of this review have been published elsewhere).[26] An evidence-based example is reviewed that challenges a perceived best practice and argues how to move the field further. A postulated best practice to increase therapy effectiveness beyond past studies is to develop new whole-arm functionally based approaches that better integrate robotic treatment with clinical practice to enhance the carryover of robot trained movements into functional tasks. Two potential approaches to deliver such functional training are (1) to train functional tasks with the robot or alternatively and (2) to aim at impairment reduction at the capacity level with different robotic modules, breaking these functional tasks into components and relying on a therapist to facilitate carryover of observed impairment gains from robotic training into functional activities.

These 2 approaches are explored, with the expectation based on the perceived best practice that a robotic treatment protocol, properly targeted to emphasize a sequence and timing of sensory and motor stimuli similar to those naturally occurring in daily life tasks, could facilitate carryover of the observed gains in motor abilities, thereby conferring greater improvements in functional recovery. This approach is a departure from, for example, the VA ROBOTICS study (discussed previously) or the Robot Assisted Training for the Upper Limb after Stroke [RATULS] study (https://research.ncl.ac.uk/ratuls/), which was based on a bottom-up approach and assumed that improvements in underlying capacities would enhance motor function during activities and tasks, leaving it to the therapist to concatenate the different impairment gains into a coherent set of functional gains. The authors envisioned, instead, that functional rehabilitation robotics might be guided by a top-down rehabilitation approach, in which a person's identified goals for task performance are used in conjunction with our evaluation data to establish a treatment plan. Robotic technology would not only provide remediation for impairments at the capacity or body function levels (eg, strength and isolated movement) but also provide task-specific, intensive therapy for impaired body functions (eg, coordination of limb movement) that underlie task performance or activities. Although this top-down rationale is in line with current therapy views, there is some evidence that questions this view and raises the possibility that the opposite might be correct. For example, Platz[27] has shown that therapy aiming at impairment reduction seems to lead to better outcomes than functional/Bobath training for inpatients with severe impairment.

As a first step toward applying this top-down approach to rehabilitation robotics, the authors wanted to investigate the effects of different robotic therapy approaches on subjects' ability to reach, grasp, and release with a paretic arm and hand. The authors compared the effects of repetitive upper limb reaching training to a protocol in which integrated reach, grasp, and release training was implemented, hypothesizing that training the shoulder and elbow, wrist, and hand together (transport of the arm to the target and grasping/releasing an actual or a virtual object) should lead to better outcomes than simple training for one of the components of this functional task, namely transport of the arm (reaching or pointing to the target). Remarkably, the functionally based approach, which integrated training of limb transport with grasp/release, did not outperform the impairment-based approach training of limb transport in isolation.[26]

Expanding this idea further, Reinkensmeyer[28] used a novel a 6-DOFs exoskeleton (BONES [**Fig. 3**]) that allows movement of the upper limb to assist in rehabilitation.

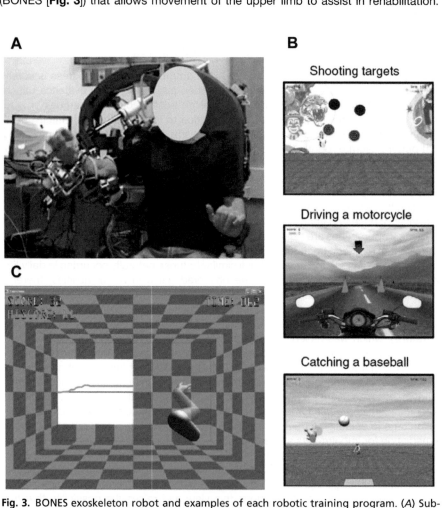

Fig. 3. BONES exoskeleton robot and examples of each robotic training program. (*A*) Subject training on BONES, (*B*) examples of games played during multijoint functional robotic training, and (*C*) example of single joint robotic training (shoulder flexion/extension). (*Courtesy of* D. Reinkensmeyer, MD, University of California, Irvine, CA; with permission.)

His objectives were to evaluate the impact of training with BONES on function of the affected upper limb and to assess whether multijoint functional robotic training would translate into greater gains in arm function than single-joint robotic training also conducted with BONES. He used a crossover design and tested 20 community-dwelling volunteers with mild to moderate chronic stroke. Each subject experienced 3 sessions per week, for 4 weeks, of multijoint functional training and single joint training (8 weeks total) with the order of presentation of the different approaches randomized.[28] Training with the robotic exoskeleton resulted in significant improvements in Box and Block Test, Fugl-Meyer Assessment, Wolf Motor Function Test, Motor Activity Log, and quantitative measures of strength and speed of reaching, and these improvements were sustained at the 3-month follow-up. Comparing the effect of type of training on the gains obtained, however, no significant difference was noted between multijoint functional and single-joint impairment training programs. These results confirmed those reported by Krebs and colleagues[26] and Platz and colleagues.[27] They suggest that multijoint functional training is not decisively superior to impairment training. This observation was further corroborated in an RCT using the ArmeoPower (Hocoma, Volketswil, Switzerland) and functional training, which achieved an advantage of only 0.78 points on the Fugl-Meyer assessment over usual care as practice in Switzerland (inferior results as compared to many studies employing impairment-based training).[14] This challenges the idea that functionally oriented games and training are key elements for improving behavioral outcomes; perhaps breaking it down is better.[29]

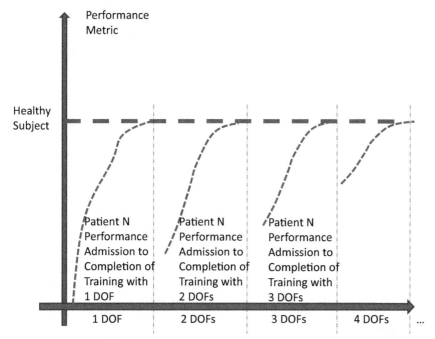

Fig. 4. The paradox of diminishing number of DOFs. The figure sketches the progression of Patient N with severe impairment, who should start training in a rehabilitation robotic device with the smallest number of DOFs that provide challenge and some level of success. Training should be enhanced to a robotic device with additional DOFs only when a ceiling effect is observed.

THE PARADOX OF THE DIMINISHING NUMBER OF DEGREES OF FREEDOM

The authors' work on multijoint functionally based robotic therapy leads to an additional question: How many DOFs should a robot provide for a particular patient? Because the evidence is sparse, these speculations should be taken with the appropriate caveats, but the authors strongly believe in what one author (ES) describes as the paradox of the diminishing number of DOFs. The paradox is that to reduce a person's impairment and increase motor control on a larger number of DOFs, the number of DOFs of the devices in which they train might need to be reduced. The paradox can be best explained in **Fig. 4**. A patient with severe impairment should train in a rehabilitation robotic device with the smallest number of DOFs that provides challenge and some level of success. Training should be enhanced to a robotic device with additional DOFs only when a ceiling effect is observed. The paradox also holds for assistive technology.

SUMMARY

In the authors' opinion, robotics are not a general panacea for stroke recovery; for clinically effective training, there should be a mandatory number of movements per session along the lines of the 10,000 hours of practice required to attain expert athlete levels of physical performance. Interactive robot–delivered therapy achieved 1000 to-and-from movements per 45 minutes of therapy session, far in excess of the 45 movement attempts under standard care.[15] Furthermore, VA ROBOTICS represents the tipping point of upper extremity robotic therapy. The authors contend that robotic therapy for the upper extremity that involves an interactive high-intensity, intention-driven therapy based on motor learning principles and assist as needed leads to better outcomes than usual care in chronic stroke (and probably with even a greater impact for subacute strokes). Moreover, this treatment modality is now practical to implement in the clinical realm. But much remains to be answered and researched.

How to tailor therapy for a particular patient's needs is still not known. The example presented in this article based on evidential data suggests that many of the perceived best practices (such as delivering functionally based rehabilitation approaches instead of impairment-based approaches) need to be carefully examined; the authors' results did not support this hypothesis. The authors speculate that until a minimum set of body functions is present, intensive robotic training might serve patients better if it focuses on impairment—in line with the paradox of the diminishing number of DOFs—leaving the functional integration of those gains for a later phase under the supervision of a therapist.

The situation is less bright for the lower extremity. Although it neither data nor with AHA or VA/DOD statements that robotic for lower extremity is still in its infancy cannot be argue, the authors believe that the field can mature and demonstrate its promise for lower extremity rehabilitation. The authors and other research groups are working toward such a goal of properly understanding the neuroscientific basis of gait and stroke recovery and of exploring creative solutions to move robotic therapy for the lower extremity to the same standing as upper extremity. Whether for the upper or lower extremities, therapeutic robotics is still a work in progress.

REFERENCES

1. Krebs HI, Hogan N. Robotic therapy: the tipping point. Am J Phys Med Rehabil 2012;91:S290–7.
2. Christensen CM, Suárez FF, Utterback JM. Strategies for survival in fast-changing industries. Cambridge (MA): International Center for Research on the

Management of Technology, Sloan School of Management, Massachusetts Institute of Technology; 1996.

3. Christensen CM. The innovator's dilemma: when new technologies cause great firms to fail. Boston: Harvard Business School Press; 1997.

4. Gladwell M. The tipping point: how little things can make a big difference. 1st edition. Boston: Little, Brown; 2000.

5. Aisen ML, Krebs HI, Hogan N, et al. The effect of robot-assisted therapy and rehabilitative training on motor recovery following stroke. Arch Neurol 1997;54: 443–6.

6. Kwakkel G, Kollen BJ, Krebs HI. Effects of robot-assisted therapy on upper limb recovery after stroke: a systematic review. Neurorehabil Neural Repair 2008;22: 111–21.

7. Norouzi-Gheidari N, Archambault PS, Fung J. Effects of robot-assisted therapy on stroke rehabilitation in upper limbs: systematic review and meta-analysis of the literature. J Rehabil Res Dev 2012;49:479–96.

8. Mehrholz J, Hadrich A, Platz T, et al. Electromechanical and robot-assisted arm training for improving generic activities of daily living, arm function, and arm muscle strength after stroke. Cochrane Database Syst Rev 2012;(6):CD006876.

9. Miller EL, Murray L, Richards L, et al, American Heart Association Council on Cardiovascular Nursing and the Stroke Council. Comprehensive overview of nursing and interdisciplinary rehabilitation care of the stroke patient: a scientific statement from the American Heart Association. Stroke 2010;41:2402–48.

10. Management of Stroke Rehabilitation Working Group. VA/DOD Clinical practice guideline for the management of stroke rehabilitation. J Rehabil Res Dev 2010; 47:1–43.

11. Lo AC, Guarino PD, Richards LG, et al. Robot-assisted therapy for long-term upper-limb impairment after stroke. N Engl J Med 2010;362:1772–83.

12. Wolf SL, Winstein CJ, Miller JP, et al. Effect of constraint-induced movement therapy on upper extremity function 3 to 9 months after stroke: the EXCITE randomized clinical trial. JAMA 2006;296:2095–104.

13. Duncan PW, Sullivan KJ, Behrman AL, et al. Body-weight-supported treadmill rehabilitation after stroke. N Engl J Med 2011;364:2026–36.

14. Klamroth-Marganska V, Blanco J, Campen K, et al. Three-dimensional, task-specific robot therapy of the arm after stroke: a multicentre, parallel-group randomised trial. Lancet Neurol 2014;13(2):159–66.

15. Lang CE, Macdonald JR, Reisman DS, et al. Observation of amounts of movement practice provided during stroke rehabilitation. Arch Phys Med Rehabil 2009;90:1692–8.

16. Volpe BT, Lynch D, Rykman-Berland A, et al. Intensive sensorimotor arm training mediated by therapist or robot improves hemiparesis in patients with chronic stroke. Neurorehabil Neural Repair 2008;22:305–10.

17. Page SJ, Fulk GD, Boyne P. Clinically important differences for the upper-extremity Fugl-Meyer Scale in people with minimal to moderate impairment due to chronic stroke. Phys Ther 2012;92:791–8.

18. Lin JH, Hsu MJ, Sheu CF, et al. Psychometric comparisons of 4 measures for assessing upper-extremity function in people with stroke. Phys Ther 2009;89:840–50.

19. Wagner JM, Rhodes JA, Patten C. Reproducibility and minimal detectable change of three-dimensional kinematic analysis of reaching tasks in people with hemiparesis after stroke. Phys Ther 2008;88:652–63.

20. Dobkin BH. Progressive staging of pilot studies to improve phase iii trials for motor interventions. Neurorehabil Neural Repair 2009;23:197–206.

21. Wagner TH, Lo AC, Peduzzi P, et al. An economic analysis of robot-assisted therapy for long-term upper-limb impairment after stroke. Stroke 2011;42:2630–2.

22. Hornby TG, Campbell DD, Kahn JH, et al. Enhanced gait-related improvements after therapist- versus robotic-assisted locomotor training in subjects with chronic stroke: a randomized controlled study. Stroke 2008;39:1786–92.

23. Hidler J, Nichols D, Pelliccio M, et al. Multicenter randomized clinical trial evaluating the effectiveness of the Lokomat in subacute stroke. Neurorehabil Neural Repair 2009;23:5–13.

24. Duncan PW, Sullivan KJ, Behrman AL, et al. Protocol for the Locomotor Experience Applied Post-stroke (LEAPS) trial: a randomized controlled trial. BMC Neurol 2007;7:39.

25. Dobkin BH, Duncan PW. Should body weight-supported treadmill training and robotic-assistive steppers for locomotor training trot back to the starting gate? Neurorehabil Neural Repair 2012;26:308–17.

26. Krebs HI, Mernoff S, Fasoli SE, et al. A comparison of functional and impairment-based robotic training in severe to moderate chronic stroke: a pilot study. Neuro-Rehabilitation 2008;23:81–7.

27. Platz T, Eickhof C, van Kaick S, et al. Impairment-oriented training or Bobath therapy for severe arm paresis after stroke: a single-blind, multicentre randomized controlled trial. Clin Rehabil 2005;19:714–24.

28. Milot MH, Spencer SJ, Chan V, et al. A crossover pilot study evaluating the functional outcomes of two different types of robotic movement training in chronic stroke survivors using the arm exoskeleton BONES. J Neuroeng Rehabil 2013; 10:112.

29. Klein J, Spencer SJ, Reinkensmeyer DJ. Breaking it down is better: haptic decomposition of complex movements aids in robot-assisted motor learning. IEEE Trans Neural Syst Rehabil Eng 2012;20:268–75.

The Split-Belt Walking Paradigm

Exploring Motor Learning and Spatiotemporal Asymmetry Poststroke

Erin E. Helm, DPT[a], Darcy S. Reisman, PT, PhD[b],*

KEYWORDS

- Stroke • Motor learning • Locomotion • Split-belt • Adaptation

KEY POINTS

- The split-belt paradigm can be used to examine motor learning or potentially as a rehabilitation intervention after stroke.
- After stroke, patients retain the ability to adapt their walking pattern to new constraints.
- Locomotor adaptation and learning may be slowed after stroke.
- Exaggeration of spatial gait asymmetries using the split-belt treadmill results in improved spatial gait symmetry.

INTRODUCTION

Stroke is the leading cause of long-term disability in the United States, with approximately 795,000 people experiencing a new or recurrent stroke each year.[1] A primary concern of individuals experiencing a stroke is the ability to regain ambulatory function.[2] Moreover, improved ambulatory function after stroke is linked to increased community participation, improved cardiovascular fitness, and decreased risk of stroke recurrence.[1] As such, gait retraining is a major component of rehabilitation.[3]

Gait after stroke is characterized by pronounced asymmetry.[4] Following stroke, individuals increase reliance on the nonparetic lower extremity in static standing as well as during ambulation. This results in a shortened nonparetic swing phase and

Funding from NIH grant 1R01HD078330-01A, 5R01HD078330.
Disclosures: The authors declare no material financial interests that relate to this research.
[a] Biomechanics and Movement Science Program, University of Delaware, 540 South College Avenue, Newark, DE 19716, USA; [b] Biomechanics and Movement Science Program, Department of Physical Therapy, University of Delaware, 540 South College Avenue, Newark, DE 19716, USA
* Corresponding author. University of Delaware, 540 South College Avenue, Newark, DE 19713.
E-mail address: dreisman@udel.edu

increased stance phase on the nonparetic lower extremity. The resulting spatiotemporal asymmetries (stance time, swing time, and step length asymmetries) are well documented in individuals after stroke.[4,5] Step length asymmetry, in particular, has been shown to influence other gait deviations. By taking a shorter nonparetic step, the propulsive force of the paretic limb is decreased, thereby limiting forward propulsion of the body.[6] Step length asymmetry and its associated gait deviations have been linked to decreased walking speed[6,7] and efficiency,[8] as well as decreased dynamic balance,[9] thereby limiting safe functional ambulation. Various novel rehabilitation interventions have attempted to target these asymmetries to improve safe locomotion. In particular, several studies have utilized principles of motor learning to target specific gait deviations utilizing a split-belt treadmill.[10–13]

The split-belt treadmill has 2 independent belts, one under each leg, so that subjects can walk with belts moving at the same speed, tied, or with the belts moving at different speeds, split-belt. By splitting the treadmill belt speeds in a 2 to 1 ratio, the paradigm requires both neurologically intact subjects[14] and subjects after stroke[10] to alter their coordination while walking. Initially, both spatial and temporal characteristics of step symmetry are altered; however, over a period of 10 to 15 minutes, this asymmetry will be reduced with the use of trial-and-error practice.[10,11,14] When returning the treadmill to a normal walking condition or a tied-belt configuration, both neurologically intact subjects and poststroke subjects demonstrate after effects, with a reversal of the initial asymmetry induced by the split-belt treadmill configuration. The presence of this after effect indicates that the nervous system has learned and stored a new locomotor pattern.[10,14,15] The use of trial-and-error practice, or adaptation, to a perturbing environment provides important insight into the ability of the poststroke central nervous system (CNS) to temporarily store and recall a motor memory.

Thus, the split-belt treadmill paradigm allows exploration of various aspects of motor learning, including adaptation and retention of a novel locomotor pattern, but also allows exploration of the capacity of the nervous system for error recognition and correction. Recent evidence suggests exaggeration of poststroke gait asymmetry using the split-belt treadmill can lead to after effects, resulting in a more symmetric pattern of walking on the treadmill as well as over ground.[10,11] With repeated exposure to split-belt treadmill walking subjects after stroke demonstrate longer-term improvements in step length symmetry.[12,16] Consequently, the split-belt treadmill can be utilized to facilitate improvements in asymmetric gait after stroke, or can be utilized as a specific probe of motor learning. This article discusses the current role of the split-belt treadmill in the examination of locomotor learning as well as a potential therapeutic tool for intervention in individuals after stroke.

ADAPTATION

Research employing principles of motor learning, specifically adaptation, have recently gained interest because of the ability to target specific gait abnormalities in individuals after stroke.[10–12,17] Within these studies, adaptation may be defined as the process of modifying or adjusting an already well-learned movement or motor skill based on error feedback.[15] This process of adaptation occurs over a period of trial-and-error practice in response to novel task demands.[15,18] Given this definition, motor adaptation can be considered as 1 specific component of motor skill learning. Once fully adapted, storage of a new motor pattern within the CNS is reflected through after effects. Upon removal of the stimulus, the subject is not able to retrieve the previous motor behavior.[19,20] The subject must de-adapt, during a period of continued practice without the perturbation, in order to return to his or her previous baseline motor performance.[20,21]

Given that motor adaptation involves relearning an already well known movement pattern, the process strongly reflects the relearning process of subjects after stroke early within a therapeutic intervention. As a short-term learning process, adaptation has gained interest within motor learning research, particularly locomotor learning. Locomotor adaptation affords the ability to learn and unlearn a given locomotor pattern rapidly depending on the environment, allowing for flexibility and efficiency.[17] The capacity of the nervous system to adapt to and store a new locomotor pattern that approximates an already stored walking pattern may provide insight into the ability of the damaged nervous system to regain a more normal walking pattern.[10,20,22]

When subjects are asked to walk on a split-belt treadmill, participants with chronic stroke and neurologically intact participants demonstrate an immediate reaction in which the leg on the slow belt will immediately spend more time in stance, and the fast leg will spend less time in stance to accommodate the difference in belt speeds.[10,14] When the belts are returned to normal conditions, tied belts, subjects immediately return stance times to the baseline walking pattern. Additional intralimb characteristics, including swing time, stride length, and intralimb joint kinematics, appear to demonstrate a similar pattern of reactive change to the split-belt treadmill condition with absence of adaptation and after effects.[10,14] These reactive changes require utilization of peripheral feedback and do not appear to rely on adaptive processes as indicated by lack of after effects.[10,14] In contrast, interlimb gait parameters of step length, double support time, and center of oscillation have been found to change slowly during locomotor adaptation and demonstrate appreciable after effects.[14] Specifically, step length asymmetry exaggerated by the split-belt paradigm requires a period of trial-and-error practice in order to reduce this asymmetry toward baseline. During the split-belt condition, an adaptive response occurs via feedforward changes in interlimb coordination in order to allow a return to normal step symmetry, despite the treadmill belts going 2 different speeds.[10,14] When the belts are returned to tied, neurologically intact subjects demonstrate step asymmetry in the opposite direction, while chronic stroke subjects may demonstrate an improved symmetry relative to baseline.

In patients after stroke, improved step length symmetry is only achieved through exaggeration of the subjects' initial step length asymmetry.[10] Specifically, an individual with stroke who ambulates with a longer paretic step length relative to the nonparetic step will walk on the split-belt treadmill with the paretic leg on the slow belt. When the treadmill is set to a 2 to 1 speed ratio, split-belt, the subject will initially walk with an even longer paretic step than demonstrated with baseline tied belt walking, thus exaggerating his or her step length asymmetry or error. Over a period of 10 to 15 minutes, individuals after stroke are able to reduce this asymmetry. When the belts are returned to the tied belt condition, after effects are evident, with subjects maintaining a more symmetric walking pattern.[10] The improved gait pattern also transfers to overground walking.[11] As in a true adaptation paradigm, however, the improved symmetry is short-lived, and subjects return to baseline asymmetry within several minutes. Despite the brevity of improved symmetry, the current findings demonstrate that individuals after stroke maintain the ability to ambulate with a more symmetric walking pattern.[10,11]

The studies presented demonstrate that individuals after stroke retain the basic capacity to adapt their walking pattern to novel environmental conditions. Recent locomotor adaptation studies also indicate, however, that the rate of adaptation is slowed after stroke.[13,23] Rate deficits appear to be specific to spatial rather than temporal gait parameters in those after stroke.[13] Differences in adaptation rates of temporal versus spatial characteristics of gait have been previously demonstrated in neurologically intact subjects.[24] Specifically, Malone and Bastian demonstrated that neurologically intact subjects walking on a split-belt treadmill were able to adapt limb phasing at a rate twice that of step length.[24] In addition, temporal characteristics of gait appear to be much more resistant to manipulations of practice structure[24] as well as developmental stage.[25] Young children demonstrate rates of adaption of center of oscillation and step length symmetry that improve with age, while rates of limb phase adaptation are similar regardless of age.[25] These differences in temporal versus spatial gait characteristics have been postulated to be caused by differing sites of neural control,[21,26] with temporal characteristics thought to be under subcortical control.

Recent exploration of locomotor adaptation in neurologically intact subjects utilizing the split-belt treadmill highlight additional constructs that may be utilized to enhance the rate of adaptation of spatial parameters after stroke. Providing visual feedback in order to allow conscious correction of step symmetry during split-belt adaptation in neurologically intact subjects resulted in an increased rate of adaptation, however also increased the rate of de-adaptation, thereby limiting the potential for increased retention of the split-belt pattern.[24] Performance of a secondary task while walking on the split-belt treadmill, however, resulted in a decreased rate of adaptation and de-adaptation, thereby allowing enhanced retention of the split-belt pattern. It is currently unknown whether this paradigm could be utilized in those after stroke given that individuals after stroke demonstrate difficulties with interference between cognitive tasks and motor control activities including gait.[27] Further research identifying specific task parameters that may improve or limit adaptation and retention of a novel locomotor pattern are required in order to develop targeted and effective interventions in those after stroke.

Although individuals with stroke retain the basic ability to adapt to the split-belt treadmill, recent evidence indicates that damage to the cerebellum, whether due to stroke or other causes, interferes with this adaptive capacity.[22] When exposed to the split-belt walking condition, patients with cerebellar lesions are able to make reactive, feedback-driven changes to intralimb characteristics including stride length, stance, and swing time. Subjects with cerebellar damage, however, are unable to utilize trial-and-error practice to adapt characteristics of interlimb coordination that require feedforward, predictive changes in gait.[22] Similar to previously cited studies, Morton and Bastian indicated that differing levels of locomotor adaptability, feedforward versus reactive, may be under separate neural control. Given that the control of motor learning is suggested to occur in multiple brain areas that may be affected by stroke, it is plausible that specific deficits in locomotor adaptation may be a result of deficits in acquisition of a motor skill within particular damaged cortical areas.

RETENTION

Motor learning can be defined as a set of processes associated with practice or experience leading to relatively permanent changes in skilled behavior.[28] To learn a motor skill requires increased practice over longer time periods and may be influenced by offline learning, consolidation, and long-term storage processes along with various cognitive processes including attention and decision making.[17] Restoration of movement function after stroke is thought to be a function of motor learning or relearning.[29] However, the optimal characteristics of learning that promote functional recovery of walking are not well defined for the poststroke population.

Few studies have examined the motor learning capability of individuals after stroke,[11,13,23,30–32] with most evidence confined to the upper extremity.[30–37] Winstein and colleagues[31] 1999 demonstrated that those with chronic stroke retain the ability to utilize augmented feedback in a manner similar to neurologically intact controls to learn a novel upper extremity task; however, they demonstrate greater errors and increased variability in their movements compared with controls. Platz and colleagues[32] also demonstrated that patients after stroke retain the ability to learn both simple and complex upper extremity motor tasks compared with neurologically intact controls. Subjects after stroke, however, demonstrated increased variability in their movements and increased errors, and required increased time for performance during skill acquisition of a more complex maze coordination task and peg board task.[32] These studies highlight the capability of patients after stroke to perform and retain a novel motor task with use of the upper extremity. They, also, however, call attention to an increase in variability and error during motor performance, in comparison to neurologically intact controls. It is plausible that this increased error and slowed performance may be increasingly detrimental in more complex functional tasks, such as locomotion, which may require increased practice to achieve learning and retention of the motor skill.

The capacity to learn a novel walking pattern has been explored in both neurologically intact people[14,21,38] and individuals following stroke[10,11] utilizing the split-belt treadmill during single sessions of adaptation. The split-belt treadmill has also recently been used to characterize longer-term motor learning.[13,26] To assess longer-term motor learning, participants are asked to walk on the split-belt treadmill over the course of days. If participants have learned something about how to walk on the split-belt treadmill, with each subsequent day of exposure the participant will be less perturbed by the split-belt condition and will therefore demonstrate less initial asymmetry.[26] In addition, it would be expected that with each day, the time required to reduce the asymmetry and achieve a more stable pattern of locomotion would be reduced, indicating a faster rate of readaptation. Through evaluation of the rate and magnitude of learning one can determine whether subjects can successfully learn a novel walking pattern specific to the split-belt treadmill.

Tyrell and colleagues[13] had subjects with chronic stroke and age and sex-matched neurologically intact controls participate in 15 minutes of split-belt walking at a 2 to 1 speed ratio for 5 consecutive days. Retention of the newly learned walking pattern was assessed each day and with a final 15-minute split-belt treadmill session after 2 days without exposure to the split-belt treadmill. Similar to previously cited studies,[10,11] they found that those with chronic stroke retain the ability to acquire a novel locomotor pattern through adaptation to an exaggeration of step length asymmetry. Subjects after stroke also demonstrated similar retention of the split-belt locomotor pattern on the sixth day of split-belt practice. However, compared with neurologically intact controls, subjects after stroke demonstrated a slowed rate of adaptation to the split-belt paradigm on the initial day of practice as well as a slowed rate of readaptation and reduction in initial step asymmetry over the course of 5 days. These results are similar to previously evidenced results in the upper extremity,[31,32] as well as a recent locomotor adaptation paradigm.[23] Savin and colleagues[23] required subjects with hemiparesis as well as neurologically intact controls to overcome a novel swing phase resistance during treadmill walking. They found that both neurologically intact and chronic stroke subjects were able to adapt both temporal and spatial parameters of gait. Those with chronic stroke, however, differed in the rate of adaptation, requiring increased repetition compared with controls. This study did not examine the rate of learning over subsequent days.

Currently, the study by Tyrell and colleagues[13] is the only study to demonstrate that learning over multiple days, in addition to acquisition in a single session, of a novel locomotor pattern is slowed in individuals after stroke. The study, however, also indicates that although slowed, if given sufficient practice, individuals with chronic stroke can achieve gains through locomotor learning similar to neurologically intact individuals. In the animal model, the amount of practice needed to directly influence task-dependent neuroplastic changes and demonstrate significant improvements in stepping quality is greater than 1000 steps per session.[39] Corroborating this effect, Moore and colleagues[40] previously demonstrated a dose–response relationship between the amount of stepping practice and improved community ambulation in individuals after stroke. Despite the apparent dose–response relationship, patients often receive a limited amount of locomotor practice within a physical therapy session.[40] This inconsistency highlights a crucial role for empirical evaluation of optimal motor learning strategies that may be utilized for efficient and effective locomotor rehabilitation.

TRAINING

Although preserved, a more symmetric, and possibly more efficient,[8] safe,[9] and speedy[6,7] gait pattern is not easily achieved in individuals after stroke. Within the split-belt treadmill paradigm, after effects resulting in improved symmetry are only achieved when the initial step length asymmetry is exaggerated and returns to baseline asymmetry. Previous use of error augmentation has been shown to be effective at targeting specific movement deficits following stroke.[10,11,23,41] The exaggeration of asymmetry, or error, is critical, because it provides the nervous system with a cue to correct the gait deviation induced by the split-belt paradigm.[10,11] Error augmentation may be particularly useful for those with chronic stroke whose gait deviations are now perceived as normal by the nervous system.[17] By providing an exaggeration of the locomotor asymmetry, the split-belt paradigm draws attention to the error in order to correct the gait asymmetry.

Recent studies have assessed whether short-term improvements in step length asymmetry could be capitalized upon with repetitive split-belt treadmill training in order to produce longer-term improvements in gait after stroke.[12,16] Utilizing an error augmentation strategy, a single participant trained 3 days per week for 4 weeks, with each training session consisting of 6 5-minute bouts of split belt treadmill walking.[16] The belt configuration during split-belt walking was set so that the participant's baseline step length asymmetry would be exaggerated. Utilizing the after effect of improved step length symmetry, the participant practiced walking overground for 5 minutes following each split-belt walking session. Improved step length symmetry during overground walking was reinforced with verbal cuing from the physical therapist. Following 4 weeks of treadmill training, the participant demonstrated an increase in self-selected and fastest walking speed, which was maintained at 1 month follow-up. Gait analysis comparison from pre- to post-treadmill training revealed that step length asymmetry improved from 21% asymmetry at baseline to 9% after training. Decrements in step length asymmetry continued at 1 month follow-up to 7% asymmetry.[16] Expanding upon these results, Reisman and colleagues[12] trained 12 subjects with chronic stroke with the identical paradigm as described previously (**Table 1**). Across the 12 subjects, step length asymmetry improved significantly from baseline to after testing (**Fig. 1**A). In addition, subjects demonstrated a difference between step length asymmetry at baseline and 1- and 3-month follow-up evaluations that approached significance. In order to identify responders to the intervention, a double baseline evaluation was employed to assess day-to-day differences in step length asymmetry. Seven participants demonstrated a change in step length asymmetry greater than day-to-day variability (responders) from before training to after training,

Table 1
Split-belt training paradigm

Baseline	Baseline	Training (3 Sessions/wk × 4 wk)								After Testing	1-mo Follow-up	3-mo Follow-up
		Split-Belt Treadmill Training							Overground Training			
		Bout 1	Bout 2	Bout 3	Bout 4	Bout 5	Bout 6					
Overground walking	Overground walking	5 min	5 min	5 min	5 min	5 min	5 min		5–10 min	Overground walking	Overground walking	Overground walking
Functional testing	Functional testing									Functional testing	Functional testing	Functional testing

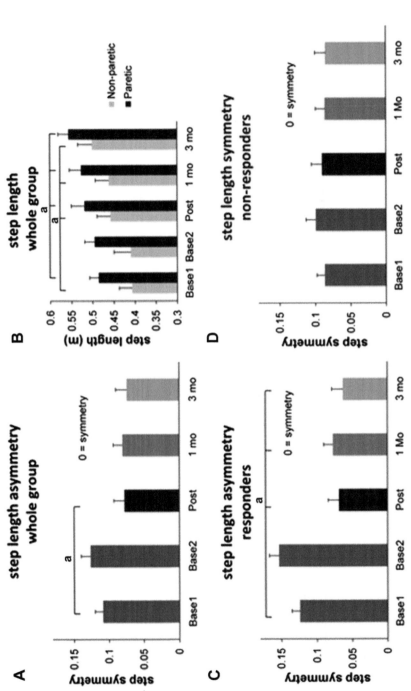

Fig. 1. Step length during overground walking measured at each baseline session (Base1, Base2), at post-training (Post) and at 1 and 3 months after training (1 mo and 3 mo respectively). (*A*) Step length asymmetry for the entire group (n = 12). (*B*) Step length asymmetry in the group identified as responders based on their pre- to post-training change in asymmetry (n = 7). (*D*) Step length asymmetry in the group identified as nonresponders based on their pre- to post-training change in asymmetry (n = 5). ᵃ Indicates *P*<.05. (*From* Reisman DS, McLean H, Keller JA, et al. Repeated split-belt treadmill training improves post-stroke step length asymmetry. Neurorehabil Neural Repair 2013;27:460–68; with permission.)

while 5 participants did not (nonresponders) (see **Fig. 1**C, D, respectively). The improvements in step length symmetry occurred as a result of an increased step length bilaterally, with a relatively larger change on the extremity with the shorter step at baseline (see **Fig. 1**B). A decreased step length on the extremity with a longer step would have also provided an improved step length bilaterally; however, the improvements achieved through increased step length provides increased functionality, given the association between increased step length and increased walking speed in post-stroke walking interventions.[42] It is important to note, however, that the only gait parameter demonstrating long-term change (ie, step length asymmetry) was targeted specifically by the split-belt intervention through exaggeration of baseline asymmetry. Longer-term changes were not noted for double-support time, percent stance time, or overground gait speed.[12]

The previously described studies demonstrate that repetitive short-term adaptations observed in previous single-session split-belt studies can be capitalized on through repetitive practice and can lead to longer-term improvements in gait deficits after stroke. The ability to maintain an improvement in step length symmetry at 1- and 3-month follow-up suggests that the effects of training are sustainable, which is particularly important given that gait asymmetries after stroke, namely step length asymmetry, are particularly resistant to rehabilitative training.[5] These results suggest a potential therapeutic role for the split-belt treadmill in gait rehabilitation. Further empirical evaluation of poststroke motor learning strategies and an understanding of for whom this intervention is effective are required.

SUMMARY

Current evidence indicates that the split-belt treadmill may be utilized as a probe of motor learning after stroke, or as a therapeutic intervention in order to promote a more symmetric gait pattern in individuals after stroke. Existing evidence indicates that the split-belt paradigm may influence some aspects of gait to a greater degree than others. Location of neural injury, type of feedback, and task constructs, all may impact the adaptability of specific gait parameters with exposure to the split-belt paradigm. Further study is required to fully characterize the adaptive capacity of the poststroke nervous system in order to develop rational methods for improved locomotor rehabilitation.

REFERENCES

1. Go AS, Mozaffarian D, Roger VL, et al. Heart disease and stroke statistics–2014 update: a report from the American Heart Association. Circulation 2014;129: e28–292.
2. Bohannon RW, Andrews AW, Smith MB. Rehabilitation goals of patients with hemiplegia. Int J Rehabil Res 1998;11:181–3.
3. Jette DU, Latham NK, Smout RJ, et al. Physical therapy interventions for patients with stroke in inpatient. Phys Ther 2005;85:238–48.
4. Patterson KK, Gage WH, Brooks D, et al. Evaluation of gait symmetry after stroke: a comparison of current methods and recommendations for standardization. Gait Posture 2010;31(2):241–6.
5. Patterson KK, Parafianowicz I, Danells CJ, et al. Gait asymmetry in community-ambulating stroke survivors. Arch Phys Med Rehabil 2008;89(2):304–10.
6. Balasubramanian CK, Bowden MG, Neptune RR, et al. Relationship between step length asymmetry and walking performance in subjects with chronic hemiparesis. Arch Phys Med Rehabil 2007;88(1):43–9.

7. Olney SJ, Griffin MP, McBride ID. Temporal, kinematic, and kinetic variables related to gait speed in subjects with hemiplegia: a regression approach. Phys Ther 1994;74(9):872–85. Available at: http://www.ncbi.nlm.nih.gov/pubmed/8066114. Accessed February 6, 2015.

8. Awad LN, Palmer JA, Pohlig RT, et al. Walking speed and step length asymmetry modify the energy cost of walking after stroke. Neurorehabil Neural Repair 2014. http://dx.doi.org/10.1177/1545968314552528.

9. Lewek MD, Bradley CE, Wutzke CJ, et al. The relationship between spatiotemporal gait asymmetry and balance in individuals with chronic stroke. J Appl Biomech 2014;30(1):31–6.

10. Reisman DS, Wityk R, Silver K, et al. Locomotor adaptation on a split-belt treadmill can improve walking symmetry post-stroke. Brain 2007;130(Pt 7):1861–72.

11. Reisman DS, Wityk R, Silver K, et al. Split-belt treadmill adaptation transfers to overground walking in persons poststroke. Neurorehabil Neural Repair 2009;23(7):735–44.

12. Reisman DS, McLean H, Keller J, et al. Repeated split-belt treadmill training improves poststroke step length asymmetry. Neurorehabil Neural Repair 2013;27(5):460–8.

13. Tyrell CM, Helm E, Reisman DS. Learning the spatial features of a locomotor task is slowed after stroke. J Neurophysiol 2014;112(2):480–9.

14. Reisman DS, Block HJ, Bastian AJ. Interlimb coordination during locomotion: what can be adapted and stored? J Neurophysiol 2005;94(4):2403–15.

15. Martin TA, Keating JG, Goodkin HP, et al. Throwing while looking through prisms: II. Specificity and storage of multiple gaze–throw calibrations. Brain 1996;119(4):1199–211.

16. Reisman DS, McLean H, Bastian AJ. Split-belt treadmill training poststroke: a case study. J Neurol Phys Ther 2010;34(4):202–7.

17. Reisman DS, Bastian AJ, Morton SM. Neurophysiologic and rehabilitation insights from the split-belt and other locomotor adaptation paradigms. Phys Ther 2010;90(2):187–95.

18. Tseng Y-W, Diedrichsen J, Krakauer JW, et al. Sensory prediction errors drive cerebellum-dependent adaptation of reaching. J Neurophysiol 2007;98(1):54–62.

19. Shadmehr R, Mussa-Ivaldi FA. Adaptive representation of dynamics during learning of a motor task. J Neurosci 1994;14(5 Pt 2):3208–24. Available at: http://www.ncbi.nlm.nih.gov/pubmed/8182467. Accessed July 19, 2014.

20. Bastian AJ. Understanding sensorimotor adaptation and learning for rehabilitation. Curr Opin Neurol 2008;21(6):628–33.

21. Torres-Oviedo G, Vasudevan E, Malone L, et al. Locomotor adaptation. Prog Brain Res 2011;191:65–74.

22. Morton SM, Bastian AJ. Cerebellar contributions to locomotor adaptations during split-belt treadmill walking. J Neurosci 2006;26(36):9107–16.

23. Savin DN, Tseng S-C, Whitall J, et al. Poststroke hemiparesis impairs the rate but not magnitude of adaptation of spatial and temporal locomotor features. Neurorehabil Neural Repair 2013;27(1):24–34.

24. Malone LA, Bastian AJ. Thinking about walking: effects of conscious correction versus distraction on locomotor adaptation. J Neurophysiol 2010;103(4):1954–62.

25. Vasudevan EVL, Torres-Oviedo G, Morton SM, et al. Younger is not always better: development of locomotor adaptation from childhood to adulthood. J Neurosci 2011;31(8):3055–65.

26. Malone LA, Vasudevan EVL, Bastian AJ. Motor adaptation training for faster relearning. J Neurosci 2011;31(42):15136–43.

27. Haggard P, Cockburn J, Cock J, et al. Interference between gait and cognitive tasks in a rehabilitating neurological population. J Neurol Neurosurg Psychiatry 2000; 69(4):479–86. Available at: http://www.pubmedcentral.nih.gov/articlerender.fcgi? artid=1737140&tool=pmcentrez&rendertype=abstract. Accessed January 27, 2015.
28. Schmidt RA. Motor Control and Learning: A Behavioral Emphasis. 2nd edition. Champaign, IL: Human Kinetics; 1988.
29. Nudo RJ. Adaptive plasticity in motor cortex: implications for rehabilitation after brain injury. J Rehabil Med 2003;(41 Suppl):7–10. Available at: http://www.ncbi.nlm.nih.gov/pubmed/12817650. Accessed February 17, 2015.
30. Hanlon RE. Motor learning following unilateral stroke. Arch Phys Med Rehabil 1996;77:811–5.
31. Winstein CJ, Merians AS, Sullivan KJ. Motor learning after unilateral brain damage. Neuropsychologia 1999;37(8):975–87. Available at: http://www.ncbi.nlm.nih.gov/pubmed/10426521. Accessed August 25, 2014.
32. Platz T, Denzler P, Kaden B, et al. Motor learning after recovery from hemiparesis. Neuropsychologia 1994;32(10):1209–23. Available at: http://www.ncbi.nlm.nih.gov/pubmed/7845561.
33. Pohl PS, McDowd JM, Filion DL, et al. Implicit learning of a perceptual-motor skill after stroke. Phys Ther 2001;81(11):1780–9. Available at: http://www.ncbi.nlm.nih.gov/pubmed/11694171. Accessed August 25, 2014.
34. Boyd LA, Vidoni ED, Wessel BD. Motor learning after stroke: is skill acquisition a prerequisite for contralesional neuroplastic change? Neurosci Lett 2010;482(1): 21–5.
35. Vidoni ED, Boyd LA. Preserved motor learning after stroke is related to the degree of proprioceptive deficit. Behav Brain Funct 2009;5:36.
36. Meehan SK, Randhawa B, Wessel B, et al. Implicit sequence-specific motor learning after subcortical stroke is associated with increased prefrontal brain activations: an fMRI study. Hum Brain Mapp 2011;32(2):290–303.
37. Boyd LA, Winstein CJ. Implicit motor-sequence learning in humans following unilateral stroke: the impact of practice and explicit knowledge. Neurosci Lett 2001; 298(1):65–9.
38. Savin DN, Tseng S-C, Morton SM. Bilateral adaptation during locomotion following a unilaterally applied resistance to swing in nondisabled adults. J Neurophysiol 2010;104(6):3600–11.
39. Cha J, Heng C, Reinkensmeyer DJ, et al. Locomotor ability in spinal rats is dependent on the amount of activity imposed on the hindlimbs during treadmill training. J Neurotrauma 2007;24(6):1000–12.
40. Moore JL, Roth EJ, Killian C, et al. Locomotor training improves daily stepping activity and gait efficiency in individuals poststroke who have reached a "plateau" in recovery. Stroke 2010;41(1):129–35.
41. Patton JL, Stoykov ME, Kovic M, et al. Evaluation of robotic training forces that either enhance or reduce error in chronic hemiparetic stroke survivors. Exp Brain Res 2006;168(3):368–83.
42. Ada L, Dean CM, Hall JM, et al. A treadmill and overground walking program improves walking in persons residing in the community after stroke: a placebo-controlled, randomized trial. Arch Phys Med Rehabil 2003;84(10):1486–91. Available at: http://www.ncbi.nlm.nih.gov/pubmed/14586916. Accessed February 18, 2015.

Integrating Mental Practice with Task-specific Training and Behavioral Supports in Poststroke Rehabilitation
Evidence, Components, and Augmentative Opportunities

Heather T. Peters, MOT, OTR/L[a],*, Stephen J. Page, PhD, MS, OTR/L, FAHA, FACRM[b]

KEYWORDS

- Mental practice • Motor imagery • Stroke • The PRACTICE principles
- Rehabilitation

KEY POINTS

- Mental practice involves mental rehearsal of physical movements without the use of physical practice.
- Mental practice has been shown to increase motor learning and performance in a variety of clinical and performance-related environments.
- Mental practice elicits the same neural and muscular events as physical practice. Therefore, if used repetitively, its use is thought to increase poststroke skill reacquisition.
- The PRACTICE (part-whole practice, repetitive and goal focused, activities that are salient, client driven, train practically, impairments addressed, challenge regularly, and emphasize accomplishments) principles can be used as a guide to structure the contents of mental and physical practice.
- Noninvasive brain stimulation can be used adjunctively with mental practice.

Disclosures: None.
[a] B.R.A.I.N. Laboratory (Better Rehabilitation and Assessment for Improved Neuro-recovery), Department of Occupational Therapy, The Ohio State University, 453 West 10th Avenue, Suite 443, Columbus, OH 43210, USA; [b] B.R.A.I.N. Laboratory (Better Rehabilitation and Assessment for Improved Neuro-recovery), Department of Occupational Therapy, The Ohio State University, 453 West 10th Avenue, Suite 406, Columbus, OH 43210, USA
* Corresponding author.
E-mail address: Heather.tanksley@osumc.edu

Phys Med Rehabil Clin N Am 26 (2015) 715–727
http://dx.doi.org/10.1016/j.pmr.2015.06.004
1047-9651/15/$ – see front matter © 2015 Elsevier Inc. All rights reserved.
pmr.theclinics.com

Stroke remains a leading cause of death and one of the most costly and burdensome diseases.[1–3] For example, the 2010 Global Burden of Disease Study estimated that there were 16.9 million people who had experienced a first-ever stroke, 33 million stroke survivors, and 102 million disability-adjusted life-years lost in that year alone.[4] Moreover, despite organized efforts to prevent and treat stroke more quickly and effectively, since 1990 there has been continued growth in the overall incidence and mortality of stroke.[4]

The global impact of stroke and the rapidly expanding number of stroke survivors with residual disabilities[4] provide impetus for the development of rehabilitative approaches that increase poststroke function. In response, several rehabilitative regimens have been tested, with the most efficacious therapies[5–7] encouraging survivors to practice functionally and repetitively (termed repetitive task-specific practice [RTP]). RTP seems to be a critical factor in poststroke plasticity and functional increases.[8] For example, in stroke survivors with minimally impaired upper extremities (UEs), constraint-induced movement therapy increases UE use and function[5,7] by integrating RTP with behavioral strategies that encourage paretic limb use. Similarly, among survivors with moderate UE impairments (people with no active movement in their paretic wrists and fingers) RTP augmented by electrical stimulation enables active participation in UE motor practice, and significantly increases paretic UE use and function.[9–12]

Informed by these promising findings, and based on decades of motor learning, neuroplasticity, and cognitive behavior training literature, we recently proposed the PRACTICE principles,[13] which speak to the ways in which RTP should ideally be integrated into poststroke care. Specific components of the PRACTICE principles are as follows: (1) part-whole practice should be used, with an eye toward realistic task analysis, (2) repetitive and goal focused, (3) activities should be salient, (4) client driven, (5) train in a practical way, (6) impairments should be addressed, (7) challenge regularly and appropriately, and (8) emphasize accomplishments. One of the concepts elucidated by the PRACTICE principles is the ability of the client to easily access and meaningfully engage in RTP (ie, train in a practical fashion). This principle speaks to the match of a regimen's practice parameters with the abilities and physical activity tolerance of the client (eg, are the parameters too intensive and/or too long in duration for the client to tolerate? Does the regimen use equipment that the client and/or the clinic cannot easily integrate into care?), as well as the physical proximity and accessibility of the resources needed to fully implement the regimen. Such practical considerations are important in ensuring full client participation and high fidelity with the regimen to facilitate neural and motor changes. However, they are not always embraced by contemporary approaches, such as those mentioned earlier, which often require intensive parameters and/or expensive equipment that is only available at specialized rehabilitation and academic medical centers. For instance, in the largest trial to date of constraint-induced movement therapy, subjects could only tolerate about two-thirds of the assigned 6 hours of RTP before fatigue set in.[12]

In response to these limitations, this laboratory was the first to apply mental practice (MP) to increase learning and outcomes in stroke,[14] later showing that MP use increases paretic UE use and function.[15,16] More recently, our work has shown that MP use causes the same cortical changes as physical practice in survivors of stroke.[17] The regimen has also been extended to other poststroke impairments and neurologic conditions,[18–20] and our pioneering findings have been replicated by others around the world.[21–26] The critical advantage of MP compared with newer but less pragmatic rehabilitative approaches (and even some conventional rehabilitative therapies) is its use of cognitive rehearsal without the use of physical practice or voluntary physical movement attempts by the client. Instead, the client listens to an audio file that elucidates the goal-directed actions to be performed, and/or watches a video depicting these movements. Restated, during MP, the individual is cognitively rehearsing RTP. These straightforward requirements allow MP to be performed with minimal direct supervision, minimal expense, and in virtually any environment with no specialized equipment. Moreover, a variety of laboratories have confirmed that MP use activates the same neural areas and musculature as physical practice of the same tasks,[27–30] providing a strong scientific rationale for cognitively rehearsing a skill to simulate conditions brought about by RTP. This finding is important because, in some clinical situations, mental rehearsal may be a safer and/or better justified clinical option than engaging in physical practice because of the client's impairments (eg, when it is unsafe for a client to physically practice ambulation).

Given its implementation advantages compared with many physically based practice approaches and its strong scientific bases, the overall goal of this article is to review the considerations associated with the clinical implementation of MP. Specifically, this article begins by briefly discussing literature supporting MP use, including current MP work occurring at this laboratory. It then describes the basic components of clinical MP regimens with the goal of facilitating increased integration of MP into clinical practice. In addition, it concludes with a discussion of future directions and emerging applications designed to enhance MP outcomes. Most of discussion focuses on motor impairments, because this is the primary area of MP investigation in the stroke population, and because motor impairments are frequent and especially disabling.

EMPIRICAL SUPPORT FOR MENTAL PRACTICE

Although there is a growing body of evidence for the impact of MP on lower extremity function,[31–34] most efforts to date have targeted UE motor recovery.[6,14,17,21–24,34–40] Results and methods from selected cited trials are included in **Table 1**. Specifically, research gathered from these trials suggests that MP combined with RTP is the most efficacious approach, resulting in greater increases in UE motor function than RTP alone.[6,14,21,23,24,34,35,37] In addition to these significant gains in UE function, Liu and colleagues[21] showed that MP combined with RTP may also facilitate increased translation of learned motor skills to new environments. Based on promising results from controlled trials, several sites have also implemented MP alongside rehabilitative therapies in clinical settings (eg, inpatient rehabilitation[21,23,37]) with patients in the acute/subacute phase of recovery, finding significant gains in performance of activities of daily living (ADLs)[21,23] and UE function[21,23,37] for those receiving MP alongside conventional therapy compared with conventional therapy alone. In addition to significant improvements on aforementioned motor-based and activity-based outcome measures, evidence also suggests that MP combined with RTP results in improved UE kinematics,[15] increased cortical representation of the affected hemisphere,[17] efficacy when combined with other therapies (eg, modified constraint-induced therapy[40]), and more frequent paretic UE use.[16] Building on this work, our laboratory is now leading a multicenter, randomized controlled trial examining the effect of MP and RTP in chronic, hemiparetic stroke. This is the first multicenter trial to investigate the effect of an MP regimen not only on affected UE outcomes and impairment but also on cortical reorganization in the ipsilesional motor cortex.

CONSIDERATIONS FOR INTEGRATING MENTAL PRACTICE INTO CLINICAL ENVIRONMENTS

Stroke rehabilitation is ultimately focused on regaining the ability to perform valued ADLs to facilitate maximal independence in the community. As such, rehabilitation

Table 1
Selected, randomized controlled trials of MP in UE rehabilitation

Author, Year	Study Objective	Study Design, Participants	Intervention	Primary Outcome Measures	Results
Liu et al,[37] 2004	Determine efficacy of MP in promoting UE motor relearning	Design: prospective, randomized controlled trial Participants: 46 acute inpatients, >60 y old	15 sessions (1 h/d for 3 wk) of either MP and therapy or conventional therapy only	Trained and untrained tasks, FM and CTT	MP group improved significantly on trained (P<.005) and untrained (P<.001). MP group improved significantly on CTT (P<.005) but not on FM
Page et al,[6] 2007	Determine efficacy of MP in increasing function and use of affected UE in chronic stroke	Design: randomized, placebo-controlled trial Participants: 32 patients with chronic stroke, average time poststroke = 3.6 y	30 min of traditional therapy 2 d/wk for 6 wk and either 30-min MP or relaxation session	UE section of the FM and ARAT	MP group increased significantly on the FM (+6.7 vs +1.0, P<.0001) and ARAT (+7.8 vs +0.44, P<.0001) compared with sham
Muller et al,[22] 2007	Determine efficacy of MP in increasing hand function	Design: multiple baseline, randomized controlled trial Participants: 17 patients (6 women; mean age, 62 y) with severe hemiparesis	4 wk of mental rehearsal of a nonsequential finger opposition task, motor execution of a nonsequential finger opposition task, or conventional therapy	Pinch/grip strength, Jebsen Hand Function Test, Barthel Index, and European Stroke Scale	MP and motor groups showed statistically significant gains on Jebsen Hand Function Test and pinch/grip strength compared with the control group
Page et al,[41] 2009	Determine efficacy of MP and mCIT on UE function	Design: randomized controlled trial Participants: 10 patients with chronic stroke (7 men). Mean age = 61.4 ± 3.02 y. Age range = 48–79 y Average time after stroke = 28.5 mo	MP (30 min/d) and mCIT or mCIT alone; both interventions 3×/wk for 10 wk	ARAT and FM	mCIT + MP group showed significantly greater increases on the FM (+7.8 vs +4.1, P = .01) and ARAT (+15.4 vs 8.4, P<.001) immediately following and 3-months after intervention

Study	Purpose	Design/Participants	Intervention	Outcome Measures	Results
Liu et al,[21] 2009	Determine effect of MP on generalization of learned task skills to trained and untrained tasks in new environments	Design: randomized controlled trial Participants: 35 patients with acute stroke	MP and traditional rehabilitation or traditional rehabilitation alone; both provided 1 h/d for 3 wk	Gains in task performance	MP participants improved performance significantly on 4 out of 5 trained tasks ($P = .001–.026$) vs improvement on 1 trained task ($P = .021$) in control group. MP participants improved performance on 3 out of 5 trained ($P = .025$) and 2 out of 3 untrained tasks ($P = .042$) in new environment
Bovend'Eert et al,[38] 2010	Investigate feasibility of the integration of MP into occupational and physical therapy rehabilitation	Design: single-blind, randomized controlled trial Participants: 50 patients with stroke, brain injury, or multiple sclerosis in inpatient or outpatient rehabilitation (>18 y old)	6 wk of traditional rehabilitation and MP traditional rehabilitation only	Goal Attainment Scaling, Barthel Index, Rivermead Mobility Index, Nottingham Extended ADL, ARAT and Timed up and Go	Gains measured in both groups on all outcome measures, but no significant differences in outcome measures between groups
Riccio et al,[23] 2010	Investigate effect of MP on functional UE recovery after stroke	Design: randomized, single-blind crossover study Participants: 36 patients with stroke with UE hemiparesis	Convention rehabilitation (3 h a day, 5 d a week) followed by 3 wk of conventional therapy with additional 60 min of MP. A separate group received the same intervention in reverse order	Motricity Index (UE section), Arm Function Test–Functional Ability Scale and time	The conventional + MP group at the 3-wk crossover point showed statistically significant improvement compared with the control group at the 3-wk crossover point on all outcome measures. There were no significant differences between groups at the end of treatment period

(continued on next page)

Table 1
(continued)

Author, Year	Study Objective	Study Design, Participants	Intervention	Primary Outcome Measures	Results
Letswaart et al,[39] 2011	Examine the effect of MP on UE function in stroke	Design: multicenter, randomized controlled trial Participants: 121 patients with stroke. Average time post stroke <3 months	Traditional rehabilitation 3 d/wk for 45 min. Participants additionally received MP, nonmotor mental rehearsal, or usual care with no mental rehearsal	ARAT, grip strength (dynamometry), timed manual dexterity performance	No significant changes between groups were seen on any outcome measures
Page et al,[35] 2011	Compare efficacy of 20-min, 40-min, and 60-min sessions of MP on UE function after stroke	Design: single-blind, multiple baseline, randomized controlled trial Participants: 29 patients with chronic stroke	20-min, 40-min, or 60-min MP + RTP sessions or RTP + audiotaped sham intervention	FM and ARAT	Duration of MP predicted changes in FM scores, with the 60-min duration group showing the largest increases (+5.4). The 20-min duration showed the greatest gains in ARAT scores (changes were nonsignificant). Subjects who received MP, regardless of dose, showed larger increases than those in the control group, but differences were not statistically significant

Abbreviations: ADL, activities of daily living; ARAT, Action Research Arm test; CTT, Color Trails Test; FM, Fugl-Meyer; mCIT, modified constraint-induced therapy.

professionals typically target reacquisition of the UE motor skills (ie, strength, range of motion, coordination) necessary to perform these tasks. As previously highlighted, research has consistently shown the efficacy of MP when combined with RTP in modulating cortical plasticity and increasing poststroke motor function. Despite these facts, MP remains a promising adjunct that has not yet been incorporated consistently into clinical practice. To address this gap, this article provides a guide for the structuring of an MP and RTP regimen in a rehabilitative setting.

Mental Practice for Upper Extremity Retraining

A typical MP regimen consists of 2 components: (1) mental rehearsal and (2) physical practice.

The Physical Practice Component

As mentioned previously, RTP is the most commonly used physical practice approach that is combined with MP because of its efficacy in increasing UE motor function. Typically, RTP interventions used in this laboratory are provided 3 days per week for a period of 6 to 10 weeks, with each treatment session lasting 30 to 60 minutes. Not only has this dosage been shown to be efficacious in increasing UE outcomes[6,14,17,23,34,35] but this also aligns well with the typical duration of therapy in an outpatient setting, making it advantageous compared with other paradigms that require higher duration parameters[5] with only incrementally larger UE motor changes than those that are observed with MP. In integrating MP into clinical settings, it is necessary to identify particular areas of UE deficit and establish mutually agreed on goals around which to center therapy. This approach is typically accomplished by conducting an evaluation (which is common in most rehabilitative environments) but also by including an informal interview or the use of a more formal measure (eg, Canadian Occupational Performance Measure[41]) that specifically identifies the client's goals and quantifies the client's satisfaction and performance of those targeted tasks. Inclusion of the client in the goal-setting process ensures a client-driven approach, which addresses not only the physical but also the psychosocial aspects of patient care. Further, this practice increases the likelihood that activities performed in therapy are meaningful and motivating, which we have found increases compliance with the treatment protocol. Once these goals are established, the rehabilitation team implements a treatment plan based on activities that are of interest to the client. Integration of the client into the goal-setting process is supported by other researchers,[42] and can even be integrated into billing of patient education and/or therapy time blocks. However, the use of salient, client-centered goals is not necessarily incorporated into many conventional UE rehabilitative approaches, such as Neurodevelopmental Therapy[43] and Proprioceptive Neuromuscular Facilitation,[44] in which the therapy contents depend largely on the therapist's ascertainment of clients' deficits and needs with little input from the client.

Per the PRACTICE principles,[13] RTP also involves the repetition of movements that are functionally based (eg, turning pages in a book, bringing a cup to the mouth), context specific (ie, real world), and challenging, because these components are essential to driving neuroplasticity.[42,45] Although performance of entire tasks (or whole performance of similar tasks) is often used as a practice ingredient in clinical settings, depending on the patient's level of impairment, this type of practice may be overly difficult and result in poor technique, frustration, and/or poor compliance. Thus, it is often more efficacious to break tasks into smaller components to be practiced repetitively before attempting task completion, and such part-whole practice is supported by decades of motor learning research.[46] For example, if a patient's goal is to feed independently, it is often beneficial to repetitively practice isolated components of feeding (eg, grasp and release of the utensil, bringing the spoon to the chin) before progressing to self-feeding. After performing these movement attempts, it is also important to routinely assess the difficulty of the task (eg, asking the patient to rate task difficulty from 1–10) and to regrade the task accordingly to achieve the just right challenge and maximize difficulty without making the task overly challenging. Most studies incorporating RTP[6,14,16,17,21,37] have included 3 to 5 different tasks per session, allowing for adequate repetitions of each activity to facilitate increased motor learning and skill acquisition.

Behavioral support

In addition, to encourage regimen compliance, a variety of forms of behavioral supports are used by this laboratory on a routine basis to encourage and motivate clients during therapies, and to increase the likelihood of carryover to real-world environments. These supports include (1) home use logs, which document UE use but also serve as a reminder for the client to be cognizant of paretic UE reintegration; (2) use of behavioral contracts, which require clients to agree to fully participate in the regimen to the best of their ability but also stipulate specific and/or unique aspects of the RTP, such as whether they are to wear a restrictive device on the less affected UE to encourage paretic UE use, and/or the use of specific home exercises. These contracts can be brandished by the therapist daily or weekly to remind the client and/or care partner of the commitment to which they have agreed. (3) Self-efficacy training, in which the client's feelings of self-efficacy while using the paretic UE are regularly assessed. Self-efficacy training is often followed by problem-solving techniques that the client can use at home or that are used in therapy to increase feelings of self-efficacy, which, in turn, are expected to positively affect UE use, neuroplasticity, and ultimately UE motor function. These and other behavioral supports are integrated into our RTP programs on a case-by-case basis and are discussed in greater detail in other work by this laboratory.[7]

The Mental Practice Component

Following intensive RTP, patients typically report to another room where they mentally rehearse the tasks that have just been physically practiced. Across most MP literature, patients typically perform MP while sitting in a quiet environment in order to minimize environmental distractions.[6,14,16,17,23,34,35] The importance of this environmental aspect should not be ignored, because a peaceful area to conduct these sessions, in which the patient can concentrate on instructions contained in the MP audio files without distraction or interruption, constitutes an essential component of any clinical MP intervention.

In this laboratory, MP is typically administered using 1 of 2 methods: (1) using an audio file; or (2) orally, guided by the therapist. Most UE motor studies have used audio files, because this ensures consistency of the intervention being provided across subjects, but also ensures consistent delivery of the intervention without using a busy clinician's time. Further, the advent and ease of mp3 files constitute an especially promising development because their portability allows sessions to be conducted in a clinical setting or from the client's community setting. MP audio files may range from 10 minutes[34] to 60 minutes[23] in length with the mental rehearsal of tasks comprising only a portion of the total duration. As this laboratory has shown, shorter dosages ($\leq$30 minutes) tend to be as efficacious[6,12,14,16,17,34,35,40] as longer dosages, with the latter being less plausible in a clinical setting. Thus, using a 30-minute audio file as a framework, the audio sequences typically begin with ~5 minutes of progressive relaxation, asking patients to contract and relax their muscles while imagining themselves in a relaxing place (eg, the beach). It is suggested that this period of relaxation serves as a primer for MP, helping to later increase attention and vividness of the imagery.[47] This portion is followed by ~20 minutes of guided motor imagery of the activities performed in therapy. Essential to the efficacy of MP is the assurance that the patient is provided with guided, polysensory cues[48] that match the recently performed motor tasks. For example, if the focus of that day's therapy session was grasping and bringing a utensil to the mouth, the imagery should take the client through the movements and sensations associated with that task (eg, the sensation of the cup in the hand, the fingers and elbow flexing to grasp and bring the cup toward the mouth). Several tasks can be included in 1 session, provided that many mental repetitions of each task are completed to facilitate motor learning and that the regimen does not become too demanding on the patient. The file ends with ~5 minutes of relaxation, allowing the patient to refocus into the room.[6,12,14,16,17,34,35,40]

FUTURE DIRECTIONS FOR MENTAL PRACTICE RESEARCH AND INTEGRATION
The Window of Mental Practice Administration

Although numerous studies have examined the potential role of MP in stroke rehabilitation, several questions relating to its optimal use remain unanswered. One such question is whether MP administered more subacutely or acutely (ie, in the days or weeks after stroke) elicits a larger treatment effect than when used in the chronic stages of stroke (ie, in the months and years after stroke), because of greater levels of endogenous plasticity that are thought to exist earlier postictus. In one of the largest MP trials to date, Letswaart and colleagues[39] investigated the effect of inpatient subacute rehabilitation that was augmented by either MP, nonmotor rehearsal, or no mental rehearsal in 121 stroke survivors. Contrary to most UE MP studies described herein, results showed no differences in UE function changes between the groups. However, subjects enrolled in this study were also concurrently engaged in a multitude of treatments, as is common in the days and weeks after stroke. Thus, the results of this study should be taken with caution and more research on the subacute administration of MP is justified. As part of one of the author's training grants (SJP), this laboratory recently completed a carefully controlled study of ≈30 subjects greater than 3 months and less than 12 months postictus who were administered MP as an adjunct to a well-controlled UE intervention, and results are pending at the time of writing of this article.

Mental Practice Augmented by Noninvasive Brain Stimulation

In addition to augmenting rehabilitation with MP, the opportunity also exists to enhance MP with other treatments to maximize its efficacy. One notable example is transcranial magnetic stimulation (TMS), a type of noninvasive brain stimulation that delivers brief magnetic pulses through the scalp into the brain, resulting in depolarization of targeted neural networks. This technology is being increasingly used diagnostically and therapeutically in acute[49,50] and chronic[51,52] stroke clinical trials, and has been shown to be efficacious in both increasing motor function through increased neuronal firing (ie, increased motor-evoked potentials [MEPs]) as well as decreasing the neural input needed to evoke a muscle contraction (ie, decreased motor thresholds). Much like other imaging techniques, TMS has also been used to investigate the underlying mechanisms at work during MP.[53–55] These trials used TMS to measure MEPs at rest, during mental rehearsal, and during physical performance. Results from these trials consistently showed greater activation of the motor cortex during MP than during rest and verified that areas of activation are the same when mentally versus physically rehearsing.[53–55]

In addition to its diagnostic capabilities, TMS can also be used as an adjunctive therapy technique through repetitive stimulation (repetitive TMS) of desired areas (eg, the area of the cortex controlling the hand). Many studies have shown the efficacy of TMS as a therapeutic tool in improving UE motor function both in acute/subacute[54,55] and chronic[51,52] populations. Further, a similar form of noninvasive brain stimulation, transcranial direct current stimulation (tDCS), has been shown to increase MEPs produced during MP.[56] tDCS applied concurrently with MP in healthy subjects resulted in increased motor function.[57] Despite these capabilities, neither TMS nor tDCS has been used as an assessment tool or therapeutic tool with MP regimens in the poststroke population. Given these promising initial results, noninvasive brain stimulation may constitute a promising adjunct to a poststroke MP regimen and future research in this area is warranted.

SUMMARY

UE motor dysfunction is a common and disabling deficit experienced by most stroke survivors. Despite improved patient care and awareness of stroke risk factors, stroke incidence continues to increase. As such, there is a growing need for efficacious interventions to address the large group of survivors experiencing UE motor deficits. Over the past 15 years, countless studies have shown the efficacy of MP when combined with RTP. However, at this time, MP is not being incorporated consistently into clinical practice. Based on the extensive empirical evidence, ease of implementation, and applicability to poststroke care, we recommend implementation of MP into the clinical setting using the suggestions provided herein. Further, future areas of research include focusing on optimal timing for MP delivery and possible adjunctive therapies to maximize MP efficacy.

REFERENCES

1. Krishnamurthi RV, Feignin VL, Forouzanfar MH, et al. Global and regional burden of first-ever ischaemic and haemorrhagic stroke during 1990–2010: findings from the Global Burden of Disease Study 2010. Lancet Glob Health 2013;1:e259–81.
2. Lozano R, Naghavi M, Foreman K, et al. Global and regional mortality from 235 causes of death for 20 age groups in 1990 and 2010: a systematic analysis for the Global Burden of Disease Study 2010. Lancet 2012;380:2095–128.
3. Murray CJ, Vos T, Lozano R, et al. Disability-adjusted life years (DALYs) for 291 diseases and injuries in 21 regions, 1990–2010: a systematic analysis for the Global Burden of Disease Study 2010. Lancet 2012;380:2197–223.
4. Feigin VL, Forouzanfar MH, Mensah GA, et al. Global and regional burden of stroke during 1990–2010: findings from the Global Burden of Disease Study 2010. Lancet 2014;383:245–54.
5. Wolf SL, Winstein CJ, Miller JP, et al. Effect of constraint-induced movement therapy on upper extremity function 3 to 9 months after stroke: the EXCITE randomized clinical trial. JAMA 2006;296:2095–104.
6. Page SJ, Levine P, Leonard A. Mental practice in chronic stroke: results of a randomized, placebo controlled trial. Stroke 2007;38:1293–7.
7. Page SJ, Boe S, Levine P. What are the "ingredients" of modified constraint-induced therapy? An evidence based review, recipe, and recommendations. Restor Neurol Neurosci 2013;31:299–309.
8. Nudo RJ. Plasticity. NeuroRx 2006;3:420–7.
9. Dunning K, Berberich A, Albers B, et al. A four-week, task-specific neuroprosthesis program for a person with no active wrist or finger movement because of chronic stroke. Phys Ther 2008;88:397–405.

10. Hill-Hermann V, Strasser A, Albers B, et al. Task-specific, patient-driven neuro-prosthesis training in chronic stroke: results of a 3-week clinical study. Am J Occup Ther 2008;62:466–72.
11. Page SJ, Maslyn S, Hermann VH, et al. Activity-based electrical stimulation training in a stroke patient with minimal movement in the paretic upper extremity. Neurorehabil Neural Repair 2009;23:595–9.
12. Page SJ, Levin L, Hermann V, et al. Longer versus shorter daily durations of electrical stimulation during task specific practice in moderately impaired stroke. Arch Phys Med Rehabil 2012;2:200–6.
13. Page SJ, Peters H. Mental practice: applying motor PRACTICE and neuro-plasticity principles to increase upper extremity function. Stroke 2014;45: 3454–60.
14. Page SJ. Imagery improves upper extremity motor function in chronic stroke patients: a pilot study. Occ Ther J Res 2000;20:200–15.
15. Hewitt TE, Ford K, Levine P, et al. Reaching kinematics to measure motor changes after mental practice in stroke. Top Stroke Rehabil 2007;14:23–9.
16. Page SJ, Levine P, Leonard AC. Effects of mental practice on affected limb use and function in chronic stroke. Arch Phys Med Rehabil 2005;86:399–402.
17. Page SJ, Szaflarski JP, Eliassen J, et al. Cortical plasticity following motor skill learning during mental practice in stroke. Neurorehabil Neural Repair 2009;23: 382–8.
18. Sharp KG, Gramer R, Butler L, et al. Effect of overground training augmented by mental practice on gait velocity in chronic, incomplete spinal cord injury. Arch Phys Med Rehabil 2014;95:615–21.
19. Page SJ, Harnish SM. Thinking about better speech: mental practice for stroke-induced motor speech impairments. Aphasiology 2012;26:127–42.
20. Grooms D, Page SJ, Onate J. Cortical control of jump landing in anterior cruciate ligament reconstructed individuals. Abstract submitted to 7th World Congress of Biomechanics. Boston, July 6, 2014.
21. Liu KP, Chan CC, Wong RS, et al. A randomized controlled trial of mental imagery augment generalization of learning in acute poststroke patients. Stroke 2009;40: 2222–5.
22. Muller K, Butefisch CM, Seitz RJ, et al. Mental practice improves hand function after chronic stroke. Restor Neurol Neurosci 2007;25:501–11.
23. Riccio I, Iolascon G, Barillari MR, et al. Mental practice is effective in upper limb recovery after stroke: a randomized single-blind cross-over study. Eur J Phys Rehabil Med 2010;46:19–25.
24. Lee MM, Cho HY, Song CH. The mirror therapy program enhances upper-limb motor recovery and motor function in acute stroke patients. Am J Phys Med Rehabil 2012;91:689–96.
25. Decety J. Do imagined and executed actions share the same neural substrate? Brain Res Cogn Brain Res 1996;3:87–93.
26. Decety J. The neurophysiological basis of motor imagery. Behav Brain Res 1996; 77:45–52.
27. Decety J, Ingvar DH. Brain structures participating in mental simulation of motor behavior: a neuropsychological interpretation. Acta Psychol 1990;73: 13–34.
28. Weiss T, Hansen E, Beyer L, et al. Activation processes during mental practice in stroke patients. Int J Psychophysiol 1994;17:91–100.
29. Ito M. Movement and thought: identical control mechanisms by the cerebellum. Trends Neurosci 1993;16:453–4.

30. Malouin F, Richards CL, Durand A, et al. Added value of mental practice combined with a small amount of physical practice on the relearning of rising and sitting post-stroke: a pilot study. J Neurol Phys Ther 2009;33:195–202.

31. Braun SM, Beurskens AJ, Kleynen M, et al. A multicenter randomized controlled trial to compare subacute 'treatment as usual' with and without mental practice among persons with stroke in Dutch nursing homes. J Am Med Dir Assoc 2012;13:e1–7.

32. Hosseini SA, Fallahpour M, Sayadi M, et al. The impact of mental practice on stroke patients' postural balance. J Neurol Sci 2012;15:263–7.

33. Schuster C, Butler J, Andrews B, et al. Comparison of embedded and added motor imagery training in patients after stroke: results of a randomised controlled pilot trial. Trials 2012;13:11.

34. Page SJ, Levine P, Sisto SA, et al. Mental practice combined with physical practice for upper-limb motor deficit in subacute stroke. Phys Ther 2001;81: 1455–62.

35. Page SJ, Dunning K, Hermann V. Longer versus shorter mental practice sessions for affected upper extremity movement after stroke: a randomized controlled trial. Clin Rehabil 2011;25:627–37.

36. Dijkerman HC, Letswaart M, Johnston M, et al. Does motor imagery training improve hand function in chronic stroke patients? A pilot study. Clin Rehabil 2004;18:538–49.

37. Liu KP, Chan CC, Lee TM, et al. Mental imagery for promoting relearning for people after stroke: a randomized controlled trial. Arch Phys Med Rehabil 2004;85:1403–8.

38. Bovend'Eert TJ, Dawes H, Sackley C, et al. An integrated motor imagery program to improve functional task performance in neurorehabilitation: a single-blind randomized controlled trial. Arch Phys Med Rehabil 2010;91:939–46.

39. Letswaart M, Johnston M, Dijkerman HC, et al. Mental practice with motor imagery in stroke recovery: randomized controlled trial of efficacy. Brain 2011;134:1373–86.

40. Page SJ, Levine P, Khoury JC. Modified constraint-induced therapy combined with mental practice: thinking through better motor outcomes. Stroke 2009;40: 551–4.

41. Law M, Baptiste S, McColl M, et al. The Canadian occupational performance measure: an outcome measure for occupational therapy. Can J Occup Ther 1990;57:82–7.

42. Kleim JA, Jones TA. Principles of experience-dependent neuroplasticity: implications for rehabilitation after brain damage. J Speech Lang Hear Res 2008;51: S225–39.

43. Bobath B. Adult hemiplegia evaluation and treatment. London: Butterworth; 1990.

44. Radomski MV, Trombley CA. Occupational therapy for physical dysfunction. Philadelphia: Lippincott Williams & Wilkins; 2007.

45. Dobkin B. Strategies in rehabilitation. Lancet 2004;3:528–36.

46. Schmitt R and Lee T. Motor control and learning: a behavioral emphasis. Champaign, IL: Human Kinetics; 2011.

47. Murphy SM. Imagery interventions in sport. Med Sci Sports Exerc 1994;26: 486–94.

48. Paivio A. Cognitive and motivational functions of imagery in human performance. Can J Appl Sport Sci 1985;10:22S–8S.

49. Kehdr EM, Abdel-Fadeil MR, Farghali A, et al. Role of 1 and 3 Hz repetitive transcranial magnetic stimulation on motor function recovery after acute ischaemic stroke. Eur J Neurol 2009;16:1323–30.

50. Liepert J, Zittel S, Weiller C. Improvement of dexterity by single session low-frequency repetitive transcranial magnetic stimulation over the contralesional motor cortex in acute stroke: a double-blind placebo controlled crossover trial. Restor Neurol Neurosci 2007;25:461–5.

51. Takeuchi N, Chuma T, Matsuo Y, et al. Repetitive transcranial magnetic stimulation of contralesional primary motor cortex improves hand function after stroke. Stroke 2005;36:2681–6.

52. Kim YH, You SH, Ko MH, et al. Repetitive transcranial magnetic stimulation–induced corticomotor excitability and associated motor skill acquisition in chronic stroke. Stroke 2006;37:1471–6.

53. Facchini S, Muellbacher W, Battaglia F, et al. Focal enhancement of motor cortex excitability during motor imagery: a transcranial magnetic stimulation study. Acta Neurol Scand 2002;105:146–51.

54. Izumi SI, Findley TW, Ikai T, et al. Facilitatory effect of thinking about movement on motor-evoked potentials to transcranial magnetic stimulation of the brain. Am J Phys Med Rehabil 1995;74:262–8.

55. Cicinelli P, Marconi B, Zaccagnini M, et al. Imagery-induced cortical excitability changes in stroke: a transcranial magnetic stimulation study. Cereb Cortex 2006;16:247–53.

56. Quartarone A, Morgante F, Bagnato S, et al. Long lasting effects of transcranial direct current stimulation on motor imagery. Neuroreport 2004;15:1287–91.

57. Foerster A, Rocha S, Wiesiolek C, et al. Site-specific effects of mental practice combined with transcranial direct current stimulation on motor learning. Eur J Neurosci 2012;37:786–9.

Neuromuscular Electrical Stimulation for Motor Restoration in Hemiplegia

Jayme S. Knutson, PhD[a,b,c,*], Michael J. Fu, PhD[a,c,d],
Lynne R. Sheffler, MD[a,b,c], John Chae, MD[a,b,c]

KEYWORDS

- Stroke rehabilitation • Upper limb hemiplegia • Neuroplasticity • Medical device
- Electrical stimulation therapy

KEY POINTS

- Hemiparesis following stroke is associated with significant upper and lower limb impairment, activity limitation, and reduced quality of life.
- Neuromuscular electrical stimulation as a motor relearning tool reduces upper and lower limb motor impairment following stroke.
- Neuromuscular electrical stimulation as a neuroprosthesis improves ambulation function of stroke survivors but not more than the standard of care ankle-foot orthoses.
- Research is needed to more firmly establish the effects of electrical stimulation on upper limb activity limitations and quality of life.
- The benefit of upper limb neuromuscular electrical stimulation modalities relative to alternative therapies or standard of care remains to be fully elucidated.

INTRODUCTION

Motor impairment is common after stroke and directly impacts the stroke survivor's function and quality of life. Neuromuscular electrical stimulation (NMES) may reduce disability by improving recovery of volitional movement (therapeutic effect) or by

Disclosure: Dr J.S. Knutson and Dr J. Chae are co-inventors on the contralaterally controlled neuromuscular electrical stimulation patent assigned to Case Western Reserve University, Patent 8,165,685: System and Method for Therapeutic Neuromuscular Electrical Stimulation.
[a] MetroHealth Rehabilitation Institute, MetroHealth System, 4229 Pearl Road, Cleveland, OH 44109, USA; [b] Department of Physical Medicine and Rehabilitation, Case Western Reserve University, 2109 Adelbert Road, Cleveland 44106, OH, USA; [c] Cleveland FES Center, Louis Stokes Department of Veterans Affairs Medical Center, 10701 East Blvd., Cleveland, OH 44106, USA; [d] Department of Electrical Engineering and Computer Science, Case Western Reserve University, 10900 Euclid Ave., Cleveland, OH 44106, USA
* Corresponding author. Department of Physical Medicine and Rehabilitation, Case Western Reserve University, MetroHealth Rehabilitation Institute of Ohio, 4229 Pearl Road, Suite 5N, Cleveland, OH 44109.
E-mail address: Jsk12@case.edu

Phys Med Rehabil Clin N Am 26 (2015) 729–745
http://dx.doi.org/10.1016/j.pmr.2015.06.002
1047-9651/15/$ – see front matter © 2015 Elsevier Inc. All rights reserved.

assisting and replacing lost volitional movement (neuroprosthetic effect). This article describes NMES treatment modalities for upper and lower limb stroke rehabilitation and summarizes the research literature regarding the therapeutic and neuroprosthetic efficacy of those modalities. The scope of this article is limited to NMES interventions that produce limb movement by direct stimulation of the peripheral nerves or motor points of target muscles for the purpose of restoring motor function and, therefore, does not cover somatosensory electrical stimulation,[1] electrical stimulation for post-stroke shoulder pain,[2] or brain stimulation modalities.[3]

NEUROMUSCULAR ELECTRICAL STIMULATION FUNDAMENTALS

NMES is the use of electrical current to produce contractions of paralyzed or paretic muscles. Lower motor neurons to target muscles must be intact for NMES to effectively produce muscle contractions; therefore, NMES is usually only applicable to patients whose paralysis or paresis is caused by upper motor neuron injury (eg, stroke, spinal cord injury, and so forth). NMES can be applied to paretic muscles with surface electrodes positioned on the skin over the motor points of target muscles or with electrodes that are implanted near or on the muscle motor points or nerves that innervate target muscles. The electrical current generated by most NMES devices can be characterized as a waveform of pulses having a particular pulse frequency, width, and amplitude. Adjusting the pulse parameters can modulate the strength of evoked muscle contraction. Typically, the stimulation frequency is set between 12 and 50 Hz; the strength of the muscle contraction is modulated by changing either the pulse amplitude (typically 0–100 mA) or pulse width (typically 0–300 μs).

An NMES device fundamentally consists of electrodes that are connected to a stimulator and a controller (**Fig. 1**). A pair of electrodes constitutes a stimulus channel. Surface (ie, transcutaneous) electrodes, percutaneous intramuscular wire electrodes, and implanted epimysial, intramuscular or nerve cuff electrodes may be used. The stimulator (ie, pulse generator) may have a controller built into it or have a separate controller attached or wirelessly linked to it. The controller regulates the timing and intensity of stimulation delivered through one or multiple stimulus channels. Input to the stimulator's controller may be via buttons, switches, and/or various types of external or implanted sensors or recording (eg, electromyographic) electrodes.

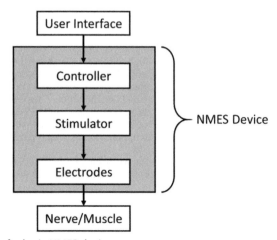

Fig. 1. Diagram of a basic NMES device.

PURPOSES OF NEUROMUSCULAR ELECTRICAL STIMULATION FOR UPPER AND LOWER LIMB REHABILITATION AFTER STROKE

Paresis is the inability or decreased ability to volitionally activate motor units and is one of the most common manifestations of stroke.[4] Clinically, paresis presents as muscle weakness and reduced speed of activation and the inability to generate functionally useful movement of the involved limb. Lang and associates[5] studied the relative strengths of the associations between specific upper limb impairments and function and concluded that paresis was the strongest contributor to the loss of function. In the upper limb, the combination of paresis, loss of fractionated movements, flexor hypertonia, and somatosensory abnormalities often manifest as difficulty extending the elbow and opening the hand in a functional manner, which severely limits the functional work space. At 6 months after a stroke, about 65% of patients still cannot incorporate the affected arm and hand into their daily activities.[6] Therefore, NMES for upper limb stroke rehabilitation is usually applied to the elbow, wrist, and/or hand extensor muscles.

In the lower limb, paresis, along with the inability to grade muscle contractions, poor motor coordination, poor endurance, spasticity, and impaired balance have significant consequences on ambulation.[7] At 6 months after a stroke, approximately 30% of stroke survivors are unable to walk unassisted.[8] A major contributor to impaired ambulation is the inability to dorsiflex the ankle during the swing phase of the gait. Diminished ankle dorsiflexion, knee flexion, or hip flexion can result in the inability to clear the floor with the affected limb during the swing phase of the gait, resulting in difficult and unsafe ambulation or nonambulation. Patients frequently use compensatory strategies, such as circumduction, hip hiking, or vaulting, to clear the toes. An ankle-foot orthosis (AFO) is the standard of care for foot drop; but because AFOs limit ankle mobility, they may actually inhibit recovery of dorsiflexion. Therefore, NMES has been used to improve ankle dorsiflexion and a more normal gait pattern.

Various NMES modalities have been used for upper and lower limb motor relearning after a stroke. Motor relearning is defined as the reacquisition of motor skills following central nervous system injury. NMES can be used as a motor relearning tool by enabling stroke survivors with significant paresis to participate in goal-oriented repetitive movement therapy. The NMES-mediated task must be repetitive, novel, volitionally controlled, and functionally relevant.[9–11] Although stroke survivors may use an NMES motor relearning system to assist execution of daily activities, its primary intent is training, such that improved functional use of the hemiparetic limb is maintained when the system is *not being used*. Improved upper limb function or ambulation that remains after an NMES device has been used is called a *therapeutic effect*.

For patients who are in the chronic phase of stroke and in whom motor relearning strategies have been exhausted, NMES may be used as a neuroprosthesis. The primary intent of a neuroprosthesis is to enable patients to execute functional tasks with the affected upper limb or walk *while using the device* as part of routine daily living. Improved function that is realized while using an NMES device is called a *neuroprosthetic effect*.

NEUROMUSCULAR ELECTRICAL STIMULATION MODALITIES FOR UPPER LIMB REHABILITATION

Cyclic NMES uses a 1- or 2-channel stimulator to activate the wrist and/or finger and thumb extensors in a repetitive (cyclic) fashion via surface electrodes placed on the forearm over the motor points of those muscles. Cyclic NMES devices typically have a menu of on/off cycle settings from which to choose. Once the device is set up and switched on, the stimulation automatically ramps on and off according to a selected duty cycle, with patients not having to exert any simultaneous effort. Patients do not control the timing or intensity of cyclic stimulation (**Table 1**); therefore, this modality is not typically used to mediate functional task practice.

Cyclic NMES has been shown in several randomized controlled trials (RCTs) of *acute and subacute* hemiplegic patients to reduce upper limb motor impairment (eg, increase in strength, upper limb Fugl-Meyer score, and so forth) relative to controls.[12–16] Some studies reported an enduring effect over 2 to 6 months,[12,13,15,16] whereas others found that the effect was not sustained beyond the treatment period.[14] Some studies found that the positive effects on impairment did not translate to significant improvements in basic self-care tasks or upper limb function (ie, functional independent measure score, action research arm test [ARAT]) relative to controls,[13,14] whereas other studies did show significant, though sometimes transient, improvements in function relative to controls.[12,17] The beneficial effects of cyclic NMES seem to be more apparent in patients who have some residual movement at baseline.[12,18] In a study of 95 subacute patients, initial motor severity (ie, baseline Fugl-Meyer score) was identified as the most significant predictor of improvement in upper limb function after 4 weeks of cyclic NMES.[17] Studies of cyclic NMES in *chronic* hemiplegia have typically been relatively small case series designs (ie, no control group) but have also demonstrated improvements in various upper limb motor impairment measures.[18,19]

Electromyographic (EMG)-triggered NMES attempts to make stimulated hand opening coincide with the patients' own effort to open the hand. Surface EMG recording electrodes are placed over the wrist and/or finger extensors of the paretic side to detect EMG signals when patients attempt to open the hand. When the processed EMG signal surpasses a preset threshold, electrical stimulation ramps on to a preset stimulation intensity that produces full hand opening. After several seconds, the stimulation turns off and the patients are prompted with visual and/or audio cues to try to open the hand again, repeating the EMG-triggered NMES cycle. Thus, EMG-triggered stimulation facilitates repetitive and volitionally initiated exercises of the hemiparetic upper extremity and provides cutaneous and proprioceptive feedback time-locked to each attempted movement,[20] which may be important for motor relearning.[21] Like cyclic NMES, EMG-triggered NMES is not typically used to mediate functional task practice because the intensity and duration of stimulation are not controlled by the patients (see **Table 1**). Because EMG-triggered NMES requires patients to be able to produce discernable EMG signals consistently, it may not be applicable to the most severely impaired patients.[21]

EMG-triggered NMES has been shown to improve upper limb motor *impairment*. An early case series study of 69 chronic patients reported improvement in wrist active range of motion and extensor EMG activity in response to EMG-triggered NMES

Table 1				
Degree of patient control for different upper limb NMES modalities				
Patients Have Real-time Control of the Following:	**Cyclic NMES**	**EMG-Triggered NMES**	**Switch-Triggered NMES**	**Contralaterally Controlled NMES**
Timing of NMES	No	Onset only	Yes	Yes
Intensity of NMES	No	No	No	Yes

Abbreviation: EMG, electromyographic.

integrated with conventional therapy.[21] The participants who received a greater dosage (ie, sessions per week) of EMG-triggered NMES had greater increases in voluntary extensor EMG amplitude. RCTs in chronic hemiplegia also show that EMG-triggered NMES improved performance on one or more measures of motor impairment (eg, Fugl-Meyer score, Box and Blocks score, extensor and grip strength) as compared with conventional therapy, though not all studies agree on which outcomes improve relative to controls.[22–25] Most of the trials in chronic patients did not assess upper limb *function* (ie, activity limitation) or the persistence of effect. In acute and subacute patients, an RCT showed greater improvement on impairment measures but not on upper limb function relative to conventional therapy[20]; but another study showed the opposite: improvement on function (ie, ARAT) but not on impairment measures relative to usual care.[26] Nearly all of the RCTs of EMG-triggered NMES have had small sample sizes (ie, <10 per group); like cyclic NMES, the improvements relative to controls are generally modest and of questionable clinical relevance.

Although EMG-triggered NMES might be expected to improve upper limb movement and function more than cyclic NMES,[27] several RCTs that directly compared the two treatments showed no significant difference in the outcomes of cyclic and EMG-triggered NMES, whether in chronic[28,29] or subacute[30] subjects. Explanations for why no differences in outcomes were found between cyclic and EMG-triggered NMES include: (1) EMG-triggered NMES may not require enough active involvement (ie, patients only trigger stimulation, not control duration or intensity) to create a large enough contrast with cyclic NMES.[28] (2) The cyclic NMES group may have also been exerting effort during stimulation, further reducing the contrast between the two treatments.[28] (3) With EMG-triggered NMES, any time delays between the attempt to extend the wrist and fingers and the initiation of stimulation may negate any neurophysiologic advantage the treatment might have had over cyclic NMES.

Switch-triggered NMES is a modality intended to facilitate functional task practice. Switches (or button presses) allow patients[31] or the therapist[32] to control both the initiation and termination of stimulation sequences (ie, the timing of the stimulated movement; see **Table 1**) with button presses so that the device can be used in assisting task practice during therapy sessions.[33] The intensity of stimulation is not controlled by patients but is preset. The Bioness H200 (Bioness Inc, Valencia, CA) is an example of a switch-triggered device that stimulates finger and thumb extensors and flexors through surface electrodes that are mounted inside a wrist-forearm orthosis, which also houses the stimulator. Patients turn the stimulation on and off to the extensors and flexors by pressing buttons on a separate control unit with their unaffected hand. Stimulation sequences that produce different hand opening and closing postures can be programmed and selected to match the task to be performed. Significant therapeutic effects were reported on several measures of motor impairment (eg, Box and Blocks score, Ashworth score) and function (eg, timed Jebsen-Taylor Hand Function tasks) in chronic patients after 5 weeks of home exercise and task practice with the Bioness H200.[34] Several follow-up RCTs in acute[33,35] and subacute[31] patients found that switch-triggered NMES with therapy had greater improvements than therapy alone on measures of spasticity, wrist extension, Box and Blocks score, Fugl-Meyer score, and timed tasks. Although the Bioness H200 can be used as a neuroprosthesis and has been shown to have a significant neuroprosthetic effect,[36] it is typically used and studied as a motor relearning tool.

Another switch-triggered NMES approach uses stimulation only as needed to assist first with repetitive reaching tasks (stimulating shoulder and elbow muscles) and then with grasping tasks (stimulating wrist, finger, and thumb muscles), progressively decreasing the use of NMES as patients improve.[37] The treating therapist uses button switches to activate the stimulation sequences that are needed to perform tasks. Greater therapeutic effects were measured in acute patients who had 12 to 16 weeks of this switch-triggered NMES approach as compared with patients who received conventional task-specific occupational therapy.[32]

Sensor- and EMG-*controlled* NMES modalities use controllers that are designed to let patients control the timing *and* intensity of stimulation to their hand in a way that can be fluid with task practice, which may result in greater sensorimotor integration and superior motor relearning (ie, therapeutic effects). Such systems may also be suitable as neuroprostheses to assist with activities of daily living. Indeed, the earliest NMES devices for upper limb stroke rehabilitation used a sensor mounted to the contralateral shoulder to let patients proportionally control the intensity of stimulation to the forearm extensors as they practiced tasks.[38] Electrogoniometers, bend sensors, touch-sensitive mats, and accelerometers are among the external sensors that have been incorporated into NMES systems for upper limb stroke rehabilitation.[39–42] Researchers also continue to explore the use of EMG signals from the impaired upper limb to not merely *trigger* the onset of a preset intensity and duration of stimulation but also to *control* the intensity and timing of stimulation.[43,44] A challenge for EMG-controlled NMES modalities is that the effort required from patients to contract the muscle that operates the controller may induce flexor synergies or hypertonia, which can overpower the electrical stimulation of extensors and result in reduced degrees of stimulated hand opening.[43,45]

Contralaterally controlled NMES is a unique version of sensor-controlled stimulation that uses movement from the unimpaired side to control the timing and intensity of stimulation to the paretic side (see **Table 1**).[42] The hand system consists of a glove with bend sensors worn on the *nonparetic* hand and a multichannel stimulator that delivers stimulation to the *paretic* hand extensors with an intensity that is proportional to the degree of opening of the glove (**Fig. 2**). This modality enables repetitive hand opening exercise and functional task practice with the paretic hand. The control strategy gives the user intimate proportional control of the stimulation intensity without requiring any residual movement or EMG signals from the paretic hand. Therefore, the likelihood of triggering flexor synergy patterns may be less than sensor-controlled or EMG-controlled stimulation devices that require control signals from the paretic limb. Contralaterally controlled NMES produced larger improvements in maximum voluntary finger extension and other measures of upper extremity impairment and activity limitation than cyclic NMES in an RCT of subacute patients.[46]

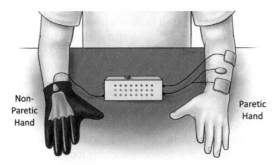

Non-
Paretic
Hand

Paretic
Hand

Fig. 2. Contralaterally controlled NMES system, an example of a sensor-controlled NMES modality. Volitional opening of the nonparetic hand wearing an instrumented glove produces a proportional intensity of stimulation to the paretic hand, giving patients control of the timing and intensity of NMES.

NEUROMUSCULAR ELECTRICAL STIMULATION MODALITIES FOR LOWER LIMB REHABILITATION

Cyclic, EMG-triggered, and contralaterally controlled NMES applied to paretic lower limb muscles while patients are seated or side-lying has been evaluated for therapeutic effects. In a randomized placebo-controlled trial of 46 acute hemiplegic subjects, cyclic NMES was applied to the quadriceps, hamstring, tibialis anterior, and medial gastrocnemius in an activation sequence that mimicked normal gait while the subjects were side-lying with their lower extremity supported by a sling.[47] Significantly greater improvement in ankle dorsiflexion torque and EMG activity and significantly less spasticity and cocontraction were demonstrated after 3 weeks of multichannel cyclic NMES as compared with the control group. Also, a significantly greater percentage of subjects in the cyclic NMES group were able to complete a timed walking task by the end of the 3-week treatment and 5 weeks later as compared with the control group. EMG-triggered NMES of paretic ankle dorsiflexors has been shown to have positive effects on ankle strength, range of motion, balance, and ambulation in chronic patients.[21,48,49] Contralaterally controlled NMES, whereby patients controlled the intensity of stimulation to the paretic ankle dorsiflexors by dorsiflexion of their nonparetic ankle while seated, was first tested in a case series[50] and later in an RCT.[51] Contralaterally controlled NMES was shown to increase lower extremity Fugl-Meyer score, maximum dorsiflexion angle and moment while seated, and performance on the modified Emory Functional Ambulation Profile in chronic patients, but not more than cyclic NMES.

Liberson and associates[52] first describes applying NMES to the paretic ankle dorsiflexors (ie, peroneal nerve) *during* the swing phase of the gait in 1961. The common peroneal nerve was stimulated with a pair of electrodes, one placed just below the head of the fibula and the other over the tibialis anterior. A heel switch worn in the shoe of the paretic side turned the stimulation on when the foot was lifted off the ground and turned the stimulation off at heel strike and during the stance phase of the gait. Currently, there are 3 surface electrode NMES systems for preventing foot drop during gait approved by the Food and Drug Administration: the Odstock Dropped-Foot Stimulator (Odstock Medical Limited, Salisbury, UK), WalkAide (Innovative Neurotronics Inc, Austin, TX), and Bioness L300 Foot Drop System (Bioness Inc, Valencia, CA). These devices use either a heel switch or a tilt sensor below the knee to synchronize the timing of stimulation to the swing phase of the gait (**Fig. 3**).[53,54] Two multichannel foot-drop systems with implanted electrodes and stimulator have the CE mark in Europe. One is a dual-channel device developed by the University of Twente (Netherlands) that stimulates the deep and superficial branches of the common peroneal nerve for better control of ankle dorsiflexion, eversion, and inversion.[55] The other is a 4-channel device developed at Aalborg University (Denmark) and uses a 4-channel nerve cuff electrode surgically placed around the common peroneal nerve.[56]

Peroneal nerve stimulation (PNS) during gait has positive neuroprosthetic and therapeutic effects on ambulation. *Neuroprosthetic* effects have been shown in several case series studies and several RCTs, with outcome measures ranging from gait kinematic and spatiotemporal parameters to metabolic cost indices.[53,54,57–59] According to a systematic review, there is a positive neuroprosthetic effect of PNS on walking speed.[60] A recent multicenter clinical trial of 99 chronic patients showed that after 42 weeks of PNS during gait, 67% of participants had a gain of 0.1 m/s or greater (the minimal clinically important difference) in comfortable gait speed when walking with PNS.[61] *Therapeutic* effects associated with PNS during gait have also been

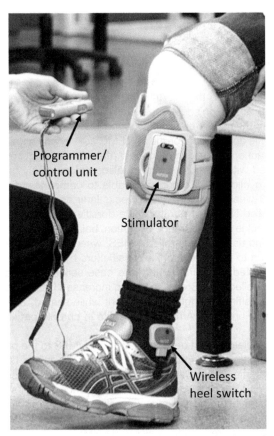

Fig. 3. Example of a peroneal nerve stimulator with a wireless heel switch for dorsiflexion of the paretic ankle during gait. (*Courtesy of* Bioness, Inc, Valencia, CA; with permission.)

observed since the earliest studies. That is, PNS during gait produces not only positive neuroprosthetic effects (ie, the effects on gait observed when the stimulator is on) but also carryover or therapeutic effects after the device has been turned off. Such effects have been observed in multiple case series studies and include improvements in ambulation function, normalization of EMG muscle activation patterns, emergence of EMG signals in previously silent muscles, and decreased cocontraction of antagonist muscles.[52–54,62–67] After 30 weeks of PNS during gait, 29% of 99 patients with chronic stroke had a therapeutic effect on comfortable walking speed of 0.1 m/s or greater.[61]

The research on PNS during gait has progressed to RCTs comparing the effects of PNS to standard of care, which is an AFO. In order for PNS to challenge standard-of-care practice, definitive evidence would be necessary to show that PNS provides either an equivalent neuroprosthetic effect on walking or a superior therapeutic effect restoring volitional gait. Four large clinical trials have recently been published comparing PNS with AFO. Sheffler and colleagues[68] compared the therapeutic effects of 12 weeks of PNS and AFO on lower limb impairment, ambulation, and quality of life in 110 chronic patients and found significant but similar *therapeutic* effects on ambulation and quality of life from both PNS and AFO. Kluding and colleagues[69] compared the effects of 30 weeks of PNS and AFO in 197 chronic patients and found both groups to improve similarly on walking speed with their assigned device (*neuroprosthetic* effect). They also noted significant but similar *therapeutic* effects on walking speed for both groups. Everaert and colleagues[70] enrolled 121 patients who were less than 1 year after a stroke and found similar improvements in walking speed between PNS and AFO groups. Bethoux and colleagues[71] reported a 30-site study that enrolled 495 patients with chronic stroke who wore a PNS device or an AFO for 6 months. Both groups had significant improvements in gait velocity while wearing their device (AFO or PNS), but no between-group differences were found.

Based on these 4 large RCTs, PNS during gait for 12 to 30 weeks can have significant therapeutic effects on functional mobility and walking speed. Wearing the PNS device can further increase walking speed and walking endurance beyond the therapeutic effects. However, no significant differences were found between PNS and AFO on walking speed or functional ambulation, although questionnaires showed that patients preferred PNS over AFO with respect to long-term use, all-day use, confidence on inclines, and ease of donning/doffing.[70]

Because gait deviation in hemiplegia is not limited to ankle dysfunction, multichannel stimulation systems have been investigated for therapeutic effects. Early work used surface electrodes and demonstrated improvements in qualitative and quantitative measures of gait after training with a 6-channel surface system that activated ankle dorsiflexion and plantar flexion, knee flexion and extension, and hip extension.[72,73] However, as the number of electrodes increases, surface systems become increasingly difficult to implement because of the difficulty of donning and doffing of multiple electrodes, pain of stimulation, and poor repeatability of electrode placement and muscle contractions. Therefore, multichannel percutaneous systems have also been explored for motor relearning.[74] A single-blinded RCT of 32 patients with chronic stroke demonstrated that multichannel percutaneous NMES-mediated ambulation training in combination with body weight–supported treadmill training (BWSTT) improved gait components and knee flexion coordination more than BWSTT without NMES[75] and that the gains were maintained at 6 months after treatment.[76]

PERIPHERAL AND CENTRAL EFFECTS OF NEUROMUSCULAR ELECTRICAL STIMULATION IN STROKE REHABILITATION

The mechanisms by which NMES reduces motor impairment and activity limitation have not been fully elucidated, but therapeutic effects are probably caused by a combination of peripheral and central effects. Peripheral effects of NMES include increase in contractile force and fatigue resistance,[77,78] increase in muscle mass,[79] reduction of edema,[80] conversion of fast-twitch fast-fatiguing glycolytic type II muscle fibers to slow-twitch fatigue-resistant oxidative type I muscle fibers,[78] and enhanced hyperemic arterial response and endothelium-dependent cutaneous vasodilation.[81] These peripheral effects can reverse disuse atrophy and may explain in part some improvements patients who have had a stroke experience after various NMES treatments.

Some NMES treatments may also affect the central nervous system and how it controls movement. For example, NMES may promote motor relearning by uniquely providing an artificial way of ensuring synchronized presynaptic and postsynaptic activity (Hebbian plasticity), especially if the electrical stimulation is paired with simultaneous voluntary effort that activates the residual upper motor neurons.[82] Indeed, cortical excitability, as assessed by measuring motor-evoked potentials (MEPs) in response to transcranial magnetic stimulation, has been shown to increase more when NMES is paired with voluntary muscle contraction than with NMES alone.[83]

This finding suggests that the effect of NMES on cortical excitability is improved by concurrent voluntary cortical drive. Whether the increase in cortical excitability is caused by changes at the spinal level, cortical reorganization, or both is unclear. Several researchers have hypothesized that EMG-triggered NMES may produce functional cortical reorganization by inducing long-term potentiation in sensorimotor cortex caused by proprioceptive and cutaneous afferent feedback occurring concurrently with attempted movements.[20,21,23] A regimen of EMG-triggered NMES to the upper extremity has been shown to increase metabolic activity (measured by PET) in the *contralesional* supplementary motor area, primary motor cortex, and primary somatosensory cortex,[84] and to increase the intensity of hand related cortical activity (measured by fMRI) in *contralesional* somatosensory cortex.[24] In contrast, a shift in the laterality index toward the *ipsilesional* sensorimotor cortex was shown after EMG-triggered NMES[22]; brain cortical perfusion (measured by near-infrared spectroscopy) was greater in the *ipsilesional* sensorimotor cortex *during* EMG-controlled NMES than during cyclic NMES or voluntary attempts to extend the wrist and fingers.[85]

There is also evidence that, when unpaired with voluntary effort, NMES may produce changes in the brain. For example, progressively increasing the intensity of surface NMES of the quadriceps muscle from sensory threshold to maximum motor response produced proportional increases in cortical activity in specific areas of interest, including primary somatosensory and motor cortices, as shown by functional MRI (fMRI).[86] Another study showed that stimulation of the common peroneal nerve at 25 Hz with intensities greater than the motor threshold for 30 minutes while seated at rest increased the MEP in the tibialis anterior by 50% at a transcranial magnetic stimulation (TMS) intensity that initially gave a half-maximum MEP. This effect was evident after 10 minutes of stimulation and persisted for at least 30 minutes after the stimulation ended.[87] Follow-up experiments provided evidence that the increase in excitability did not occur at the level of motorneurons but rather at the cortical level.[87,88] Long-term use of a foot-drop stimulator has been found to increase both MEPs elicited by TMS and maximum voluntary contraction of the tibialis anterior in patients who have had a stroke, evidence that regular use of a PNS device strengthens activation of motor cortical areas and their residual descending connections.[89]

These studies and others provide mounting evidence that there is a cortical component to NMES, but more studies are needed to elucidate the precise mechanisms at work under specific NMES modalities and patient characteristics.

EMERGING DIRECTIONS FOR NEUROMUSCULAR ELECTRICAL STIMULATION IN STROKE REHABILITATION

New NMES techniques for upper and lower limb stroke rehabilitation continue to be developed, especially those that use sensors to trigger stimulation when patients achieve some minimum volitional movement.[41,90,91] It is highly doubtful that any single NMES modality used in isolation from other motor rehabilitation therapies will lead to substantial motor recovery. Therefore, there is a growing trend toward combining NMES with other emerging therapeutic strategies that have shown promise. Examples include combining NMES with mirror therapy,[92] repetitive transcranial magnetic stimulation,[93] constraint-induced movement therapy,[94] robot-assisted movement therapy,[95] motor imagery,[30,84] bilateral movement training,[96] virtual reality games,[97] transcranial direct current stimulation,[98] and BWSTT.[76,99] Perhaps the best stroke rehabilitation program would have a defined sequence of therapies and combination therapies that become suitable for patients who have had a stroke as they progress from severe impairment to complete motor recovery, NMES being an important component in the slate of rehabilitation therapies and techniques.

Currently, a clinically viable upper extremity neuroprosthesis for daily long-term use as an assistive device is not available for persons with hemiparesis. Implantable microstimulator[39,100] or multichannel implantable pulse generator[43] approaches may be suitable for patients who have had a stroke who have been carefully screened for prohibitive flexor hypertonia. But most patients will not be able to realize a robust neuroprosthetic effect unless a means of suppressing flexor hypertonia is incorporated. Emerging technology that uses nerve cuff electrodes to deliver high-frequency stimulus waveforms to block action potentials in nerves may prove capable of suppressing hypertonia.[101] Adding such spasticity suppressing stimulation to an NMES system could considerably improve its neuroprosthetic effect and widen its applicability.

As more NMES modalities and technology continue to emerge, more clinical research studies will be needed. With some exceptions, most of the NMES efficacy studies to date have been relatively small and, therefore, limited in power to make strong conclusions. Large RCTs comparing different NMES modalities as well as comparing NMES with the standard of care are still needed. Studies aimed at elucidating the mechanisms of NMES-mediated recovery (ie, specific effects on the central nervous system) could lead to treatment optimization. Also studies are needed to define the optimum treatment dose and the most likely responders for any given NMES modality.

REFERENCES

1. Conforto AB, Cohen LG, dos Santos RL, et al. Effects of somatosensory stimulation on motor function in chronic cortico-subcortical strokes. J Neurol 2007; 254:333–9.
2. Wilson RD, Gunzler DD, Bennett ME, et al. Peripheral nerve stimulation compared with usual care for pain relief of hemiplegic shoulder pain: a randomized controlled trial. Am J Phys Med Rehabil 2014;93:17–28.
3. Harvey RL, Stinear JW. Cortical stimulation as an adjuvant to upper limb rehabilitation after stroke. PM R 2010;2:S269–78.
4. Sathian K, Buxbaum LJ, Cohen LG, et al. Neurological principles and rehabilitation of action disorders: common clinical deficits. Neurorehabil Neural Repair 2011;25:21S–32S.
5. Lang CE, Bland MD, Bailey RR, et al. Assessment of upper extremity impairment, function, and activity after stroke: foundations for clinical decision making. J Hand Ther 2013;26:104–14 [quiz: 115].
6. Dobkin BH. Rehabilitation after stroke. N Engl J Med 2005;352:1677–84.
7. Eng JJ, Tang PF. Gait training strategies to optimize walking ability in people with stroke: a synthesis of the evidence. Expert Rev Neurother 2007;7:1417–36.
8. Kelly-Hayes M, Beiser A, Kase CS, et al. The influence of gender and age on disability following ischemic stroke: the Framingham study. J Stroke Cerebrovasc Dis 2003;12:119–26.
9. Nudo RJ, Plautz EJ, Frost SB. Role of adaptive plasticity in recovery of function after damage to motor cortex. Muscle Nerve 2001;24:1000–19.
10. Kleim JA, Barbay S, Nudo RJ. Functional reorganization of the rat motor cortex following motor skill learning. J Neurophysiol 1998;80:3321–5.
11. Plautz EJ, Milliken GW, Nudo RJ. Effects of repetitive motor training on movement representations in adult squirrel monkeys: role of use versus learning. Neurobiol Learn Mem 2000;74:27–55.

12. Powell J, Pandyan AD, Granat M, et al. Electrical stimulation of wrist extensors in poststroke hemiplegia. Stroke 1999;30:1384–9.
13. Chae J, Bethoux F, Bohine T, et al. Neuromuscular stimulation for upper extremity motor and functional recovery in acute hemiplegia. Stroke 1998;29: 975–9.
14. Rosewilliam S, Malhotra S, Roffe C, et al. Can surface neuromuscular electrical stimulation of the wrist and hand combined with routine therapy facilitate recovery of arm function in patients with stroke? Arch Phys Med Rehabil 2012;93: 1715–21.e1.
15. Hsu SS, Hu MH, Wang YH, et al. Dose-response relation between neuromuscular electrical stimulation and upper-extremity function in patients with stroke. Stroke 2010;41:821–4.
16. Lin Z, Yan T. Long-term effectiveness of neuromuscular electrical stimulation for promoting motor recovery of the upper extremity after stroke. J Rehabil Med 2011;43:506–10.
17. Hsu SS, Hu MH, Luh JJ, et al. Dosage of neuromuscular electrical stimulation: is it a determinant of upper limb functional improvement in stroke patients? J Rehabil Med 2012;44:125–30.
18. Hendricks HT, IJzerman MJ, de Kroon JR, et al. Functional electrical stimulation by means of the 'Ness Handmaster Orthosis' in chronic stroke patients: an exploratory study. Clin Rehabil 2001;15:217–20.
19. Santos M, Zahner LH, McKiernan BJ, et al. Neuromuscular electrical stimulation improves severe hand dysfunction for individuals with chronic stroke: a pilot study. J Neurol Phys Ther 2006;30:175–83.
20. Francisco G, Chae J, Chawla H, et al. Electromyogram-triggered neuromuscular stimulation for improving the arm function of acute stroke survivors: a randomized pilot study. Arch Phys Med Rehabil 1998;79:570–5.
21. Fields RW. Electromyographically triggered electric muscle stimulation for chronic hemiplegia. Arch Phys Med Rehabil 1987;68:407–14.
22. Shin HK, Cho SH, Jeon HS, et al. Cortical effect and functional recovery by the electromyography-triggered neuromuscular stimulation in chronic stroke patients. Neurosci Lett 2008;442:174–9.
23. Cauraugh J, Light K, Kim S, et al. Chronic motor dysfunction after stroke: recovering wrist and finger extension by electromyography-triggered neuromuscular stimulation. Stroke 2000;31:1360–4.
24. Kimberley TJ, Lewis SM, Auerbach EJ, et al. Electrical stimulation driving functional improvements and cortical changes in subjects with stroke. Exp Brain Res 2004;154:450–60.
25. Kraft GH, Fitts SS, Hammond MC. Techniques to improve function of the arm and hand in chronic hemiplegia. Arch Phys Med Rehabil 1992;73:220–7.
26. Bello AI, Rockson BE, Olaogun MO. The effects of electromyographic-triggered neuromuscular electrical muscle stimulation on the functional hand recovery among stroke survivors. Afr J Med Med Sci 2009;38:185–91.
27. de Kroon JR, Ijzerman MJ, Chae J, et al. Relation between stimulation characteristics and clinical outcome in studies using electrical stimulation to improve motor control of the upper extremity in stroke. J Rehabil Med 2005;37:65–74.
28. de Kroon JR, Ijzerman MJ. Electrical stimulation of the upper extremity in stroke: cyclic versus EMG-triggered stimulation. Clin Rehabil 2008;22:690–7.
29. Boyaci A, Topuz O, Alkan H, et al. Comparison of the effectiveness of active and passive neuromuscular electrical stimulation of hemiplegic upper extremities: a randomized, controlled trial. Int J Rehabil Res 2013;36:315–22.

30. Hemmen B, Seelen HA. Effects of movement imagery and electromyography-triggered feedback on arm hand function in stroke patients in the subacute phase. Clin Rehabil 2007;21:587–94.
31. Ring H, Rosenthal N. Controlled study of neuroprosthetic functional electrical stimulation in sub-acute post-stroke rehabilitation. J Rehabil Med 2005;37: 32–6.
32. Thrasher TA, Zivanovic V, McIlroy W, et al. Rehabilitation of reaching and grasping function in severe hemiplegic patients using functional electrical stimulation therapy. Neurorehabil Neural Repair 2008;22:706–14.
33. Alon G, Levitt AF, McCarthy PA. Functional electrical stimulation enhancement of upper extremity functional recovery during stroke rehabilitation: a pilot study. Neurorehabil Neural Repair 2007;21:207–15.
34. Alon G, Sunnerhagen KS, Geurts AC, et al. A home-based, self-administered stimulation program to improve selected hand functions of chronic stroke. NeuroRehabilitation 2003;18:215–25.
35. Alon G, Levitt AF, McCarthy PA. Functional electrical stimulation (FES) may modify the poor prognosis of stroke survivors with severe motor loss of the upper extremity: a preliminary study. Am J Phys Med Rehabil 2008;87:627–36.
36. Alon G, McBride K, Ring H. Improving selected hand functions using a noninvasive neuroprosthesis in persons with chronic stroke. J Stroke Cerebrovasc Dis 2002;11:99–106.
37. Popovic MR, Thrasher TA, Zivanovic V, et al. Neuroprosthesis for retraining reaching and grasping functions in severe hemiplegic patients. Neuromodulation 2005;8:58–72.
38. Merletti R, Acimovic R, Grobelnik S, et al. Electrophysiological orthosis for the upper extremity in hemiplegia: feasibility study. Arch Phys Med Rehabil 1975; 56:507–13.
39. Burridge JH, Turk R, Merrill D, et al. A personalized sensor-controlled microstimulator system for arm rehabilitation poststroke. Part 2: objective outcomes and patients' perspectives. Neuromodulation 2011;14:80–8 [discussion: 88].
40. Merrill DR, Davis R, Turk R, et al. A personalized sensor-controlled microstimulator system for arm rehabilitation poststroke. Part 1: system architecture. Neuromodulation 2011;14:72–9 [discussion: 79].
41. Mann G, Taylor P, Lane R. Accelerometer-triggered electrical stimulation for reach and grasp in chronic stroke patients: a pilot study. Neurorehabil Neural Repair 2011;25:774–80.
42. Knutson JS, Harley MY, Hisel TZ, et al. Improving hand function in stroke survivors: a pilot study of contralaterally controlled functional electric stimulation in chronic hemiplegia. Arch Phys Med Rehabil 2007;88:513–20.
43. Knutson JS, Chae J, Hart RL, et al. Implanted neuroprosthesis for assisting arm and hand function after stroke: a case study. J Rehabil Res Dev 2012;49: 1505–16.
44. Thorsen R, Cortesi M, Jonsdottir J, et al. Myoelectrically driven functional electrical stimulation may increase motor recovery of upper limb in poststroke subjects: a randomized controlled pilot study. J Rehabil Res Dev 2013;50: 785–94.
45. Makowski N, Knutson J, Chae J, et al. Interaction of poststroke voluntary effort and functional neuromuscular electrical stimulation. J Rehabil Res Dev 2013;50: 85–98.
46. Knutson JS, Harley MY, Hisel TZ, et al. Contralaterally controlled functional electrical stimulation for upper extremity hemiplegia: an early-phase randomized

clinical trial in subacute stroke patients. Neurorehabil Neural Repair 2012;26: 239–46.

47. Yan T, Hui-Chan CW, Li LS. Functional electrical stimulation improves motor recovery of the lower extremity and walking ability of subjects with first acute stroke: a randomized placebo-controlled trial. Stroke 2005;36:80–5.

48. Chae J, Fang ZP, Walker M, et al. Intramuscular electromyographically controlled neuromuscular electrical stimulation for ankle dorsiflexion recovery in chronic hemiplegia. Am J Phys Med Rehabil 2001;80:842–7.

49. Barth E, Herrman V, Levine P, et al. Low-dose, EMG-triggered electrical stimulation for balance and gait in chronic stroke. Top Stroke Rehabil 2008;15:451–5.

50. Knutson JS, Chae J. A novel neuromuscular electrical stimulation treatment for recovery of ankle dorsiflexion in chronic hemiplegia: a case series pilot study. Am J Phys Med Rehabil 2010;89:672–82.

51. Knutson JS, Hansen K, Nagy J, et al. Contralaterally controlled neuromuscular electrical stimulation for recovery of ankle dorsiflexion: a pilot randomized controlled trial in patients with chronic post-stroke hemiplegia. Am J Phys Med Rehabil 2013;92:656–65.

52. Liberson WT, Holmquest HJ, Scot D, et al. Functional electrotherapy: stimulation of the peroneal nerve synchronized with the swing phase of the gait of hemiplegic patients. Arch Phys Med Rehabil 1961;42:101–5.

53. Burridge JI I, Taylor PN, Hagan SA, et al. The effects of common peroneal stimulation on the effort and speed of walking: a randomized controlled trial with chronic hemiplegic patients. Clin Rehabil 1997;11:201–10.

54. Stein RB, Chong S, Everaert DG, et al. A multicenter trial of a foot drop stimulator controlled by a tilt sensor. Neurorehabil Neural Repair 2006;20:371–9.

55. Kottink AI, Hermens HJ, Nene AV, et al. A randomized controlled trial of an implantable 2-channel peroneal nerve stimulator on walking speed and activity in poststroke hemiplegia. Arch Phys Med Rehabil 2007;88:971–8.

56. Burridge JH, Haugland M, Larsen B, et al. Phase II trial to evaluate the ActiGait implanted drop-foot stimulator in established hemiplegia. J Rehabil Med 2007; 39:212–8.

57. Merletti R, Andina A, Galante M, et al. Clinical experience of electronic peroneal stimulators in 50 hemiparetic patients. Scand J Rehabil Med 1979;11:111–21.

58. Granat MH, Maxwell DJ, Ferguson AC, et al. Peroneal stimulator; evaluation for the correction of spastic drop foot in hemiplegia. Arch Phys Med Rehabil 1996; 77:19–24.

59. Sabut SK, Sikdar C, Mondal R, et al. Restoration of gait and motor recovery by functional electrical stimulation therapy in persons with stroke. Disabil Rehabil 2010;32:1594–603.

60. Kottink AI, Oostendorp LJ, Buurke JH, et al. The orthotic effect of functional electrical stimulation on the improvement of walking in stroke patients with a dropped foot: a systematic review. Artif Organs 2004;28:577–86.

61. O'Dell MW, Dunning K, Kluding P, et al. Response and prediction of improvement in gait speed from functional electrical stimulation in persons with poststroke drop foot. PM R 2014;6:587–601 [quiz: 601].

62. Taylor PN, Burridge JH, Dunkerley AL, et al. Clinical use of the Odstock dropped foot stimulator: its effect on the speed and effort of walking. Arch Phys Med Rehabil 1999;80:1577–83.

63. Robbins SM, Houghton PE, Woodbury MG, et al. The therapeutic effect of functional and transcutaneous electric stimulation on improving gait speed in stroke patients: a meta-analysis. Arch Phys Med Rehabil 2006;87:853–9.

64. Stefancic M, Rebersek M, Merletti R. The therapeutic effects of the Ljublijana functional electrical brace. Eur Medicophys 1976;12:1–9.

65. Carnstam B, Larsson LE, Prevec TS. Improvement of gait following functional electrical stimulation. I. Investigations on changes in voluntary strength and proprioceptive reflexes. Scand J Rehabil Med 1977;9:7–13.

66. Kljajic M, Malezic M, Acimovic R, et al. Gait evaluation in hemiparetic patients using subcutaneous peroneal electrical stimulation. Scand J Rehabil Med 1992;24:121–6.

67. Stein RB, Everaert DG, Thompson AK, et al. Long-term therapeutic and orthotic effects of a foot drop stimulator on walking performance in progressive and nonprogressive neurological disorders. Neurorehabil Neural Repair 2010;24:152–67.

68. Sheffler LR, Taylor PN, Gunzler DD, et al. Randomized controlled trial of surface peroneal nerve stimulation for motor relearning in lower limb hemiparesis. Arch Phys Med Rehabil 2013;94:1007–14.

69. Kluding PM, Dunning K, O'Dell MW, et al. Foot drop stimulation versus ankle foot orthosis after stroke: 30-week outcomes. Stroke 2013;44:1660–9.

70. Everaert DG, Stein RB, Abrams GM, et al. Effect of a foot-drop stimulator and ankle-foot orthosis on walking performance after stroke: a multicenter randomized controlled trial. Neurorehabil Neural Repair 2013;27:579–91.

71. Bethoux F, Rogers HL, Nolan KJ, et al. The effects of peroneal nerve functional electrical stimulation versus ankle-foot orthosis in patients with chronic stroke: a randomized controlled trial. Neurorehabil Neural Repair 2014;28:688–97.

72. Bogataj U, Gros N, Kljajic M, et al. The rehabilitation of gait in patients with hemiplegia: a comparison between conventional therapy and multichannel functional electrical stimulation therapy. Phys Ther 1995;75:490–502.

73. Stanic U, Acimovic-Janezic R, Gros N, et al. Multichannel electrical stimulation for correction of hemiplegic gait. Scand J Rehabil Med 1978;10:75–92.

74. Daly JJ, Barnicle K, Kobetic R, et al. Electrically induced gait changes post stroke, using an FNS system with intramuscular electrodes and multiple channels. J Neurol Rehabil 1993;7:17–25.

75. Daly JJ, Roenigk K, Holcomb J, et al. A randomized controlled trial of functional neuromuscular stimulation in chronic stroke subjects. Stroke 2006;37:172–8.

76. Daly JJ, Zimbelman J, Roenigk KL, et al. Recovery of coordinated gait: randomized controlled stroke trial of functional electrical stimulation (FES) versus no FES, with weight-supported treadmill and over-ground training. Neurorehabil Neural Repair 2011;25:588–96.

77. Peckham PH, Mortimer JT, Marsolais EB. Alteration in the force and fatigability of skeletal muscle in quadriplegic humans following exercise induced by chronic electrical stimulation. Clin Orthop Relat Res 1976;(114):326–33.

78. Gondin J, Brocca L, Bellinzona E, et al. Neuromuscular electrical stimulation training induces atypical adaptations of the human skeletal muscle phenotype: a functional and proteomic analysis. J Appl Physiol (1985) 2011;110:433–50.

79. Arija-Blazquez A, Ceruelo-Abajo S, Diaz-Merino MS, et al. Effects of electromyostimulation on muscle and bone in men with acute traumatic spinal cord injury: a randomized clinical trial. J Spinal Cord Med 2014;37(3):299–309.

80. Meijer JW, Voerman GE, Santegoets KM, et al. Short-term effects and long-term use of a hybrid orthosis for neuromuscular electrical stimulation of the upper extremity in patients after chronic stroke. J Rehabil Med 2009;41:157–61.

81. Wang JS, Chen SY, Lan C, et al. Neuromuscular electric stimulation enhances endothelial vascular control and hemodynamic function in paretic

upper extremities of patients with stroke. Arch Phys Med Rehabil 2004;85: 1112–6.

82. Rushton DN. Functional electrical stimulation and rehabilitation–an hypothesis. Med Eng Phys 2003;25:75–8.

83. Khaslavskaia S, Sinkjaer T. Motor cortex excitability following repetitive electrical stimulation of the common peroneal nerve depends on the voluntary drive. Exp Brain Res 2005;162:497–502.

84. Hong IK, Choi JB, Lee JH. Cortical changes after mental imagery training combined with electromyography-triggered electrical stimulation in patients with chronic stroke. Stroke 2012;43:2506–9.

85. Hara Y, Obayashi S, Tsujiuchi K, et al. The effects of electromyography-controlled functional electrical stimulation on upper extremity function and cortical perfusion in stroke patients. Clin Neurophysiol 2013;124:2008–15.

86. Smith GV, Alon G, Roys SR, et al. Functional MRI determination of a dose-response relationship to lower extremity neuromuscular electrical stimulation in healthy subjects. Exp Brain Res 2003;150:33–9.

87. Knash ME, Kido A, Gorassini M, et al. Electrical stimulation of the human common peroneal nerve elicits lasting facilitation of cortical motor-evoked potentials. Exp Brain Res 2003;153:366–77.

88. Thompson AK, Stein RB, Chen XY, et al. Modulation in spinal circuits and corticospinal connections following nerve stimulation and operant conditioning. Conf Proc IEEE Eng Med Biol Soc 2006;1:2138–41.

89. Everaert DG, Thompson AK, Chong SL, et al. Does functional electrical stimulation for foot drop strengthen corticospinal connections? Neurorehabil Neural Repair 2010;24:168–77.

90. Hayward KS, Barker RN, Brauer SG, et al. SMART arm with outcome-triggered electrical stimulation: a pilot randomized clinical trial. Top Stroke Rehabil 2013; 20:289–98.

91. Chung Y, Kim JH, Cha Y, et al. Therapeutic effect of functional electrical stimulation-triggered gait training corresponding gait cycle for stroke. Gait Posture 2014;40:471–5.

92. Kim H, Lee G, Song C. Effect of functional electrical stimulation with mirror therapy on upper extremity motor function in poststroke patients. J Stroke Cerebrovasc Dis 2014;23:655–61.

93. Theilig S, Podubecka J, Bosl K, et al. Functional neuromuscular stimulation to improve severe hand dysfunction after stroke: does inhibitory rTMS enhance therapeutic efficiency? Exp Neurol 2011;230:149–55.

94. Page SJ, Levine P. Back from the brink: electromyography-triggered stimulation combined with modified constraint-induced movement therapy in chronic stroke. Arch Phys Med Rehabil 2006;87:27–31.

95. Meadmore KL, Hughes AM, Freeman CT, et al. Functional electrical stimulation mediated by iterative learning control and 3D robotics reduces motor impairment in chronic stroke. J Neuroeng Rehabil 2012;9:32.

96. Cauraugh JH, Kim S. Two coupled motor recovery protocols are better than one: electromyogram-triggered neuromuscular stimulation and bilateral movements. Stroke 2002;33:1589–94.

97. Knutson JS, Harley MY, Hisel TZ, et al. Contralaterally controlled functional electrical stimulation for stroke rehabilitation. Conf Proc IEEE Eng Med Biol Soc 2012;2012:314–7.

98. Schabrun SM, Chipchase LS, Zipf N, et al. Interaction between simultaneously applied neuromodulatory interventions in humans. Brain Stimul 2013;6:624–30.

99. Lee HJ, Cho KH, Lee WH. The effects of body weight support treadmill training with power-assisted functional electrical stimulation on functional movement and gait in stroke patients. Am J Phys Med Rehabil 2013;92:1051–9.
100. Turk R, Burridge JH, Davis R, et al. Therapeutic effectiveness of electric stimulation of the upper-limb poststroke using implanted microstimulators. Arch Phys Med Rehabil 2008;89:1913–22.
101. Kilgore KL, Bhadra N. Reversible nerve conduction block using kilohertz frequency alternating current. Neuromodulation 2014;17(3):242–54.

Stroke Rehabilitation Using Virtual Environments

Michael J. Fu, PhD[a,b,c,*], Jayme S. Knutson, PhD[b,c,d],
John Chae, MD[b,c,d,e]

KEYWORDS

- Virtual reality • Motor relearning • Hemiparesis • Neuroplasticity • Stroke

KEY POINTS

- Virtual environment interventions for motor relearning are popular and well received, but they have a small positive effect over conventional therapy.
- Common consensus is that virtual environment interventions are low risk and are likely beneficial if used as an adjunct to conventional therapy.
- There is a lack of effective and widely available virtual environment treatments for nonmotor deficits such as speech, cognitive function, and sensory dysfunction.
- Future approaches may need to strategically combine multiple interventions to address the multifaceted nature of stroke rehabilitation.

INTRODUCTION

Despite our best efforts, stroke continues to be a leading cause of acquired disability throughout the world and is responsible for approximately 102 million disability-adjusted life years annually.[1] Even more concerning to care providers, 66% of the 666,000 new stroke survivors each year may suffer chronic cognitive or physical impairment after 6 months of conventional care.[2,3]

Disclosures: M.J. Fu is supported by the Clinical and Translational Science Collaborative of Cleveland, UL1TR000439 (NIH NCATS).
[a] Department of Electrical Engineering and Computer Science, Case Western Reserve University, 2123 Martin Luther King Jr. Blvd., Cleveland, OH 44106, USA; [b] Cleveland FES Center, Case Western Reserve University, 10701 East Blvd., Cleveland, OH 44106, USA; [c] MetroHealth Rehabilitation Institute, MetroHealth System, 4229 Pearl Road, Suite N5, Cleveland, OH 44109, USA; [d] Department of Physical Medicine and Rehabilitation, Case Western Reserve University, 4229 Pearl Road, Suite N2, Cleveland, OH 44109, USA; [e] Department of Biomedical Engineering, Case Western Reserve University, 10900 Euclid Ave, 309 Wickenden Bldg, Cleveland, OH, USA
* Corresponding author. Department of Electrical Engineering and Computer Science, Case Western Reserve University, 4229 Pearl Road, Suite N5-59, Cleveland, OH 44109, USA.
E-mail address: mjf24@case.edu

Evidence for neurologic recovery through cortical reorganization[4] has led to new interventions that try to accelerate functional recovery. One promising approach uses virtual environments (VEs) in the form of video games or therapeutic tasks to train impairments. A definition of VEs is computer-simulated objects that respond to speech or motor input. Many VE therapies for stroke are now commercially available and attract intense interest.

This review focuses on VEs for stroke that are widely available outside of research programs. Those interested the broader academic field can refer to texts such as that by Dietz and Ward.[5] This article begins with the rationale for VE training along with potential mechanisms of action. It groups interventions by their targeted impairments, discusses their efficacy, and concludes with challenges for the field.

FEATURES FOR MOTOR LEARNING IN VIRTUAL ENVIRONMENTS

Human training was the first application for VEs beyond their conception as entertainment in the form of stereoscopes and video arcades. Circa 1960, VEs enhanced military flight simulators with visual information that followed pilots' head movements. Since 1990, the following features associated with promoting neuroplasticity[6] were incorporated into effective VEs for stroke rehabilitation.[7]

- Performance feedback
- Repetitive, goal-oriented tasks with variability covering a range of conditions
- Controlled environment where mistakes have minimal consequences
- Task difficulty scaled to a stroke survivor's capabilities and skill[8]
- Assist,[9] resist,[10] or repel movement and exaggerate errors[11]
- Focus on targeted skills by reducing contributions from unwanted movements[12]
- Increase motivation and engagement using features from video games[13]
- Facilitate remote social interaction with peers or therapists[12]

POTENTIAL MECHANISMS OF ACTION
Effect of Augmented Feedback on Motor Learning

There is sufficient evidence that providing stroke survivors with information about movement quality and task outcome benefits the acquisition and retention of motor skill.[14] Delivering feedback only about task measures leads to immediate improvements in the measures with no gain in movement quality. If feedback is provided only about motor performance (path deviations or compensatory behavior), participants immediately improve both task outcomes and movement quality.

Effect of Virtual Environments on Cortical Networks

Imaging reveals that visuomotor network activation occurs when both able-bodied and stroke survivors view hand motion from a virtual avatar. As the visual quality[15] and sense of immersion[16,17] increases, so does the recruitment of visuomotor networks, which is maximized when the avatar moves in synchrony with the physical hands.[17] In initial reports, recovery from VE training seems to also demonstrate similar patterns of cortical network change as observed in nonvirtual therapy.[18]

Another method of assessing the state of cortical networks is to infer motor corticospinal excitability using motor-evoked potentials induced by transcranial magnetic stimulation. In stroke survivors, lower conduction time,[19] higher baseline motor-evoked potential amplitude,[20] and greater motor-evoked potential amplitude[21] may benefit motor performance and learning. However, few studies have investigated the effect of VE interventions on corticospinal excitability. One study found that skill learning increased corticospinal excitability but not task performance.[22]

Effect of Immersion on Motor Performance

Motor performance in healthy persons improves with increased VE immersion, but few have investigated the effect of immersion on motor learning after stroke. Levels of VE immersion range from using typical PC monitors all the way to 3-dimensional (3D) goggles. Less immersion reduces movement accuracy, smoothness, and velocity, while increasing task performance time, in the healthy.[23] Stroke survivors performing reaching tasks in an immersive, head-mounted VE with a robotic exoskeleton (versus the real world) had 35% longer completion time, and increased elbow extension and horizontal shoulder abduction.[24]

IMPAIRMENTS TARGETED BY VIRTUAL ENVIRONMENT INTERVENTIONS

This section focuses on interventions commercially available in the United States.

Upper Extremity Is an Area of Focus

After the initial stroke, 80% of patients experience upper limb impairment.[25] Although 15% may have full spontaneous recovery,[26] after 6 months up to 65% cannot use their hands for activities of daily living.[3] Unsurprisingly, most VE interventions were developed for upper extremity motor training. Recent reviews consistently note that VEs are low risk and may be beneficial for motor relearning when administered as part of a physiotherapy program, but also agree that the quality of current evidence is low and that rigorous comparative studies are needed.[25,27] Costs range from $100–$200,000.

Proximal movement: shoulder and elbow

Commercial motion-controlled games made for the Wii (Nintendo of America Corp, Redmond, WA), Playstation Move (Sony Computer Entertainment Corp, San Mateo, CA), and Xbox Kinect (Microsoft Corp, Redmond, WA) use gesture-based shoulder-elbow motions as input to various sports simulations or motor coordination games. A recent review found high user acceptance, that 180 minutes per week can be safely tolerated, and no evidence for negative effects on motor function.[28]

However, evidence is weak that they are more beneficial than conventional care. Only 4 small controlled trials exist, 2 of which reported significantly improved outcomes over controls (3 points in Fugl-Myer[29] and 5.5 in the Functional Independence Measure). The current consensus is that commercial games are likely beneficial as a supplement to conventional occupational therapy.[28,30] However, noteworthy is that they do not train finger or wrist movements, difficulty levels may be unsuitable for the severely impaired, and there is no guard against using compensatory body mechanics.

Rehabilitation-specific VE systems such as IREX (GestureTek Corp, Toronto, ON, Canada), OmniVR (Accelerated Care Plus Corp, Reno, NV), and Jintronix (Jintronix Corp, Seattle, WA) use custom VEs that integrate with 3D cameras. In addition they offer task customization, movement analysis, and usage logs that game consoles cannot offer. However, meta-analysis did not find a significant advantage of clinical systems over game consoles, and no trials have directly compared clinical systems with game consoles.[25]

The largest randomized controlled trial (RCT) using systems of this type used the Virtual Reality Rehabilitation System (EU only; Khymeia Group Ltd, Noventa Padovana, Italy) on 376 stroke survivors (<12 months after stroke) for 40 sessions of 2 hours (1 hour conventional care, 1 hour VE) over 4 weeks, and found a significant effect size of 2.5 ± 0.5 points (4.9 ± 0.9 for those 3–12 months poststroke) for the Fugl-Meyer over controls that had conventional therapy.[31]

InMotion ARM (Interactive Motion Technologies Corp, Watertown, MA) is a robot that guides participants toward targets as they move its handle (like a computer mouse) in reaching tasks and games. A multicenter trial for those less than 6 months poststroke showed that 36 hours of robot therapy over 12 weeks significantly increased the Fugl-Myer by 2 points over usual care, which was not clinically meaningful.[32] Other measures were no better than usual care or dose-matched therapy. Both groups improved, but a follow-up study questioned the robot's cost-effectiveness given a $5000 premium per participant.[33]

Armeo (Hocoma Inc, Norwell, MA) Power, Spring, and Boom are exoskeletons that allow for assisted 3D arm movement in virtual tasks and games. Power uses motors to guide the arm, Spring uses passive springs to reduce arm movement effort, and Boom suspends the arm against gravity. Patients use Power first, then Spring, then Boom as they regain movement, and require less assistance for virtual task practice, although this progression has not yet been tested in clinical trials. A multisite RCT using Power on 77 chronic stroke survivors for 24 sessions of 45 minutes over 8 weeks found a significant effect of 0.78 points on the Fugl-Meyer compared with conventional care. An uncontrolled trial of Spring on chronic stroke (N = 23) for 36 hours over 12 weeks found a 5-point gain in Fugl-Myer and no change in secondary functional measures.[34]

Distal movement: hand, wrist, and fingers

Music Glove (Flint Rehabilitation Devices LLC, Irvine, CA) trains finger motion by wearing a sensor glove and touching the thumb to the other fingertips to play musical notes. A single-blinded crossover trial in 12 moderately impaired chronic stroke survivors (3 treatments, each for 6 hours over 2 weeks) showed a significant gain of 3.2 blocks on the Box and Blocks Test versus conventional care, but no gain over the game with an isometric force sensor that did not require finger motion.[35]

HandTutor (MediTouch Ltd, Netanya, Israel) uses a sensor glove to control therapy games by finger or wrist flexion/extension. A controlled trial treated 31 chronic subacute (<4 months poststroke) participants by adding 20 to 30 minutes of VE training (experiment) or conventional care (control) to usual care.[36] Results showed significant effects for primary outcomes, but were not sustained at 10 days' follow-up.

Amadeo (TyroMotion GmbH, Graz, Austria) is a hand exoskeleton that assists individual finger movement during VE training, but requires the arm to be strapped to a fixed base. An RCT with 20 acute inpatient stroke survivors had 20 treatment sessions of 40 minutes each over 4 weeks added to standard care (3 hours per day). Both usual care and robot groups had significant gains (end and 3-month follow-up), but no group effects were found.

Gait Training with Virtual Environments Have Limited Effect

Lower extremity impairment affects 75% of all stroke survivors, and only 15% regain full recovery.[26] Up to 25% will require assistive aids to walk for the rest of their lives.[26] A meta-analysis of 7 RCTs found that VE groups improved gait speed by 0.17 m/s over placebo groups and 0.15 m/s over non-VE usual walking therapy. Though promising, most studies used custom systems, and the same amount of evidence is not available for commercial systems costing $200,000 to $1 million.

LOKOMAT (Hokoma Inc) is a lower extremity exoskeleton for body-weight supported treadmill training, and can be equipped with a computer monitor for use with VE tasks to simulate walking and leg motion training. No studies examined the effect of adding VEs to this system for stroke rehabilitation, but an RCT in children with various neurologic impairments found that a soccer ball-kicking simulation increased motivation, but did not result in greater joint torques.[37]

Motek Medical BV (Amsterdam, the Netherlands) has treadmill systems that are used with wall-sized computer projection screens for immersive VE gait training. CAREN is the most immersive, with a treadmill that moves in 6° of freedom, whereas GRAIL and V-Gait are split-belt treadmills with no moving bases. One study found that adding a VE led to treadmill walking mechanics that were closer to the over-ground condition, but the differences in the VE condition were clinically negligible.[38] No controlled studies for stroke exist on the CAREN system, but case studies used artificially slow optical flow to elicit faster walking.[39]

Balance Interventions Comparable with Conventional Care

Many VE balance interventions have demonstrated positive effects, but they do not exceed controls treated with conventional care.[25,40] These interventions use a wide range of devices, including motion video games,[41] Xbox Kinect,[42] treadmills,[43] and reaching tasks.[44] Many studies used commercial games for the Wii Fit balance board, which is a force plate accessory ($100; Nintendo Corp). The games (skiing, hula-hooping, and yoga) are controlled by body-weight shifting and were shown to be feasible for both inpatient and home use.[45] Although these VE methods may not be more effective than conventional care, they have been shown to reduce therapist costs without sacrificing efficacy if prescribed appropriately for home use.[42]

Cognitive Rehabilitation Interventions Are Lacking

The efficacy of VEs for cognitive rehabilitation is a weak point in the literature, with few controlled trials and even fewer commercial interventions.[25] Those that exist cost $150 to $850. RehaCom (Hasomed GmbH, Berlin, Germany) PC software trains attention (alertness, vigilance, visual-spatial, selective, and divided), memory, executive functions, and visuomotor skills. A double-blind RCT on 36 stroke survivors (<6 months poststroke) showed significantly improved working memory and word fluency over conventional therapy after nine 30-minute sessions.[46]

"Brain games" are popular in the consumer market, but the cognitive training designed for unimpaired individuals may be unsuitable for neurologic injury. Lumosity (Lumos Labs Corp, San Francisco, CA) is a Web site that trains cognitive functions such as memory, processing speed, attention, and problem solving. Although training transfers to long-term function in healthy adults,[47] an 8-week uncontrolled trial on 5 stroke survivors (>6 months poststroke) found that 3 of the participants completed less than half of 40 self-administered home sessions of 30 minutes, and 2 did none of them. Reasons cited included fatigue and difficulty responding within the allotted time for certain tasks.[48]

Speech Rehabilitation Intervention Options Are Few

Speech therapy VEs are also lacking in evidence from controlled trials, but have consistently positive case series and cost less than $1000. AphasiaScripts (Rehabilitation Institute of Chicago, Chicago, IL) uses virtual avatars for script practice. The avatar's mouth demonstrates proper speech articulation while it converses to the patient using predefined scripts (no speech recognition). An uncontrolled trial of 20 chronic, aphasic stroke survivors showed a clinically significant decrease of 6.67 points in Communication Difficulty of the Burden of Stroke Scale after 9 weeks of home intervention for 30 minutes per day.[49]

MossTalk Words 2 (Moss Rehabilitation Research Institute, Philadelphia, PA) is PC software that trains single word production using virtual flash cards, and provides performance feedback of pronunciation accuracy using voice recognition. Four case studies spanning 17 stroke survivors all reported that 12 to 20 sessions lasting 1 hour improved untrained object-naming ability when session frequency was at least 3 to 4 per week.[50–53]

StepByStep (Steps Consulting Ltd, Acton Turville, UK) is also a flash-card–like program, but has prerecorded video of therapists pronouncing the words. It also can train spelling and sentence production, but does not have speech recognition. A single-blind controlled trial of 34 chronic stroke survivors compared 5 months of the intervention (20 minutes, 3 days per week) against no therapy. The intervention group had 19.8% greater untrained object-naming accuracy (10% was clinically significant) that did not persist at 3 months' follow-up.[54]

Spatial Neglect Is an Area of Need

VEs have been developed for assessing hemispatial neglect that may be more sensitive than manual methods,[55] but there are no widely available VE-specific interventions. One uncontrolled study demonstrated short-term improvement of far-field neglect in 6 stroke survivors (<3 months poststroke) by using a virtual reaching task with the patient's hands altered to appear in the field of neglect.[56] Others used motor training to treat neglect with the rationale of providing arousal and attention to the neglected limb. An unblinded RCT of 24 stroke survivors (<1 month poststroke) compared reaching tasks using IREX with dose-matched conventional therapy. After 5 weeks of therapy for 30 minutes per day, 5 days per week, the VE group reported greater effect in comparison with controls.[57]

Proprioception and Sensory Deficits Are Gaining Attention

Between 17% and 50% of stroke survivors experience impaired proprioception or sensation, but there are few interventions available, as treatments are passive and VEs are only used to assess deficits.[58] VEs revealed that motor recovery is strongly associated with the return of proprioception.[59] One uncontrolled study (N = 7, >1 year post stroke) showed that recovery of proprioception may be facilitated by a virtual reaching task with a custom-built planar robot providing guidance for five 1-hour sessions over 2 weeks.[32] The robot used force pulses to guide arms toward target elbow angles. All participants showed gains in perceptual acuity, but 3 of the more impaired participants did not have sustained effects at follow-up.

Sensory deficits occur in 50% of stroke survivors,[60] but few treatments exist and no VE interventions have been published. Evidence is lacking for treatments that use electrical cutaneous stimulation, and discrimination task training has little effect.[61]

CURRENT CHALLENGES

The field has advanced in the last 25 years, but there are still many questions. To begin with, the effect of VE immersion, dose, time after stroke, and severity on outcomes needs to be unraveled.[62] In addition, the use of VE-facilitated social interaction to boost motor recovery has only begun to be explored. Furthermore, it is important to advocate technology companies to design technologies suitable for neurologic impairment. Proffitt and Lange[63] recently challenged the field to also investigate the effect of presence and immersion on motor recovery as immersive displays become more accessible.

The greatest challenge is the trend in large comparative trials of treatments successful in smaller studies showing little difference compared with conventional care.[64] It is possible that larger sample sizes increase heterogeneity in impairments,

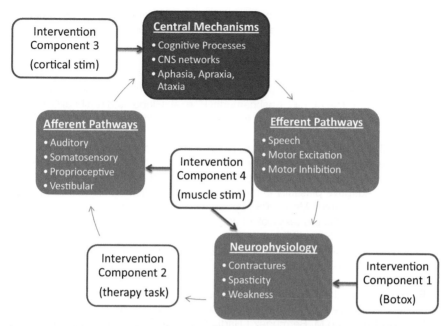

Fig. 1. General system-level framework to identify mechanistic targets for multimodal approaches to stroke rehabilitation. The unfilled boxes are example interventions that point to the processes they directly affect, which are represented by filled boxes. The contents of each process are examples and not comprehensive. Red arrows represent intervention effects, and blue arrows represent outputs from each process and input into the next process. CNS, central nervous system; stim, stimulation.

demographics, and pathophysiology.[65] The National Center for Medical Rehabilitation Research recently advocated for defining therapies' active ingredients and integrating them into treatment packages to maximize efficacy in diverse populations.[66]

This complicated task may benefit from a framework that can expand as mechanisms are defined. **Fig. 1** is therefore introduced as a potential framework, adapted from the close-loop feedback model of motor learning[67] to include placeholders for processes that are affected by stroke and can be targeted by interventions. This schema illustrates how the framework can describe an intervention package that incorporates (1) cortical stimulation to increase neuronal excitability, (2) Botox to relieve hypertonia, (3) electrical stimulation to assist hand opening, and (4) a VE to undertake therapy task practice. This approach may help define the roles and relationships that belong to each part of a treatment package. As mechanisms are found, new hypotheses may also be generated.

SUMMARY

This review focuses on the rationale, mechanisms, and availability of commercial VE stroke rehabilitation interventions. It also identifies that cognitive, proprioceptive, and sensory dysfunction are underaddressed by the field. The consensus from more than 30 RCTs is that VEs are low risk and recommended as supplements to conventional therapy. Questions to answer going forward include what mechanisms of action drive recovery and which participant groups will respond. Finally, a framework is introduced to define therapy combinations necessary to affect the heterogeneity of stroke and move the field out of the current stagnation caused by small effects in large clinical trials.

REFERENCES

1. Feigin VL, Forouzanfar MH, Krishnamurthi R, et al. Global and regional burden of stroke during 1990-2010: findings from the Global Burden of Disease Study 2010. Lancet 2014;383:245–54.
2. Go AS, Mozaffarian D, Roger VL, et al. Heart disease and stroke statistics—2014 update: a report from the American Heart Association. Circulation 2014;129:e28–292.
3. Dobkin BH. Rehabilitation after stroke. N Engl J Med 2005;352:1677–84.
4. Nudo RJ. Adaptive plasticity in motor cortex: implications for rehabilitation after brain injury. J Rehabil Med 2003;(41 Suppl):7–10.
5. Dietz V, Ward N. Oxford textbook of neurorehabilitation. Oxford (UK): Oxford University Press; 2015. p. 418.
6. Kleim JA, Jones TA. Principles of experience-dependent neural plasticity: implications for rehabilitation after brain damage. J Speech Lang Hear Res 2008; 51:S225–39.
7. Rizzo AS, Kim GJ. A SWOT analysis of the field of virtual reality rehabilitation and therapy. Presence Teleoper Virtual Environ 2005;14:119–46.
8. Da Silva Cameirão M, Bermúdez I Badia S, Duarte E, et al. Virtual reality based rehabilitation speeds up functional recovery of the upper extremities after stroke: a randomized controlled pilot study in the acute phase of stroke using the rehabilitation gaming system. Restor Neurol Neurosci 2011;29:287–98.
9. Krebs HI, Hogan N, Volpe BT, et al. Overview of clinical trials with MIT-MANUS: a robot-aided neuro-rehabilitation facility. Technol Health Care 1999;7:419–23.
10. Wu M, Landry JM, Kim J, et al. Robotic resistance/assistance training improves locomotor function in individuals poststroke: a randomized controlled study. Arch Phys Med Rehabil 2014;95:799–806.
11. Abdollahi F, Case Lazarro ED, Listenberger M, et al. Error augmentation enhancing arm recovery in individuals with chronic stroke: a randomized crossover design. Neurorehabil Neural Repair 2014;28:120–8.
12. Novak D, Nagle A, Keller U, et al. Increasing motivation in robot-aided arm rehabilitation with competitive and cooperative gameplay. J Neuroeng Rehabil 2014; 11:64.
13. Putrino D. Telerehabilitation and emerging virtual reality approaches to stroke rehabilitation. Curr Opin Neurol 2014;27:631–6.
14. Subramanian SK, Massie CL, Malcolm MP, et al. Does provision of extrinsic feedback result in improved motor learning in the upper limb poststroke? A systematic review of the evidence. Neurorehabil Neural Repair 2010;24:113–24.
15. Perani D, Fazio F, Borghese NA, et al. Different brain correlates for watching real and virtual hand actions. Neuroimage 2001;14:749–58.
16. Jäncke L, Cheetham M, Baumgartner T. Virtual reality and the role of the prefrontal cortex in adults and children. Front Neurosci 2009;3:52–9.
17. Saleh S, Adamovich SV, Tunik E. Mirrored feedback in chronic stroke: recruitment and effective connectivity of ipsilesional sensorimotor networks. Neurorehabil Neural Repair 2014;28:344–54.
18. Orihuela-Espina F, Fernández del Castillo I, Palafox L, et al. Neural reorganization accompanying upper limb motor rehabilitation from stroke with virtual reality-based gesture therapy. Top Stroke Rehabil 2013;20:197–209.

19. Vang C, Dunbabin D, Kilpatrick D. Correlation between functional and electro-physiological recovery in acute ischemic. Stroke 1999;30:2126–30.
20. Rapisarda G, Bastings E, de Noordhout AM, et al. Can motor recovery in stroke patients be predicted by early transcranial magnetic stimulation? Stroke 1996;27: 2191–6.
21. Koski L, Mernar TJ, Dobkin BH. Immediate and long-term changes in corticomotor output in response to rehabilitation: correlation with functional improvements in chronic stroke. Neurorehabil Neural Repair 2004;18:230–49.
22. Bagce HF, Saleh S, Adamovich SV, et al. Corticospinal excitability is enhanced after visuomotor adaptation and depends on learning rather than performance or error. J Neurophysiol 2013;109:1097–106.
23. Fu MJ, Hershberger AD, Sano K, et al. Effect of visuo-motor co-location on 3D Fitts' task performance in physical and virtual environments. Presence (Camb) 2012;21:305–20.
24. Levin MF, Knaut LAM, Magdalon EC, et al. Virtual reality environments to enhance upper limb functional recovery in patients with hemiparesis. Stud Health Technol Inform 2009;145:94–108.
25. Laver KE, George S, Thomas S, et al. Virtual reality for stroke rehabilitation. Cochrane Database Syst Rev 2015;(2):CD008349.
26. Hendricks HT, van Limbeek J, Geurts AC, et al. Motor recovery after stroke: a systematic review of the literature. Arch Phys Med Rehabil 2002;83:1629–37.
27. Lohse KR, Hilderman CGE, Cheung KL, et al. Virtual reality therapy for adults post-stroke: a systematic review and meta-analysis exploring virtual environments and commercial games in therapy. PLoS One 2014;9:e93318.
28. Thomson K, Pollock A, Bugge C, et al. Commercial gaming devices for stroke upper limb rehabilitation: a systematic review. Int J Stroke 2014;9:479–88.
29. Manlapaz DG, Silverio LA, Navarro JA, et al. Effectiveness of using Nintendo Wii in rehabilitation of chronic stroke patients with upper limb hemiparesis. Hong Kong Physiother J 2010;28:25.
30. Thomson K, Pollock A, Bugge C, et al. Commercial gaming devices for stroke upper limb rehabilitation: a survey of current practice. Disabil Rehabil Assist Technol 2015;1–8. http://dx.doi.org/10.3109/17483107.2015.1005031.
31. Turolla A, Dam M, Ventura L, et al. Virtual reality for the rehabilitation of the upper limb motor function after stroke: a prospective controlled trial. J Neuroengineering Rehabil 2013;10:85.
32. De Santis D, Zenzeri J, Casadio M, et al. Robot-assisted training of the kinesthetic sense: enhancing proprioception after stroke. Front Hum Neurosci 2014;8:1037.
33. Wagner TH, Lo AC, Peduzzi P, et al. An economic analysis of robot-assisted therapy for long-term upper-limb impairment after stroke. Stroke J Cereb Circ 2011; 42:2630–2.
34. Colomer C, Baldoví A, Torromé S, et al. Efficacy of Armeo® Spring during the chronic phase of stroke. Study in mild to moderate cases of hemiparesis. Neurol Barc Spain 2013;28:261–7.
35. Friedman N, Chan V, Reinkensmeyer AN, et al. Retraining and assessing hand movement after stroke using the MusicGlove: comparison with conventional hand therapy and isometric grip training. J Neuroengineering Rehabil 2014;11:76.
36. Carmeli E, Peleg S, Bartur G, et al. HandTutorTM enhanced hand rehabilitation after stroke—a pilot study. Physiother Res Int 2011;16:191–200.
37. Brütsch K, Schuler T, Koenig A, et al. Influence of virtual reality soccer game on walking performance in robotic assisted gait training for children. J Neuroengineering Rehabil 2010;7:15.

38. Sloot LH, van der Krogt MM, Harlaar J. Effects of adding a virtual reality environment to different modes of treadmill walking. Gait Posture 2014;39:939–45.
39. Lamontagne A, Fung J, McFadyen BJ, et al. Modulation of walking speed by changing optic flow in persons with stroke. J Neuroengineering Rehabil 2007;4:22.
40. Gatica-Rojas V, Méndez-Rebolledo G. Virtual reality interface devices in the reorganization of neural networks in the brain of patients with neurological diseases. Neural Regen Res 2014;9:888–96.
41. Laufer Y, Dar G, Kodesh E. Does a Wii-based exercise program enhance balance control of independently functioning older adults? A systematic review. Clin Interv Aging 2014;9:1803–13.
42. Lloréns R, Noé E, Colomer C, et al. Effectiveness, usability, and cost-benefit of a virtual reality-based telerehabilitation program for balance recovery after stroke: a randomized controlled trial. Arch Phys Med Rehabil 2015;96:418–25.e2.
43. Yang S, Hwang WH, Tsai YC, et al. Improving balance skills in patients who had stroke through virtual reality treadmill training. Am J Phys Med Rehabil 2011;90:969–78.
44. McEwen D, Taillon-Hobson A, Bilodeau M, et al. Virtual reality exercise improves mobility after stroke an inpatient randomized controlled trial. Stroke 2014;45:1853–5.
45. Morone G, Tramontano M, Iosa M, et al. The efficacy of balance training with video game-based therapy in subacute stroke patients: a randomized controlled trial. Biomed Res Int 2014;2014:580861.
46. Richter KM, Modden C, Eling P, et al. Working memory training and semantic structuring improves remembering future events, not past events. Neurorehabil Neural Repair 2015;29:33–40.
47. Willis SL, Tennstedt SL, Marsiske M, et al. Long-term effects of cognitive training on everyday functional outcomes in older adults. JAMA 2006;296:2805–14.
48. Zickefoose S, Hux K, Brown J, et al. Let the games begin: a preliminary study using attention process training-3 and Lumosity™ brain games to remediate attention deficits following traumatic brain injury. Brain Inj 2013;27:707–16.
49. Manheim LM, Halper AS, Cherney L. Patient-reported changes in communication after computer-based script training for aphasia. Arch Phys Med Rehabil 2009;90:623–7.
50. Raymer AM, Kohen FP, Saffell D. Computerised training for impairments of word comprehension and retrieval in aphasia. Aphasiology 2006;20:257–68.
51. Jokel R, Cupit J, Rochon E, et al. Relearning lost vocabulary in nonfluent progressive aphasia with MossTalk Words®. Aphasiology 2009;23:175–91.
52. Fink RB, Brecher A, Schwartz MF, et al. A computer-implemented protocol for treatment of naming disorders: evaluation of clinician-guided and partially self-guided instruction. Aphasiology 2002;16:1061–86.
53. Ramsberger G, Marie B. Self-administered cued naming therapy: a single-participant investigation of a computer-based therapy program replicated in four cases. Am J Speech lang Pathol 2007;16:343–58.
54. Palmer R, Enderby P, Cooper C, et al. Computer therapy compared with usual care for people with long-standing aphasia poststroke: a pilot randomized controlled trial. Stroke 2012;43:1904–11.
55. Barrett AM, Buxbaum LJ, Coslett HB, et al. Cognitive rehabilitation interventions for neglect and related disorders: moving from bench to bedside in stroke patients. J Cogn Neurosci 2006;18:1223–36.
56. Castiello U, Lusher D, Burton C, et al. Improving left hemispatial neglect using virtual reality. Neurology 2004;62:1958–62.

57. Kim YM, Chun MH, Yun GJ, et al. The effect of virtual reality training on unilateral spatial neglect in stroke patients. Ann Rehabil Med 2011;35:309.

58. Dukelow SP, Herter TM, Bagg SD, et al. The independence of deficits in position sense and visually guided reaching following stroke. J Neuroengineering Rehabil 2012;9:72.

59. Semrau JA, Herter TM, Scott SH, et al. Characterizing proprioceptive recovery after stroke using robotics. In: Proceedings of the Translational and Computational Motor Control 2014. 2014. Available at: https://sites.google.com/site/acmcconference/2014/12.pdf. Accessed February 25, 2015.

60. Sullivan JE, Hedman LD. Sensory dysfunction following stroke: incidence, significance, examination, and intervention. Top Stroke Rehabil 2008;15:200–17.

61. Schabrun SM, Hillier S. Evidence for the retraining of sensation after stroke: a systematic review. Clin Rehabil 2009;23:27–39.

62. Laver KE, George S, Thomas S, et al. In: Cochrane Database Syst Rev (John Wiley & Sons, Ltd, 1996). Available at: http://onlinelibrary.wiley.com/doi/10.1002/14651858.CD008349.pub3/abstract. Accessed Febraury 21, 2015.

63. Proffitt R, Lange B. Considerations in the efficacy and effectiveness of virtual reality interventions for stroke rehabilitation: moving the field forward. Phys Ther 2014;95(3):441–8.

64. Winstein C. Translating the science into neurorehabilitation practice: challenges and opportunities. 2014. Available at: http://www.asnr.com/files/ASNR_Viste%20Award_Winstein.pptx.pdf. Accessed February 24, 2015.

65. Muir KW. Heterogeneity of stroke pathophysiology and neuroprotective clinical trial design. Stroke J Cereb Circ 2002;33:1545–50.

66. Nitkin R. Support for clinical trials at the national center for medical rehabilitation research and the NIH. 2014. Available at: http://www.asnr.com/files/NitkinHandouts.pdf. Accessed February 24, 2015.

67. Magill RA. Motor learning and control: concepts and applications. New York (NY): McGraw-Hill; 2007. p. 86.

Tailoring Brain Stimulation to the Nature of Rehabilitative Therapies in Stroke

A Conceptual Framework Based on their Unique Mechanisms of Recovery

David A. Cunningham, MSc[a,b], Kelsey A. Potter-Baker, PhD[a],
Jayme S. Knutson, PhD[c], Vishwanath Sankarasubramanian, PhD[a],
Andre G. Machado, MD, PhD[d,e], Ela B. Plow, PhD, PT[a,f,*]

KEYWORDS

- Stroke • Unilateral therapy • Bilateral therapy • Noninvasive brain stimulation
- Transcranial direct current stimulation • Repetitive transcranial magnetic stimulation
- Upper limb • Motor impairment

KEY POINTS

- Noninvasive brain stimulation is typically paired with unilateral therapies of the upper limb.
- Many recent clinical trials have failed to augment rehabilitative outcomes, especially for patients with greater motor impairments.
- Bilateral therapies may offer a more feasible and neurophysiologic advantage over unilateral therapy to augment rehabilitative outcomes for patients with greater motor impairments.
- Based on mechanisms of recovery, this article discusses how to create noninvasive brain stimulation paradigms that are tailored to the individual type of therapy (unilateral or bilateral) across varying degree of impairments.

This work was supported by the National Institutes of Health (1K01HD069504) and American Heart Association (13BGIA17120055) to E.B. Plow and by the Clinical & Translational Science Collaborative (RPC2014-1067) to D.A. Cunningham.
Conflicts of Interest: A.G. Machado has the following conflicts of interest to disclose: ATI, Enspire, and Cardionomics (distribution rights from intellectual property); Spinal Modulation and Functional Neurostimulation (consultant).
[a] Department of Biomedical Engineering, Lerner Research Institute, Cleveland Clinic, 9500 Euclid Avenue, Cleveland, OH 44195, USA; [b] School of Biomedical Sciences, Kent State University, Kent, OH, USA; [c] MetroHealth Medical Center, Case Western Reserve University, Cleveland, OH, USA; [d] Center for Neurological Restoration, Neurological Institute, Department of Neurosurgery, Neurological Institute, Cleveland, OH, USA; [e] Department of Neuroscience and Biomedical Engineering, Lerner Research Institute, Cleveland, OH, USA; [f] Department of Physical Medicine & Rehabilitation, Neurological Institute, Cleveland Clinic, Cleveland, OH, USA
* Corresponding author. Biomedical Engineering, Cleveland Clinic, 9500 Euclid Avenue, ND20, Cleveland, OH 44195.
E-mail address: plowe2@ccf.org

Phys Med Rehabil Clin N Am 26 (2015) 759–774
http://dx.doi.org/10.1016/j.pmr.2015.07.001
1047-9651/15/$ – see front matter © 2015 Elsevier Inc. All rights reserved.

INTRODUCTION

Stroke is a leading cause of long-term adult disability. Although current rehabilitation strategies carry promise, gains are modest where approximately 60% to 80% of survivors continue to experience motor impairments of the upper limb well into the chronic phase of recovery.[1–3] One reason for the modest recovery of upper-limb function is the diminishing access to rehabilitation, where therapists are required to administer best practice in a limited number of sessions. To address this limitation, current research emphasizes the need for maximizing and accelerating outcomes of rehabilitation within a limited amount of time.

To augment rehabilitative benefits, use of noninvasive brain stimulation (NIBS) has become a popular topic of research. Specifically, NIBS has the potential to augment mechanisms of plasticity that underlie rehabilitation-related recovery. The most commonly used forms of NIBS in research include repetitive transcranial magnetic stimulation (rTMS) and transcranial direct current stimulation (tDCS). rTMS operates by using electromagnetic induction, wherein an insulated coiled wire is placed on the scalp. Then, at varying frequencies, the coil produces a brief and strong alternating current that induces a perpendicular spatially focused magnetic field. The magnetic field induces current, which passes unimpeded through the skull, resulting in depolarization of neurons in superficial cortices.[4] High-frequency pulses ($\geq$5 Hz) are used to facilitate excitability of the targeted cortices,[5] whereas low-frequency pulses (<1 Hz) inhibit excitability of the underlying cortices.[6] Unlike rTMS, tDCS applies current directly to the targeted regions and has emerged as a popular NIBS approach because it is simple and easy to use in conjunction with physical and occupational therapy.[7,8] Using a constant current stimulator, surface electrodes placed in saline-soaked sponges deliver low-levels of direct current (0–4 mA) to the scalp and create changes in cortical excitability.[9] Early animal studies have shown that tDCS modulates neuronal membrane potentials in the cortices, such that anodal tDCS depolarizes membrane potentials and cathodal tDCS hyperpolarizes membrane potentials.[10] As such, anodal tDCS is typically considered excitatory for the targeted region, whereas cathodal tDCS is considered inhibitory. Although the exact mechanisms are unclear, a similar directional change in excitability has been achieved in humans. Nitche and Paulus[11] have shown that anodal tDCS increases excitability and cathodal tDCS decreases cortical excitability. Based on pharmacologic studies, the likely mechanism in humans involves up-regulation of N-methyl-D-asparate receptor activity[12] and modulation of γ-aminobutyric acid (GABA)ergic neuronal activation.[13] Thus, tDCS modulates excitability and spontaneous firing rate of neurons.

The primary application of NIBS approaches in rehabilitation has involved their pairing with unilateral upper-limb therapies. Such therapies focus on intensively retraining the paretic limb and restraining or otherwise discouraging movement of the nonparetic limb. Examples include constraint-induced movement therapy, unilateral task-oriented practice, or learning involving only the paretic limb, among several others.[14–18] NIBS approaches are applied before therapy (rTMS) or during therapy (tDCS).

Despite promising early studies,[19,20] NIBS has shown somewhat limited effects to augment rehabilitative outcomes of the unilateral upper limb in more recent and larger clinical trials.[15,16,21–25] Hence, its use remains for the most part investigational. In trying to understand the failures, it seems that the benefits of NIBS plus therapy are modest, and vary considerably from patient-to-patient, failing especially in patients with greater motor impairments.[15,26] Thus, this article addresses important lingering questions that may help devise the best combinations of NIBS with rehabilitative therapies. Are mechanisms that NIBS seeks to entrain in its pairing with unilateral therapy generalizable across patients in all ranges of impairment, or do these mechanisms fail across patients with greater motor impairments? In such cases, are therapies targeting alternate mechanisms better suited for the more impaired instead?

Several groups have recently suggested the importance of bilateral behavioral therapies as alternates to unilateral upper-limb therapies, including bilateral arm training with rhythmic auditory cueing (BATRAC),[27] bilateral isokinematic training,[28] active-passive bilateral training (APBT), and contralaterally controlled functional electrical stimulation (CCFES).[29] Even though there is no direct evidence concluding whether they are better than unilateral therapies across certain ranges of severity, it is generally considered that they likely could be more efficacious for patients with greater motor impairments,[30–32] because many of the previously mentioned therapies enable the nonparetic limb to drive movement of the paretic limb. However, there is limited understanding of what mechanisms underlie bilateral therapies, which is why there is lack of discussion on how to pair NIBS with bilateral therapies. In contrast, the mechanisms underlying unilateral therapies are better understood, which is why there is considerable evidence discussing how to apply NIBS to affect outcomes of unilateral therapies. The aim of this article is to (1) compare possible mechanisms of recovery that may be engaged by unilateral and bilateral therapies, (2) explain potentially how these mechanisms may vary across ranges of damage and impairment, and (3) present a theoretic framework for how to create NIBS paradigms that are tailored to distinctly augment bilateral and unilateral therapies.

MECHANISMS OF RECOVERY UNDERLYING UNILATERAL THERAPY

Typically, coordination between limbs requires modulating motor overflow, where motor overflow refers to facilitation from the "moving" cortices to the opposing "resting" hemisphere. During unilateral movement of a limb, mirror movements can occur in the opposite resting limb if motor overflow is not regulated. Interhemispheric interactions conducted via transcallosal pathways between both hemispheres help regulate overflow. Specifically, the hemisphere contralateral to the moving limb imposes an inhibitory influence on the ipsilateral hemisphere, whereas the ipsilateral hemisphere relaxes its counterinhibition to allow for a purely unilateral movement.[33,34]

Following stroke, however, the mechanism of regulating motor overflow is disrupted, resulting in a series of events that constitutes what is commonly referred to as the interhemispheric competition model.[35–37] Based on this model, during unilateral movement of the paretic limb, the affected hemisphere weakly inhibits the unaffected hemisphere to regulate overflow (**Fig. 1**).[38–40] In turn, the "disinhibited" unaffected hemisphere overly inhibits the affected hemisphere, further weakening its excitability and the drive to move the paretic limb.[41] Such an imbalance of mutual inhibition presumably exacerbates as patients rely on using their nonparetic limb at the cost of the weak paretic limb.[42] Therefore, the typical recommendation based on the interhemispheric competition model is to unilaterally retrain the paretic limb but restrain or discourage movements of the nonparetic limb.[43–45] By intensively retraining the paretic limb, it is believed the weak affected hemisphere is facilitated, and effectively counters inhibition from the unaffected hemisphere, promoting gains in recovery of the upper limb.

COMBINING NONINVASIVE BRAIN STIMULATION WITH UNILATERAL THERAPY BASED ON THEORY OF UNDERLYING MECHANISMS

In accordance with the interhemispheric competition model, present-day NIBS approaches aim to upregulate excitability of the affected hemisphere but inhibit that of

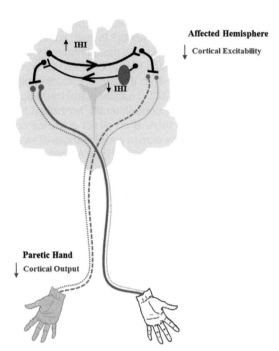

Fig. 1. Interhemispheric competition model with chronic stroke. The lesion reduces inter-hemispheric inhibition (IHI) exerted by the effect on the unaffected hemisphere. In turn, the disinhibited unaffected hemisphere generates exaggerated inhibition on the affected hemisphere, which reduces excitability and cortical drive to the paretic limb. *Dark circle* represents the lesion.

the unaffected hemisphere to enhance rehabilitative outcomes. Toward this end, multiple research groups have used high-frequency rTMS or anodal tDCS to excite the affected hemisphere or low-frequency rTMS or cathodal tDCS to inhibit the unaffected hemisphere (**Fig. 2**; for a full review see Hoyer and Celnik[46] or Sandrini and Cohen[47]). In either hemisphere, the most common target is the primary motor cortex (M1), because evidence suggests its adaptive plasticity is intimately associated with paretic upper-limb recovery.[48–50]

LIMITATIONS OF UNILATERAL THERAPIES AND ASSOCIATED NONINVASIVE BRAIN STIMULATION APPROACHES

Larger clinical trials have had limited success when replicating the early promise of pairing NIBS with unilateral therapies.[15,16,22–25,51] One possible reason for the disappointing results is that the groups were less homogenous and included patients with a wider range of impairment than in earlier smaller studies. Previous studies have discussed that pairing NIBS with unilateral therapy is less effective for the more impaired chronic stroke patients.[15,26] An important question to consider is whether the model of interhemispheric competition informing unilateral therapies and present-day NIBS approaches in the chronic stroke population is applicable across patients with greater severity. We describe three major reasons for why exciting the affected hemisphere and/or inhibiting the unaffected M1 may generalize poorly across patients with greater severity: (1) heterogeneity of stroke population, (2) extent

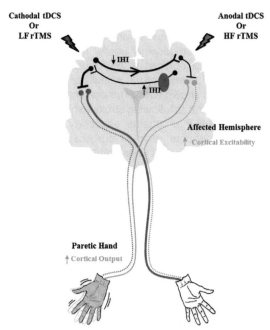

Fig. 2. Current NIBS approach. Anodal tDCS or high-frequency (HF) rTMS targets the affected hemisphere to increase the excitability of the affected hemisphere and cortical output to the paretic hand. Cathodal tDCS or low-frequency (LF) rTMS is applied to unaffected hemisphere to reduce the inhibition imposed on the affected hemisphere. *Dark circle* represents the lesion.

of damage in the affected hemisphere, and (3) the influence of the unaffected hemisphere.

Stroke Population Heterogeneity

Within the stroke population, such factors as age, location and profile of lesion, and comorbidities all show high variation.[52] Furthermore, many of these factors also contribute to the large variability in overall severity of the motor deficit, with some patients having substantial amounts of movement and others having limited movement in the paretic upper limb. Applying unilateral therapy to patients with limited movement can inherently be challenging. Specifically, because of their inability to use their paretic limb in task-based therapies, severely impaired patients are generally unable to realize the maximum benefits from unilateral therapies, which may explain why they show greater inconsistencies in benefits of NIBS. Most of these patients are unable to meet the minimal movement criteria for participation in unilateral rehabilitation, where often participants are required to have at least 20° of wrist extension and 10° extension of at least two fingers.[53] When severely impaired patients are included in trials, they do not show the same recovery as the less impaired, suggesting that unilateral behavioral therapies may be less successful and feasible for this population.[31,54,55] Therefore, current NIBS approaches combined with unilateral therapies generalize poorly across the more impaired patients because the fundamental therapy itself is inconsistently effective for this population.

Damage in the Affected Hemisphere

When patients experience hemiparesis following stroke, those with subcortical lesions typically have damage to the corticospinal tracts. The corticospinal tract originates from the primary and premotor cortices where the descending pathways synapse with lower motor neurons at the level of the spinal cord to execute volitional movements. It has previously been shown with diffusion tensor imaging that patients with poor integrity of corticospinal tracts following stroke exhibit more severe motor impairments.[56–59] Thus, it is possible that patients, especially those with severe motor impairments, do not have adequate residual corticospinal pathways that can be excited in the affected hemisphere with unilateral therapies or with current NIBS approaches. Hence, they fail to benefit from modulation of interhemispheric mechanisms of recovery for the paretic limb.[26,60]

Influence of the Unaffected Hemisphere

Several groups,[58,61–64] including our own,[57] have demonstrated that the unaffected hemisphere is not always inhibitory to the affected hemisphere as traditionally believed. Rather, it can mediate recovery when substrates in the affected hemisphere are damaged considerably and patients experience greater severity of impairment.[36] Machado and colleagues[65] show that following hemispherectomy, the unaffected hemisphere in rodent models assumes the role of the affected hemisphere, suggesting it becomes critical for recovery. In fact, rodents with large lesions experience a decline in motor function when the unaffected hemisphere is anesthetized.[61] As such, the unaffected hemisphere may provide an adaptive role through ipsilateral pathways originating from the unaffected hemisphere and innervating lower motor neurons devoted to the paretic limb. Carmel and colleagues[66] have recently demonstrated in a rodent model that electrical stimulation applied to facilitate the unaffected hemisphere promotes recovery of skilled forelimb behavior through ipsilateral pathways. Furthermore, Bachmann and colleagues[67] demonstrated in a mouse model that unilateral strokes induces axonal sprouting from the unaffected hemisphere at the level of the brainstem–spinal cord connections, with the possibility to gain control over the affected limb.

The potential adaptive role of the unaffected hemisphere in humans also aligns with these animal studies. For example, when TMS is applied transiently to disrupt the unaffected premotor cortex, patients with greater impairments experience greatest disruption in motor performance of the paretic hand, suggesting that with greater impairment, the likely role of the unaffected cortices becomes more relevant.[64] Furthermore, if NIBS is applied to inhibit the unaffected hemisphere, patients with greater impairments experience a transient decline in upper-limb motor function, suggesting that with greater impairment, unaffected cortices likely offer an adaptive potential for recovery.[68] These studies suggest that the role of the unaffected hemisphere is expressed more so with greater impairment and deficit, where its influence can be considered more adaptive than what is known typically. Although animal studies facilitating the unaffected hemisphere in models of greater damage[66] have recently supported these new views by demonstrating a causal adaptive role of the unaffected hemisphere in chronic recovery, direct evidence as to the total contribution of the unaffected hemisphere in humans remains to be seen.

The heterogeneity of the stroke population, extent of damage of the affected hemisphere, and the influence of the unaffected hemisphere may explain the shortcomings of unilateral therapies and the inconsistencies of the resultant NIBS studies. The generalizability of the theory of interhemispheric competition as a global mechanism of motor recovery following stroke thus becomes questionable. By emphasizing a single mechanism we risk creating augmentative NIBS approaches that lack flexibility to consistently serve the spectrum of stroke patients. In the same vein, we are likely to miss the advantages of potentially high-yielding therapies, such as bilateral behavioral paradigms, that might also promote recovery.

BILATERAL THERAPY AS AN ALTERNATIVE APPROACH

Bilateral approaches differ from unilateral therapies because they require moving both limbs simultaneously, either independently or in a linked manner. For example, bilateral isokinematic training[28] requires patients to move both limbs, but actions of one are not dependent or controlled by actions of the other. In contrast, Stinear and Byblow's[69] APBT, Whitall and colleagues's[27] BATRAC, and Knutson and colleagues's[29] CCFES link movements of both limbs. Using external instrumentation, such as mechanical fixations or electrical stimulation, the nonparetic limb drives the movement of the paretic limb.

Regardless of the type, bilateral therapies may provide a more feasible alternative to unilateral therapies. Because patients with severe impairments are typically unable to participate in unilateral therapies, bilateral therapies, such as APBT, BATRAC, and CCFES, where movement of the nonparetic limb drives movement of the paretic limb, could potentially provide all patients an opportunity to be involved and benefit from rehabilitation.

Although bilateral therapies may be more feasible, the important question is whether they are more efficacious than unilateral therapies. Overall, results are equivocal and seem to depend on at least the severity of motor impairment and the nature of clinical outcome of interest. For example, in a recent systematic review, van Delden and colleagues[31] concluded that bilateral therapies are as effective as unilateral therapies, but unilateral therapies still offered a slight advantage for functional independence and daily use of paretic hand across patients with mild-to-moderate impairment of the distal upper limb. In contrast, McCombe Waller and Whitall[30] argue that bilateral therapies involving repetitive reaching, as in BATRAC, offer an advantage for patients with moderate-to-severe impairments, at least in terms of proximal strength. Whether unilateral therapies improve independence and use of hand in daily life or bilateral therapies serve as a useful alternative for proximal function, their effectiveness can be best contrasted when the effect of initial impairment is balanced and the clinical goal is carefully considered.

Mechanisms of Bilateral Movement in Chronic Stroke

If indeed bilateral therapies afford greater advantage than unilateral therapies across the moderate-to-severely impaired patients, then this would suggest that their underlying mechanisms are more resilient in the presence of greater damage. Understanding these mechanisms of recovery could help derive a model that supplements the classical theory of interhemispheric competition. Here, we summarize evidence of potential mechanisms underlying bilateral therapies.

First, whether passive or active, bilateral movements could engage both hemispheres. One clear advantage would be that the unaffected hemisphere, now with evidence pointing to its adaptive and compensatory role for the more impaired patients, would naturally become engaged. Recruiting the unaffected hemisphere could indirectly facilitate the weak affected hemisphere because by symmetrically moving both limbs for a common purpose, both hemispheres become coupled.[28,70] As a result of coupling, Mudie and Matyas[28] explain, the unaffected hemisphere may offer a template of motor network recruitment to the affected hemisphere, allowing the paretic limb to learn from the nonparetic limb. This may be particularly necessary in more impaired patients where the damaged hemisphere has insufficient cortical-corticospinal resources to affect its own movement plans.

However, what is the evidence that a template could be uniquely elicited in bilateral movement? Studies with functional MRI (fMRI) show that bilateral movements elicit unique and greater activation of bilateral primary sensorimotor, premotor, and supplementary motor cortices in comparison with unilateral movements,[71] and that these distinctions amplify with therapy.[27] Patients who show the greatest recovery with BATRAC exhibit the highest gains in fMRI activation in the unaffected hemisphere, especially the unaffected premotor cortex, whereas patients who experience greater functional recovery with unilateral therapy exhibit greater activation of the premotor cortex of the affected hemisphere. Therefore, fMRI activation demonstrates that substrates recruited in bilateral movement are extensive and bihemispheric, compared with those recruited in unilateral movement.

Still, fMRI evidence alone may not be able to verify that a template of learning indeed transfers from one hemisphere to the other during bilateral movement. Studies that assess the neural basis of motor planning or functional and effective connectivity between hemispheres are needed for confirmation. As an example, TMS could reveal the neurophysiologic substrates underlying a transfer. Following stroke, one conceivable outlet for coupling and transfer of learning could involve mutual disinhibition of both hemispheres (**Fig. 3**).[72–75] Bilateral movements are in a unique position to potentiate disinhibition unlike unilateral movements because bilateral symmetric movements are considered natural and the default state of interlimb coordination.[28,70] Therefore, with bilateral synchronous movements, there is a decrease in intracortical inhibition within M1 and interhemispheric inhibition between M1s as demonstrated with TMS.[32,69,76] Release of inhibition could facilitate excitability of corticospinal output from the affected M1 and help restore the balance of mutual interhemispheric

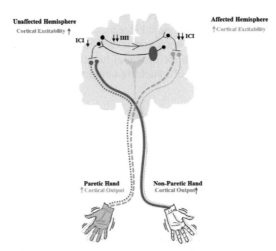

Fig. 3. Mechanisms of bilateral therapy in chronic stroke. Symmetric movements of the paretic and nonparetic limb may result in reduced intracortical inhibition (ICI) of the affected and unaffected hemisphere, and reduced interhemispheric inhibition (IHI) imposed on the affected hemisphere resulting in overall disinhibition of the corticomotor networks. *Dark circle* represents the lesion.

inhibition. Thus, it is possible that synchronous somatosensory feedback in bilateral motion, and a single set of motor commands linking bimanual movements may help upper limbs to become functionally coupled, and both hemispheres to release their inhibition on one another to allow transfer and exchange of learning.

Pathways Subserving Potential Benefits of Bilateral Therapies

Ultimately, whether it is recruitment of the unaffected hemisphere or transfer of learning via global disinhibition across hemispheres, how are these neurophysiologic effects of bilateral movements ultimately conveyed to affect the recovery of the paretic upper limb? We summarize evidence of potential pathways next (**Fig. 4**).

Spared corticomotor neuronal pool of the affected hemisphere

Sparing of corticomotor pathways in the affected hemisphere to the paretic limb depends on the severity of stroke. However, following stroke, cortical plasticity occurs such that higher motor areas (eg, the premotor cortex) can assume the role of the M1. In fact, higher-order areas have been shown to express plasticity in recovery with greater damage and impairment[77,78] and are important contributors during bilateral arm training and movements.[27,71] Thus, the release of interhemispheric and intracortical inhibition that occurs during symmetric bilateral movements may increase the motor overflow from the unaffected, "moving" cortices to the affected cortices partnering in bilateral movement.[27,32,70,79] It has previously been suggested that patients who exhibit greater motor overflow to the affected hemisphere had better motor function than those without motor overflow.[80] Thus, symmetric bilateral movements could

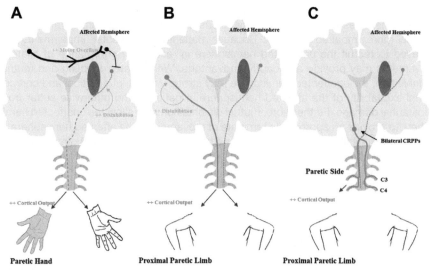

Fig. 4. Mechanisms of recovery following bilateral movement. (*A*) The affected hemisphere excitability is facilitated via release of interhemispheric and intracortical inhibition, and motor overflow from the unaffected hemisphere. (*B*) Direct ipsilateral pathways originating from the premotor cortex are thought to be facilitated following the disinhibition that occurs because of symmetric bilateral movement. The direct ipsilateral pathways synapse directly to alpha motor neurons to facilitate increased cortical output to the proximal paretic limb. (*C*) Indirect ipsilateral pathways (cortico-reticulo-propriospinal [CCRP]) synapse at the C3/C4 vertebrae to augment propriospinal neurons devoted to the proximal paretic limb.[82] *Dark circle* represents the lesion.

be powerful triggers to facilitate excitability of spared pathways originating from higher-order areas more so than unilateral movement for patients with greater motor impairment. Disinhibition and heightened excitability may help the affected hemisphere preserve as much function as possible to the affected areas (see **Fig. 4**A).[28]

Direct and indirect ipsilateral corticospinal pathways from the unaffected hemisphere
Approximately 10% to 15% of the corticospinal fibers originating from each hemisphere, primarily from the premotor cortex,[81] remain uncrossed and project directly to motor neurons devoted to the ipsilateral upper limb.[82] Several groups have noted unmasking of such ipsilateral pathways in stroke, suggesting that the ipsilateral output from the unaffected hemisphere could be beneficial for recovery.[58,64,65,82,83] Disinhibition during bilateral movements could cause ipsilateral pathways from the unaffected hemisphere to become unmasked and serve as much needed corticomotor output to the paretic limb (see **Fig. 4**B). Furthermore, aside from the direct ipsilateral pathways, nonhuman primate studies reveal that indirect ipsilateral pathways from the unaffected hemisphere are also capable of interacting with motor neurons to the paretic limb.[82] Mudie and Matyas[28] cite reticulospinal and the rubrospinal pathways as candidates to affect recovery of especially the proximal upper limb. More recently, Bradnam and colleagues[82] proposed that because cortico-reticulo-propriospinal pathways originating from the unaffected hemisphere terminate bilaterally on propriospinal neurons at the C3/C4 level of the spinal cord, the cortico-reticulo-propriospinal tract could theoretically also significantly modulate movement of the affected limb, especially in patients who have limited sparing of the corticospinal tract (see **Fig. 4**C).

Importance of Bilateral Therapy for Patients with Greater Impairment

Based on the presented possible mechanisms and pathways, it is conceivable that bilateral therapies could be more efficacious and feasible than unilateral therapies for the more impaired patients. Because patients with greater impairments are believed to recruit the unaffected hemisphere in recovery, performance of bilateral movements may provide an adaptive advantage. With greater coupling and mutual disinhibition, the unaffected hemisphere may strongly affect intracortical and corticospinal excitability of the affected hemisphere in patients who otherwise suffer from substantial damage. Furthermore, mutual disinhibition may allow the unaffected hemisphere to provide an appropriate template of movement to the affected hemisphere. It may help disinhibit "latent but existing" pathways, such as ipsilateral direct and indirect, originating from the unaffected hemisphere, which further promote motor output to the paretic limb, especially the proximal segments. Finally, disinhibition may help recruit affected and unaffected premotor cortices, importance of which we have discussed especially in the context of recovery of proximal function following stroke, a goal that is more reasonable to achieve in the severely impaired.[25]

NONINVASIVE BRAIN STIMULATION APPROACHES DURING BILATERAL THERAPY

The framework we have summarized regarding mechanisms of bilateral therapies could supply a basis for creating augmentative NIBS approaches. Bradnam and colleagues[82] previously suggested that because of the potential impact of the indirect ipsilateral corticospinal pathways, one alternative NIBS approach would be to facilitate the unaffected hemisphere to improve paretic upper-limb function. NIBS has typically been used to facilitate the affected hemisphere and inhibit the unaffected hemisphere (see **Fig. 2**). However, if NIBS was applied in the same way in conjunction with bilateral therapy as it is with unilateral therapy, we risk either negating the neurophysiologic benefit of bilateral therapy, or creating the possibility of an even greater deficit in motor function depending on the availability of the patients' motor substrates in the affected hemisphere.[68,82,84]

It is reasonable to suggest that facilitating the unaffected and the affected hemisphere together could result in an accelerative advantage when applied in conjunction with bilateral therapy because it would mimic the involvement of both hemispheres during bilateral therapy. Another compelling approach could involve recruiting the supportive role of the premotor cortex of the unaffected hemisphere in patients with greater motor impairments. When TMS is transiently applied to virtually inactivate the premotor cortex of the unaffected hemisphere, patients with greater impairments experience a greater disruption in motor performance of the paretic hand.[64] Furthermore, during bilateral movement there is greater activation of the unaffected premotor regions,[71] where following therapy there is reorganization that occurs especially in the premotor cortex.[27] Therefore, by engaging the unaffected premotor cortex with anodal tDCS or high-frequency rTMS, it is plausible to suggest that greater facilitation of the direct/indirect ipsilateral corticospinal and brainstem-mediated pathways and motor overflow to the affected hemisphere would occur.

Still, regardless of the NIBS approach, careful consideration has to be taken based on the patient's individual level of impairment.[82] Current evidence suggests patients with severe motor impairments would theoretically benefit from unaffected hemisphere excitation, whereas the mildly impaired patients may benefit to a greater degree by suppressing the unaffected hemisphere excitability in favor of the interhemispheric competition model. Still, it remains to be seen whether greater excitation of the contralesional hemisphere in severely impaired patients has an adaptive role for recovery, as indicated by a study in an animal model.[66] Future studies are needed to investigate the two approaches to compare their efficacy across varying degrees of impairment.

SUMMARY

This article discusses early evidence that bilateral therapy may be feasible and offer an alternative therapeutic advantage to unilateral therapy at least for patients with greater motor impairments. However, to date, no study has demonstrated superiority for either approach. Advances in research have demonstrated a notable shift in how scientists and therapists interpret mechanisms of recovery between patients. Many groups have begun to suggest alternative NIBS protocols and therapies (unilateral or bilateral) that challenge the one-size-fits-all approach. Even though the combinations of NIBS does show promise to maximize/accelerate functional outcomes for patients with chronic stroke, careful consideration should be taken when developing new approaches for delivering NIBS. Because of the literature presented in this review, we argue that perhaps future studies should begin to stratify patients based on individual level of impairment and type of therapy. The goal of stratification will aid in the optimization of resource allocation for current therapists and rehabilitation clinicians. Furthermore, it will take clinicians one step closer to tailoring therapy based on patients' needs.

REFERENCES

1. Broeks JG, Lankhorst GJ, Rumping K, et al. The long-term outcome of arm function after stroke: results of a follow-up study. Disabil Rehabil 1999;21(8):357–64.
2. Wilkinson PR, Wolfe CD, Warburton FG, et al. A long-term follow-up of stroke patients. Stroke 1997;28(3):507–12.

3. Coupar F, Pollock A, van Wijck F, et al. Simultaneous bilateral training for improving arm function after stroke. Cochrane Database Syst Rev 2010;(4):CD006432.

4. Terao Y, Ugawa Y. Basic mechanisms of TMS. J Clin Neurophysiol 2002;19(4): 322–43.

5. Pascual-Leone A, Valls-Sole J, Wassermann EM, et al. Responses to rapid-rate transcranial magnetic stimulation of the human motor cortex. Brain 1994;117(Pt 4):847–58.

6. Chen R, Classen J, Gerloff C, et al. Depression of motor cortex excitability by low-frequency transcranial magnetic stimulation. Neurology 1997;48(5):1398–403.

7. Schlaug G, Renga V. Transcranial direct current stimulation: a noninvasive tool to facilitate stroke recovery. Expert Rev Med devices 2008;5(6):759–68.

8. Schlaug G, Renga V, Nair D. Transcranial direct current stimulation in stroke recovery. Arch Neurol 2008;65(12):1571–6.

9. Wagner T, Fregni F, Fecteau S, et al. Transcranial direct current stimulation: a computer-based human model study. Neuroimage 2007;35(3):1113–24.

10. Purpura DP, McMurtry JG. Intracellular activities and evoked potential changes during polarization of motor cortex. J Neurophysiol 1965;28:166–85.

11. Nitsche MA, Paulus W. Excitability changes induced in the human motor cortex by weak transcranial direct current stimulation. J Physiol 2000;527(Pt 3):633–9.

12. Nitsche MA, Fricke K, Henschke U, et al. Pharmacological modulation of cortical excitability shifts induced by transcranial direct current stimulation in humans. J Physiol 2003;553(Pt 1):293–301.

13. Nitsche MA, Liebetanz D, Schlitterlau A, et al. GABAergic modulation of DC stimulation-induced motor cortex excitability shifts in humans. Eur J Neurosci 2004;19(10):2720–6.

14. Bolognini N, Vallar G, Casati C, et al. Neurophysiological and behavioral effects of tDCS combined with constraint-induced movement therapy in poststroke patients. Neurorehabil Neural Repair 2011;25(9):819–29.

15. Seniow J, Bilik M, Lesniak M, et al. Transcranial magnetic stimulation combined with physiotherapy in rehabilitation of poststroke hemiparesis: a randomized, double-blind, placebo-controlled study. Neurorehabil Neural Repair 2012;26(9): 1072–9.

16. Talelli P, Wallace A, Dileone M, et al. Theta burst stimulation in the rehabilitation of the upper limb: a semirandomized, placebo-controlled trial in chronic stroke patients. Neurorehabil Neural Repair 2012;26(8):976–87.

17. Chang WH, Kim YH, Yoo WK, et al. rTMS with motor training modulates cortico-basal ganglia-thalamocortical circuits in stroke patients. Restor Neurol Neurosci 2012;30(3):179–89.

18. Lindenberg R, Renga V, Zhu LL, et al. Bihemispheric brain stimulation facilitates motor recovery in chronic stroke patients. Neurology 2010;75(24):2176–84.

19. Hummel FC, Celnik P, Pascual-Leone A, et al. Controversy: noninvasive and invasive cortical stimulation show efficacy in treating stroke patients. Brain Stimul 2008;1(4):370–82.

20. Boggio PS, Nunes A, Rigonatti SP, et al. Repeated sessions of noninvasive brain DC stimulation is associated with motor function improvement in stroke patients. Restor Neurol Neurosci 2007;25(2):123–9.

21. Plow EB, Arora P, Pline MA, et al. Within-limb somatotopy in primary motor cortex–revealed using fMRI. Cortex 2010;46(3):310–21.

22. Hesse S, Waldner A, Mehrholz J, et al. Combined transcranial direct current stimulation and robot-assisted arm training in subacute stroke patients: an exploratory, randomized multicenter trial. Neurorehabil Neural Repair 2011;25(9):838–46.

23. Malcolm MP, Triggs WJ, Light KE, et al. Repetitive transcranial magnetic stimulation as an adjunct to constraint-induced therapy: an exploratory randomized controlled trial. Am J Phys Med Rehabil 2007;86(9):707–15.
24. Tomasevic L, Zito G, Pasqualetti P, et al. Cortico-muscular coherence as an index of fatigue in multiple sclerosis. Mult Scler 2013;19(3):334–43.
25. Plow EB, Cunningham DA, Varnerin N, et al. Rethinking stimulation of the brain in stroke rehabilitation: why higher motor areas might be better alternatives for patients with greater impairments. Neuroscientist 2014;21(3):225–40.
26. Emara T, El Nahas N, Elkader HA, et al. MRI can predict the response to therapeutic repetitive transcranial magnetic stimulation (rTMS) in stroke patients. J Vasc Interv Neurol 2009;2(2):163–8.
27. Whitall J, Waller SM, Sorkin JD, et al. Bilateral and unilateral arm training improve motor function through differing neuroplastic mechanisms: a single-blinded randomized controlled trial. Neurorehabil Neural Repair 2011;25(2):118–29.
28. Mudie MH, Matyas TA. Can simultaneous bilateral movement involve the undamaged hemisphere in reconstruction of neural networks damaged by stroke? Disabil Rehabil 2000;22(1–2):23–37.
29. Knutson JS, Harley MY, Hisel TZ, et al. Improving hand function in stroke survivors: a pilot study of contralaterally controlled functional electric stimulation in chronic hemiplegia. Arch Phys Med Rehabil 2007;88(4):513–20.
30. McCombe Waller S, Whitall J. Bilateral arm training: why and who benefits? NeuroRehabilitation 2008;23(1):29–41.
31. van Delden AE, Peper CE, Beek PJ, et al. Unilateral versus bilateral upper limb exercise therapy after stroke: a systematic review. J Rehabil Med 2012;44(2):106–17.
32. Stinear CM, Barber PA, Coxon JP, et al. Priming the motor system enhances the effects of upper limb therapy in chronic stroke. Brain 2008;131(Pt 5):1381–90.
33. Giovannelli F, Borgheresi A, Balestrieri F, et al. Modulation of interhemispheric inhibition by volitional motor activity: an ipsilateral silent period study. J Physiol 2009;587(Pt 22):5393–410.
34. Bodwell JA, Mahurin RK, Waddle S, et al. Age and features of movement influence motor overflow. J Am Geriatr Soc 2003;51(12):1735–9.
35. Nowak DA, Grefkes C, Ameli M, et al. Interhemispheric competition after stroke: brain stimulation to enhance recovery of function of the affected hand. Neurorehabil Neural Repair 2009;23(7):641–56.
36. Di Pino G, Pellegrino G, Assenza G, et al. Modulation of brain plasticity in stroke: a novel model for neurorehabilitation. Nat Rev Neurol 2014;10(10):597–608.
37. Takeuchi N, Izumi S. Noninvasive brain stimulation for motor recovery after stroke: mechanisms and future views. Stroke Res Treat 2012;2012:584727.
38. Boroojerdi B, Diefenbach K, Ferbert A. Transcallosal inhibition in cortical and subcortical cerebral vascular lesions. J Neurol Sci 1996;144(1–2):160–70.
39. Shimizu T, Hosaki A, Hino T, et al. Motor cortical disinhibition in the unaffected hemisphere after unilateral cortical stroke. Brain 2002;125(Pt 8):1896–907.
40. Ward NS, Cohen LG. Mechanisms underlying recovery of motor function after stroke. Arch Neurol 2004;61(12):1844–8.
41. Murase N, Duque J, Mazzocchio R, et al. Influence of interhemispheric interactions on motor function in chronic stroke. Ann Neurol 2004;55(3):400–9.
42. Avanzino L, Bassolino M, Pozzo T, et al. Use-dependent hemispheric balance. J Neurosci 2011;31(9):3423–8.
43. Page SJ, Levine P. Modified constraint-induced therapy in patients with chronic stroke exhibiting minimal movement ability in the affected arm. Phys Ther 2007;87(7):872–8.

44. Wolf SL, Lecraw DE, Barton LA, et al. Forced use of hemiplegic upper extremities to reverse the effect of learned nonuse among chronic stroke and head-injured patients. Exp Neurol 1989;104(2):125–32.
45. Taub E, Morris DM. Constraint-induced movement therapy to enhance recovery after stroke. Curr Atheroscler Rep 2001;3(4):279–86.
46. Hoyer EH, Celnik PA. Understanding and enhancing motor recovery after stroke using transcranial magnetic stimulation. Restor Neurol Neurosci 2011;29(6): 395–409.
47. Sandrini M, Cohen LG. Noninvasive brain stimulation in neurorehabilitation. Handbook Clin Neurol 2013;116:499–524.
48. Adkins-Muir DL, Jones TA. Cortical electrical stimulation combined with rehabilitative training: enhanced functional recovery and dendritic plasticity following focal cortical ischemia in rats. Neurol Res 2003;25(8):780–8.
49. Plautz EJ, Milliken GW, Nudo RJ. Effects of repetitive motor training on movement representations in adult squirrel monkeys: role of use versus learning. Neurobiol Learn Mem 2000;74(1):27–55.
50. Bolognini N, Pascual-Leone A, Fregni F. Using non-invasive brain stimulation to augment motor training-induced plasticity. J Neuroeng Rehabil 2009;6:8.
51. Plow EB, Carey JR, Nudo RJ, et al. Invasive cortical stimulation to promote recovery of function after stroke: a critical appraisal. Stroke 2009;40(5):1926–31.
52. Go AS, Mozaffarian D, Roger VL, et al. Heart disease and stroke statistics–2014 update: a report from the American Heart Association. Circulation 2014;129(3): e28–292.
53. Winstein CJ, Miller JP, Blanton S, et al. Methods for a multisite randomized trial to investigate the effect of constraint-induced movement therapy in improving upper extremity function among adults recovering from a cerebrovascular stroke. Neurorehabil Neural Repair 2003;17(3):137–52.
54. Bonifer N, Anderson KM. Application of constraint-induced movement therapy for an individual with severe chronic upper-extremity hemiplegia. Phys Ther 2003; 83(4):384–98.
55. Bonifer NM, Anderson KM, Arciniegas DB. Constraint-induced therapy for moderate chronic upper extremity impairment after stroke. Brain Inj 2005;19(5): 323–30.
56. Ward NS, Newton JM, Swayne OB, et al. Motor system activation after subcortical stroke depends on corticospinal system integrity. Brain 2006;129(Pt 3):809–19.
57. Cunningham DA, Machado A, Janini D, et al. The assessment of interhemispheric imbalance using imaging and non-invasive brain stimulation in patients with chronic stroke. Arch Phys Med Rehabil 2014;96(4 Suppl):S94–103.
58. Stinear CM, Barber PA, Smale PR, et al. Functional potential in chronic stroke patients depends on corticospinal tract integrity. Brain 2007;130(Pt 1): 170–80.
59. Schulz R, Park CH, Boudrias MH, et al. Assessing the integrity of corticospinal pathways from primary and secondary cortical motor areas after stroke. Stroke 2012;43(8):2248–51.
60. Nouri S, Cramer SC. Anatomy and physiology predict response to motor cortex stimulation after stroke. Neurology 2011;77(11):1076–83.
61. Biernaskie J, Szymanska A, Windle V, et al. Bi-hemispheric contribution to functional motor recovery of the affected forelimb following focal ischemic brain injury in rats. Eur J Neurosci 2005;21(4):989–99.
62. Fisher CM. Concerning the mechanism of recovery in stroke hemiplegia. Can J Neurol Sci 1992;19(1):57–63.

63. Cramer SC, Nelles G, Benson RR, et al. A functional MRI study of subjects recovered from hemiparetic stroke. Stroke 1997;28(12):2518–27.
64. Johansen-Berg H, Rushworth MF, Bogdanovic MD, et al. The role of ipsilateral premotor cortex in hand movement after stroke. Proc Natl Acad Sci U S A 2002;99(22):14518–23.
65. Machado AG, Shoji A, Ballester G, et al. Mapping of the rat's motor area after hemispherectomy: the hemispheres as potentially independent motor brains. Epilepsia 2003;44(4):500–6.
66. Carmel JB, Kimura H, Martin JH. Electrical stimulation of motor cortex in the uninjured hemisphere after chronic unilateral injury promotes recovery of skilled locomotion through ipsilateral control. J Neurosci 2014;34(2):462–6.
67. Bachmann LC, Lindau NT, Felder P, et al. Sprouting of brainstem-spinal tracts in response to unilateral motor cortex stroke in mice. J Neurosci 2014;34(9):3378–89.
68. Ackerley SJ, Stinear CM, Barber PA, et al. Combining theta burst stimulation with training after subcortical stroke. Stroke 2010;41(7):1568–72.
69. Stinear JW, Byblow WD. Rhythmic bilateral movement training modulates corticomotor excitability and enhances upper limb motricity poststroke: a pilot study. J Clin Neurophysiol 2004;21(2):124–31.
70. Byblow WD, Stinear CM, Smith MC, et al. Mirror symmetric bimanual movement priming can increase corticomotor excitability and enhance motor learning. PLoS One 2012;7(3):e33882.
71. Kloppel S, van Eimeren T, Glauche V, et al. The effect of handedness on cortical motor activation during simple bilateral movements. Neuroimage 2007;34(1):274–80.
72. Aramaki Y, Honda M, Sadato N. Suppression of the non-dominant motor cortex during bimanual symmetric finger movement: a functional magnetic resonance imaging study. Neuroscience 2006;141(4):2147–53.
73. Grefkes C, Eickhoff SB, Nowak DA, et al. Dynamic intra- and interhemispheric interactions during unilateral and bilateral hand movements assessed with fMRI and DCM. Neuroimage 2008;41(4):1382–94.
74. Maki Y, Wong KF, Sugiura M, et al. Asymmetric control mechanisms of bimanual coordination: an application of directed connectivity analysis to kinematic and functional MRI data. Neuroimage 2008;42(4):1295–304.
75. Liuzzi G, Horniss V, Zimerman M, et al. Coordination of uncoupled bimanual movements by strictly timed interhemispheric connectivity. J Neurosci 2011;31(25):9111–7.
76. Stinear JW, Byblow WD. Disinhibition in the human motor cortex is enhanced by synchronous upper limb movements. J Physiol 2002;543(Pt 1):307–16.
77. Ward N. Assessment of cortical reorganisation for hand function after stroke. J Physiol 2011;589(Pt 23):5625–32.
78. Ward NS, Brown MM, Thompson AJ, et al. Neural correlates of outcome after stroke: a cross-sectional fMRI study. Brain 2003;126(Pt 6):1430–48.
79. Staines WR, McIlroy WE, Graham SJ, et al. Bilateral movement enhances ipsilesional cortical activity in acute stroke: a pilot functional MRI study. Neurology 2001;56(3):401–4.
80. Nelles G, Cramer SC, Schaechter JD, et al. Quantitative assessment of mirror movements after stroke. Stroke 1998;29(6):1182–7.
81. Dum RP, Strick PL. The origin of corticospinal projections from the premotor areas in the frontal lobe. J Neurosci 1991;11(3):667–89.
82. Bradnam LV, Stinear CM, Byblow WD. Ipsilateral motor pathways after stroke: implications for non-invasive brain stimulation. Front Hum Neurosci 2013;7:184.

83. Netz J, Lammers T, Homberg V. Reorganization of motor output in the non-affected hemisphere after stroke. Brain 1997;120(Pt 9):1579–86.
84. Talelli P, Greenwood RJ, Rothwell JC. Exploring theta burst stimulation as an intervention to improve motor recovery in chronic stroke. Clin Neurophysiol 2007; 118(2):333–42.

Index

Note: Page numbers of article titles are in **boldface** type.

A

Acetylcholinesterase inhibitors
    in motor and speech recovery post-stroke, 683–684
Activities of daily living (ADLs)
    as predictor of functional outcome after stroke, 585–587
Adhesive capsulitis
    in HSP evaluation after stroke, 645
ADLs. *See* Activities of daily living (ADLs)
Ambulation
    as predictor of functional outcome after stroke, 587–588
Amphetamines
    in motor and speech recovery post-stroke, 672–673, 680
AOS. *See* Apraxia of speech (AOS)
Aphasia
    diagnosis of, 659
    post-stroke, 658
    treatment of, 661
Apraxia of speech (AOS)
    diagnosis of, 661
    post-stroke, 659
    treatment of, 661–663

B

Balance
    post-stroke
        virtual environments in, 751
Behavioral supports
    integrated with mental practice and task-specific training
        in post-stroke rehabilitation, **715–727** (*See also* Rehabilitation, post-stroke)
Bicipital tendinopathy
    in HSP evaluation after stroke, 645
Bilateral therapy
    post-stroke, 765–768
        mechanisms of, 765–767
        noninvasive brain stimulation during, 768–769
        pathways subserving benefits of, 767–768
        for patients with greater impairment, 768
Brain stimulation
    post-stroke
        during bilateral therapy, 768–769
        tailoring to nature of rehabilitative therapies, **759–774**

Phys Med Rehabil Clin N Am 26 (2015) 775–783
http://dx.doi.org/10.1016/S1047-9651(15)00089-3
1047-9651/15/$ – see front matter © 2015 Elsevier Inc. All rights reserved.

Brain (*continued*)
>bilateral therapy, 765–768
>combined with unilateral therapy based on theory of underlying mechanisms, 761–762
>damage in affected hemisphere and, 764
>influence of unaffected hemisphere and, 764–765
>introduction, 760–761
>limitations of unilateral therapies and associated noninvasive approaches, 762–765
>recovery mechanism underlying unilateral therapy, 761
>stroke population heterogeneity and, 763

C

Capsulitis
>adhesive
>>in HSP evaluation after stroke, 645

Center of gravity
>gait effects of, 615–617

Central hypersensitivity
>after stroke
>>in HSP evaluation, 647
>>management of, 649–650

Central poststroke pain
>HSP–related
>>after stroke, 647
>>management of, 649

Citicoline
>in motor and speech recovery post-stroke, 685–686

Cognitive rehabilitation
>post-stroke
>>virtual environments in, 751

Communication disorders
>post-stroke, **657–662**
>>AOS, 659
>>aphasia, 658
>>diagnosis of, 659–661
>>dysarthria, 658–659
>>neural control–related, 658–659
>>treatment of, 661–662

Complex regional pain syndrome (CRPS)
>after stroke
>>in HSP evaluation, 646–647
>>management of, 649

Cortical networks
>virtual environments effects on, 748–749

CRPS. See Complex regional pain syndrome (CRPS)

D

Degrees of freedom
>diminishing number of, 700

Dopaminergic agonists
    in motor and speech recovery post-stroke, 680–682
Dysarthria
    diagnosis of, 661
    post-stroke, 658–659
    treatment of, 662, 663
Dysphagia
    post-stroke, **662–667**
        described, 662
        diagnosis of, 663–667
        neural control–related, 663
        treatment of, 667

E

Elbow
    post-stroke
        virtual environments effects on, 749–750
Exercise(s)
    in HSP management after stroke, 648

F

Finger(s)
    post-stroke
        virtual environments effects on, 750
Forgetting
    as factor in upper limb motor impairment after stroke, 603–605
Functional outcome after stroke
    measures of, 584–585
    predictors of, **583–598**
        ADLs, 585–587
        ambulation, 587–588
        introduction, 583–584
        language, 592–593
        upper limb dexterity, 588–592
Functional rehabilitation
    post-stroke, 697–699

G

Gait, **611–617**
    hemiparetic, **611–623** (*See also* Hemiparetic gait)
    kinematics and kinetics of, 614–615
    normal human, **611–617**
        neural control of, 612
    spatiotemporal parameters of, 613–614
Gait cycle, **611–617**
    muscle activation during, 615–617
        center of gravity effects on, 615–617
    normal human, 613–615

Gait training
    in stroke rehabilitation
        virtual environments with, 750–751
Glenohumeral subluxation
    in HSP evaluation after stroke, 642

H

Hand(s)
    post-stroke
        virtual environments effects on, 750
Hemiparetic gait, **611–623**
    clinical assessment of, 620–621
    dynamic muscle activation in, 620
    energy costs of, 620
    introduction, 611–612
    kinematics of, 618–619
    kinetics of, 619–620
    observational assessment of, 621
    primitive locomotor patterns in, 617
    spatiotemporal parameters of, 618
Hemiplegia
    motor restoration
        NMES for, **729–745** (*See also* Neuromuscular electrical stimulation (NMES), for motor
           restoration in hemiplegia)
Hemiplegic shoulder pain (HSP)
    after stroke, **641–655**
        evaluation of, 642–647
           altered peripheral and central nervous activity, 646–647
           impaired motor control and tone changes, 642–644
           soft tissue lesions, 644–645
        introduction, 641–642
        prevalence of, 641
        treatment of, 648–651
           cause-related, 648–650
           emerging options in, 650–651
           straps/slings in, 648
HSP. *See* Hemiplegic shoulder pain (HSP)
Hypersensitivity
    central
        in HSP evaluation after stroke, 647

I

Impingement syndrome
    in HSP evaluation after stroke, 644–645

L

Language
    as predictor of functional outcome after stroke, 592–593
Learned bad use
    of affected upper limb after stroke, 602–603

Learned nonuse
    of affected upper limb after stroke, 600–602
Lithium
    in motor and speech recovery post-stroke, 686–687
Lower limb(s)
    post-stroke
        NMES for, 735–737
        robotic therapy for, 696

M

Mental practice
    integrated with task-specific training and behavioral supports
        in post-stroke rehabilitation, **715–727** (*See also* Rehabilitation, post-stroke)
Methylphenidate
    in motor and speech recovery post-stroke, 672–673, 680
Moclobemide
    in motor and speech recovery post-stroke, 686
Monoamine oxidase inhibitors
    in motor and speech recovery post-stroke, 686
Motor and speech recovery
    post-stroke
        neuropharmacology of, **671–689**
            introduction, 671–672
        pharmacologic agents in
            acetylcholinesterase inhibitors, 683–684
            amphetamines, 672–673, 680
            citicoline, 685–686
            CNS stimulators, 672–673, 680
            dopaminergic agonists, 680–682
            lithium, 686–687
            methylphenidate, 672–673, 680
            moclobemide, 686
            piracetam, 684–685
            selective serotonergic/noradrenergic reuptake inhibitors, 682–683
            studies of, 674–679
Motor control
    impaired
        HSP after stroke and, 642–644
Motor learning
    augmented feedback effects on, 748
    virtual environments in
        features for, 748
Motor performance
    immersion effects on, 749
Motor restoration
    in hemiplegia
        NMES for, **729–745** (*See also* Neuromuscular electrical stimulation (NMES))
Myofascial pain
    in HSP evaluation after stroke, 645

N

Neuromuscular electrical stimulation (NMES)
    for motor restoration in hemiplegia, **729–745**
        emerging directions for, 738–739
        fundamentals of, 730
        introduction, 729–730
        lower limb rehabilitation, 735–737
        peripheral and central effects of, 737–738
        purposes of, 731
        upper limb rehabilitation, 731–734
NMES. *See* Neuromuscular electrical stimulation (NMES)

P

Pain
    central post-stroke
        HSP–related, 647
            management of, 649
    myofascial
        in HSP evaluation after stroke, 645
    shoulder
        hemiplegic
            after stroke, **641–655** (*See also* Hemiplegic shoulder pain (HSP))
Percutaneous peripheral nerve stimulation
    in HSP management after stroke, 650–651
Peripheral nerve entrapment
    in HSP evaluation after stroke, 646
Piracetam
    in motor and speech recovery post-stroke, 684–685
Proprioception
    post-stroke
        virtual environments for, 752

R

Rehabilitation
    cognitive
        stroke rehabilitation using, 751
    post-stroke
        brain stimulation in
            tailoring of, **759–774** (*See also* Brain stimulation, post-stroke, tailoring to nature of
                rehabilitative therapies)
            integrating mental practice with task-specific training and behavioral supports in,
                715–727
            considerations for, 717–723
            empirical support for, 717
            future directions for, 723–724
            introduction, 716–717
            mental practice component in, 722–723
            physical practice component in, 721–722

speech
    stroke rehabilitation using, 751–752
Robotic therapy
    post-stroke, **691–702**
        costs related to, 695–696
        disruptive technology, 691–692
        introduction, 691–692
        lower extremity–related, 696
        results of, 693–694
        success factors, 696–697
        upper extremity–related, 692–693
Rotator cuff injury
    in HSP evaluation after stroke, 644–645

S

Scapular dyskinesis
    in HSP evaluation after stroke, 642–643
Selective serotonergic/noradrenergic reuptake inhibitors
    in motor and speech recovery post-stroke, 682–683
Sensory deficits
    post-stroke
        virtual environments for, 752
Shoulder(s)
    post-stroke
        virtual environments effects on, 749–750
Shoulder pain
    hemiplegic
        after stroke, **641–655** (*See also* Hemiplegic shoulder pain (HSP))
Sling(s)
    in HSP management after stroke, 648
Soft tissue lesions
    HSP after stroke and, 644–645
        management of, 648–649
Spasticity
    post-stroke, **625–639**
        evaluation of, 626–631
            identification of spasticity in, 626–627
            measurement tools in, 627–631
        identification of, 626–627
        introduction, 625–626
        management of, **625–639**
            combination interventions, 635–636
            nonpharmacologic, 631
            pharmacologic, 631–635
            surgical, 635
            treatment resistance/complications of, 636
        shoulder muscles–related
            in HSP evaluation, 644
            management of, 648
Spatial neglect

Spatial (*continued*)
  post-stroke
    virtual environments for, 752
Speech
  apraxia of (*See* Apraxia of speech (AOS))
Speech recovery
  post-stroke
    neuropharmacology of, **671–689** (*See also* Motor and speech recovery, post-stroke)
Speech rehabilitation
  post-stroke
    virtual environments in, 751–752
Split-belt walking paradigm
  post-stroke, **703–713**
    adaptation to, 704–706
    introduction, 703–704
    retention in, 706–708
    training in, 708–711
Strap(s)
  in HSP management after stroke, 648
Stroke
  chronic
    bilateral movement in
      mechanisms of, 765–767
  communication disorders after (*See also* Communication disorders, post-stroke)
  disability following, 703
  dysphagia after, **662–667** (*See also* Dysphagia, post-stroke)
  functional outcome after
    predictors of, **583–598** (*See also* Functional outcome after stroke, predictors of)
  functional rehabilitation after, 697–699
  hemiparetic gait after, **611–623** (*See also* Hemiparetic gait)
  HSP after, **641–655** (*See also* Hemiplegic shoulder pain (HSP))
  motor and speech recovery after
    neuropharmacology of, **671–689** (*See also* Motor and speech recovery, post-stroke)
  outcome after
    measures of, 584–585
  recovery from
    patterns of, 584–585
  rehabilitation for
    brain stimulation in
      tailoring of, **759–774** (*See also* Brain stimulation, post-stroke, tailoring to nature of rehabilitative therapies)
    virtual environments in, **747–757** (*See also* Virtual environments, stroke rehabilitation using)
  robotic therapy after, **691–702** (*See also* Robotic therapy, post-stroke)
  spasticity management after, **625–639** (*See also* Spasticity, post-stroke)
  split-belt walking paradigm after, **703–713** (*See also* Split-belt walking paradigm, post-stroke)
  upper limb motor impairment after, **599–610** (*See also* Upper limb(s), motor impairment of, after stroke)
Suprascapular nerve block
  in HSP management after stroke, 650

T

Task-specific training
    integrated with mental practice and behavioral supports
        in post-stroke rehabilitation, **715–727** (*See also* Rehabilitation, post-stroke)
Tendinopathy
    bicipital
        in HSP evaluation after stroke, 645
Tone
    changes in
        HSP after stroke and, 642–644

U

Upper limb(s)
    dexterity of
        as predictor of functional outcome after stroke, 588–592
    post-stroke
        motor impairment of, **599–610**
            clinical outcomes of, 605–606
            forgetting, 603–605
            from functional perspective, 600
            learned bad use, 602–603
            learned nonuse, 600–602
            nature of, 599–600
            therapeutic considerations, 605
        NMES in rehabilitation of, 731–734
        robotic therapy for, 692–693
        virtual environments effects on, 749–750

V

Virtual environments
    stroke rehabilitation using, **747–757**
        balance interventions, 751
        challenges related to, 752–753
        cognitive rehabilitation, 751
        gait training with, 750–751
        impairments targeted by, 749–752
        introduction, 747–748
        mechanisms of action of, 748–749
        motor learning–related, 748
        proprioception, 752
        sensory deficits, 752
        spatial neglect–related, 752
        speech rehabilitation, 751–752

W

Walking
    normal, 612–613
Wrist
    post-stroke
        virtual environments effects on, 750

United States Postal Service

Statement of Ownership, Management, and Circulation
(All Periodicals Publications Except Requestor Publications)

1. Publication Title	2. Publication Number	3. Filing Date
Physical Medicine and Rehabilitation Clinics of North America	0 0 9 - 2 4 3	9/18/15

4. Issue Frequency	5. Number of Issues Published Annually	6. Annual Subscription Price
Feb, May, Aug, Nov	4	$275.00

7. Complete Mailing Address of Known Office of Publication *(Not printer)* *(Street, city, county, state, and ZIP+4®)*

Elsevier Inc.
360 Park Avenue South
New York, NY 10010-1710

Contact Person
Stephen R. Bushing

Telephone *(Include area code)*
215-239-3688

8. Complete Mailing Address of Headquarters or General Business Office of Publisher *(Not printer)*

Elsevier Inc., 360 Park Avenue South, New York, NY 10010-1710

9. Full Names and Complete Mailing Addresses of Publisher, Editor, and Managing Editor *(Do not leave blank)*

Publisher *(Name and complete mailing address)*

Linda Belfus, Elsevier Inc., 1600 John F. Kennedy Blvd., Ste. 1800, Philadelphia, PA 19103-2899

Editor *(Name and complete mailing address)*

Jennifer Flynn-Briggs, Elsevier Inc., 1600 John F. Kennedy Blvd. Suite 1800, Philadelphia, PA 19103-2899

Managing Editor *(Name and complete mailing address)*

Barbara Cohen-Kligerman, Elsevier, Inc., 1600 John F. Kennedy Blvd. Suite 1800, Philadelphia, PA 19103-2899

10. Owner *(Do not leave blank. If the publication is owned by a corporation, give the name and address of the corporation immediately followed by the names and addresses of all stockholders owning or holding 1 percent or more of the total amount of stock. If not owned by a corporation, give the names and addresses of the individual owners. If owned by a partnership or other unincorporated firm, give its name and address as well as those of each individual owner. If the publication is published by a nonprofit organization, give its name and address.)*

Full Name	Complete Mailing Address
Wholly owned subsidiary of	1600 John F. Kennedy Blvd. Ste. 1800
Reed/Elsevier, US holdings	Philadelphia, PA 19103-2899

11. Known Bondholders, Mortgagees, and Other Security Holders Owning or Holding 1 Percent or More of Total Amount of Bonds, Mortgages, or Other Securities. If none, check box ☐ None

Full Name	Complete Mailing Address
N/A	

12. Tax Status *(For completion by nonprofit organizations authorized to mail at nonprofit rates)* *(Check one)*
The purpose, function, and nonprofit status of this organization and the exempt status for federal income tax purposes:
☐ Has Not Changed During Preceding 12 Months
☐ Has Changed During Preceding 12 Months *(Publisher must submit explanation of change with this statement)*

PS Form 3526, July 2014 [Page 1 of 3 (Instructions Page 3)] PSN 7530-01-000-9931 **PRIVACY NOTICE:** See our Privacy policy in www.usps.com

---

13. Publication Title	14. Issue Date for Circulation Data Below
Physical Medicine and Rehabilitation Clinics of North America	August 2015

15. Extent and Nature of Circulation			Average No. Copies Each Issue During Preceding 12 Months	No. Copies of Single Issue Published Nearest to Filing Date
a. Total Number of Copies *(Net press run)*			562	393
b. Legitimate Paid and/Or Requested Distribution (By Mail and Outside the Mail)	(1)	Mailed Outside County Paid/Requested Mail Subscriptions stated on PS Form 3541. *(Include paid distribution above nominal rate, advertiser's proof copies and exchange copies)*	288	202
	(2)	Mailed In-County Paid/Requested Mail Subscriptions stated on PS Form 3541. *(Include paid distribution above nominal rate, advertiser's proof copies and exchange copies)*		
	(3)	Paid Distribution Outside the Mails Including Sales Through Dealers And Carriers, Street Vendors, Counter Sales, and Other Paid Distribution Outside USPS®	101	105
	(4)	Paid Distribution by Other Classes of Mail Through the USPS (e.g. First-Class Mail®)		
c. Total Paid and/or Requested Circulation *(Sum of 15b (1), (2), (3), and (4))*		▶	389	307
d. Free or Nominal Rate Distribution (By Mail and Outside the Mail)	(1)	Free or Nominal Rate Outside-County Copies included on PS Form 3541	26	19
	(2)	Free or Nominal Rate In-County Copies included on PS Form 3541		
	(3)	Free or Nominal Rate Copies mailed at Other classes Through the USPS (e.g. First-Class Mail®)		
	(4)	Free or Nominal Rate Distribution Outside the Mail *(Carriers or other means)*	26	19
e. Total Nonrequested Distribution (Sum of 15d (1), (2), (3) and (4))			26	19
f. Total Distribution (Sum of 15c and 15e)		▶	415	326
g. Copies not Distributed (See instructions to publishers #4 (page #3))		▶	147	67
h. Total (Sum of 15f and g)			562	393
i. Percent Paid and/or Requested Circulation (15c divided by 15f times 100)		▶	93.73%	94.17%

If you are claiming electronic copies go to line 16 on page 3. If you are not claiming Electronic copies, skip to line 17 on page 3

16. Electronic Copy Circulation	Average No. Copies Each Issue During Preceding 12 Months	No. Copies of Single Issue Published Nearest to Filing Date
a. Paid Electronic Copies		
b. Total paid Print Copies (Line 15c) + Paid Electronic copies (Line 16a)		
c. Total Print Distribution (Line 15f) + Paid Electronic Copies (Line 16a)		
d. Percent Paid (Both Print & Electronic copies) (16b divided by 16c X 100)		

☐ I certify that 50% of all my distributed copies (electronic and print) are paid above a nominal price

17. Publication of Statement of Ownership
☐ If the publication is a general publication, publication of this statement is required. Will be printed in the **November 2015** issue of this publication.

18. Signature and Title of Editor, Publisher, Business Manager, or Owner

Stephen R. Bushing

Stephen R. Bushing – Inventory Distribution Coordinator

Date
September 18, 2015

I certify that all information furnished on this form is true and complete. I understand that anyone who furnishes false or misleading information on this form or who omits material or information requested on the form may be subject to criminal sanctions (including fines and imprisonment) and/or civil sanctions (including civil penalties).

PS Form 3526, July 2014 (Page 3 of 3)

Moving?

Make sure your subscription moves with you!

To notify us of your new address, find your **Clinics Account Number** (located on your mailing label above your name), and contact customer service at:

Email: journalscustomerservice-usa@elsevier.com

800-654-2452 (subscribers in the U.S. & Canada)
314-447-8871 (subscribers outside of the U.S. & Canada)

Fax number: 314-447-8029

Elsevier Health Sciences Division
Subscription Customer Service
3251 Riverport Lane
Maryland Heights, MO 63043

*To ensure uninterrupted delivery of your subscription, please notify us at least 4 weeks in advance of move.

Printed and bound by CPI Group (UK) Ltd, Croydon, CR0 4YY

21/10/2024

01777262-0001